THE BRADY
UROLOGY MANUAL

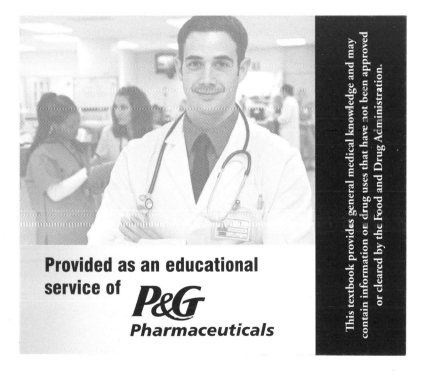

Provided as an educational service of **P&G**
Pharmaceuticals

THE BRADY UROLOGY MANUAL

EDITOR

J Kellogg Parsons MD MHS
University of California
San Diego School of Medicine
La Jolla, CA
USA

ASSOCIATE EDITOR

E James Wright MD
James Buchanan Brady Urological Institute
The Johns Hopkins Medical Institutions
Baltimore, MD
USA

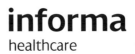

© 2006 Informa UK Ltd

First published in the United Kingdom in 2006 by Informa Healthcare, Telephone House, 69-77 Paul Street, London W1T 3JH. Informa Healthcare is a trading division of Informa UK Ltd. Registered Office: 37/41 Mortimer Street, London W1T 3JH. Registered in England and Wales Number 1072954.

Tel: ˆ44 (0)20 7017 6000
Fax· ˆ44 (0)20 7017 6699
Email: info.medicine@tandf.co.uk
Website: www.tandf.co.uk/medicine

Second printing 2007

Although every effort has been made to ensure that drug doses and other information are presented accurately in this publication, the ultimate responsibility rests with the prescribing physician. Neither the publishers nor the authors can be held responsible for errors or for any consequences arising from the use of information contained herein. For detailed prescribing information or instructions on the use of any product or procedure discussed herein, please consult the prescribing information or instructional material issued by the manufacturer.

A CIP record for this book is available from the British Library.
Library of Congress Cataloging-in-Publication Data

Data available on application

ISBN 10: 1 84184 481 0
ISBN 13: 978 1 84184 481 7

Distributed in North and South America by
Taylor & Francis
6000 Broken Sound Parkway, NW, (Suite 300)
Boca Raton, FL 33487, USA

Within Continental USA
Tel: 1 800 272 7737; Fax: 1 800 374 3401

Outside Continental USA
Tel: 561 994 0555; Fax: 561 361 6018
Email: orders@crcpress.com

Distributed in the rest of the world by
Thomson Publishing Services
Cheriton House
North Way
Andover, Hampshire SP10 5BE, UK
Tel: +44 (0)1264 332424
Email: tps.tandfsalesorder@thomson.com

Composition by J&L Composition, Filey, North Yorkshire
Printed and bound in India by Replika Press Pvt. Ltd.

Contents

Emergency urology

Practical principles

Contributors

Mohamad E Allaf MD
James Buchanan Brady Urological
Institute
The Johns Hopkins Medical
Institutions
Baltimore, MD
USA

Trinity J Bivalacqua MD PhD
James Buchanan Brady Urological
Institute
The Johns Hopkins Medical
Institutions
Baltimore, MD
USA

Mark L Gonzalgo MD PhD
Assistant Professor
James Buchanan Brady Urological
Institute
The Johns Hopkins Medical
Institutions
Baltimore, MD
USA

Matthew B Gretzer MD
Assistant Professor of Clinical Surgery
University of Arizona Health Sciences
Center
Tucson, AZ
USA

Misop Han MD MS
Assistant Professor
James Buchanan Brady Urological
Institute
The Johns Hopkins Medical
Institutions
Baltimore, MD
USA

David J Hernandez MD
James Buchanan Brady Urological
Institute
The Johns Hopkins Medical
Institutions
Baltimore, MD
USA

Benjamin H Lowentritt MD
Division of Urology
University of Maryland Medical
System
Baltimore, MD
USA

Danil V Makarov MD
James Buchanan Brady Urological
Institute
The Johns Hopkins Medical
Institutions
Baltimore, MD
USA

Jennifer Miles-Thomas MD
James Buchanan Brady Urological
Institute
The Johns Hopkins Medical
Institutions
Baltimore, MD
USA

Caleb P Nelson MD MPH
James Buchanan Brady Urological
Institute
The Johns Hopkins Medical
Institutions
Baltimore, MD
USA

Matthew E Nielsen MD
James Buchanan Brady Urological
Institute
The Johns Hopkins Medical
Institutions
Baltimore, MD
USA

Ganesh S Palapattu MD
Assistant Professor of Urology
University of Rochester Medical
Center
Rochester, NY
USA

Alan Partin MD PhD
Professor and Director
James Buchanan Brady Urological
Institute
The Johns Hopkins Medical
Institutions
Baltimore, MD
USA

J Kellogg Parsons MD MHS
University of California
San Diego School of Medicine
La Jolla, CA
USA

Peter Pinto MD
Urologic Oncology Branch
National Cancer Institute
Bethesda, MD
USA

Wilmer B Roberts MD PhD
James Buchanan Brady Urological
Institute
The Johns Hopkins Medical
Institutions
Baltimore, MD
USA

Craig Rogers MD
James Buchanan Brady Urological
Institute
The Johns Hopkins Medical
Institutions
Baltimore, MD
USA

Edward M Schaeffer MD
James Buchanan Brady Urological
Institute
The Johns Hopkins Medical
Institutions
Baltimore, MD
USA

Ioannis M Varkarakis MD PhD FEBU
Lecturer
2nd Department of Urology
University of Athens
Athens
Greece

Andrew A Wagner MD
James Buchanan Brady Urological
Institute
The Johns Hopkins Medical
Institutions
Baltimore, MD
USA

Christopher A Warlick MD PhD
James Buchanan Brady Urological
Institute
The Johns Hopkins Medical
Institutions
Baltimore, MD
USA

E James Wright MD
Assistant Professor
James Buchanan Brady Urological
Institute
The Johns Hopkins Medical
Institutions
Baltimore, MD
USA

Foreword

The Brady Urology Manual represents the combined input of many Brady urology residents and fellows and the scholarly coordination of one: J Kellogg Parsons MD MHS, known to all as Kelly. We all owe special appreciation to Kelly for undertaking this effort and for bringing it to fruition.

Medical students, nurses, residents, fellows, and faculty preparing for recertification will find reading this handbook a must. When a quick, concise, and updated review of a urological disease or situation is needed on the way to the Emergency Room or the Operating Room, this handbook will serve as your number one 'lifeline'.

I plan to use this book as a teaching aide for medical students and residents to not only inform them about the art and science of urology but also to excite them about our field. I hope that you find this text as useful in your education and practice.

Alan W Partin MD PhD
Professor and Director
James Buchanan Brady Urological Institute
The Johns Hopkins Medical Institutions
Baltimore, MD, USA

Preface

When I was a junior resident, scrambling between operating rooms, hospital floors, outpatient clinics, and ERs, abruptly swerving from one clinical scenario to the next, I resolved to develop an easy-to-use, convenient reference manual written *by* urology trainees *for* urology trainees.

The Brady Urology Manual combines basic principles of epidemiology, pathophysiology, and treatment in a concise, accessible format. It emphasizes general concepts and presents practical approaches to common problems. It is not intended as a comprehensive compendium of urological knowledge, or as a definitive guide for diagnosis and treatment, but as a practical review and quick reference manual for selected topics.

To expedite information retrieval, each chapter is similarly formatted and preceded by summaries of the most salient points.

This book represents the hard work of an exceptional group of individuals with whom I have had the privilege to work: the residents, visiting residents, and fellows of the James Buchanan Brady Urological Institute of the Johns Hopkins Medical Institutions. The strengths of this book belong to them, the shortcomings to me.

I am also indebted to my co-editor, E James Wright MD, and to Alan W Partin MD PhD – teachers, role models, and friends, without whom this book would not have been possible.

Finally, I am deeply grateful to Patrick C Walsh MD, an extraordinary mentor, whose ability to inspire excellence is exceeded only by his passion for teaching it.

J Kellogg Parsons MD MHS
University of California
San Diego School of Medicine

Infections of the urinary tract

David J Hernandez

SUMMARY

- Urinary tract infection (UTI) is a common disorder that may affect any portion of the urinary tract.
- Bladder infections include uncomplicated cystitis, recurrent uncomplicated cystitis, complicated cystitis, pyocystitis, and emphysematous cystitis.
- Kidney infections include acute and chronic pyelonephritis, acute lobar nephronia, pyonephrosis, emphysematous pyelonephritis, xanthogranulomatous pyelonephritis, and renal abscesses.
- Prostatitis may be acute, chronic, chronic non-bacterial (i.e. chronic pelvic pain syndrome), and asymptomatic.
- Pregnant women should be screened and treated for asymptomatic bacteriuria.
- *Candida* is the most common fungal infection of the urinary tract. In addition to antifungal therapy, symptomatic infections should be treated with removal or replacement of urinary tract hardware.
- Atypical infections of the genitourinary (GU) tract include tuberculosis (TB), schistosomiasis, echinococcosis, and filariasis.

GENERAL INFORMATION

EPIDEMIOLOGY

- Urinary tract infections affect 30% of women 20–40 years old.
- Account for 1.2% of all clinic visits by women and 0.6% by men per year.
- 80% of nosocomial UTIs are secondary to an indwelling urethral catheter.
- 90% of recurrent UTIs are caused by reinfection with different organisms.
- Prevalence of bacteriuria ~3.5%, increasing with age, institutionalization or hospitalization, previous UTIs, and concurrent disease.
- Annual health care expenditures for UTIs >$1 billion in the United States·
  - annual health care expenditures for nosocomial UTIs ~ $500 million.
- >7 million office visits and >1 million hospital admissions per year.

DEFINITIONS

- *UTI*: inflammatory response of the urothelium to bacterial invasion.
- *Bacteriuria*: presence of bacteria in the urine.
- *Pyuria*: presence of white blood cells (WBCs) in the urine; indicates an inflammatory response of the urothelium to bacterial invasion.
  - *Bacteriuria without pyuria*: suggests bacterial colonization without active infection.
  - *Pyuria without bacteriuria*: suggests presence of genitourinary TB, stones, *Chlamydia*, or cancer.
- *Funguria*: presence of fungus in the urine.
- *Acute pyelonephritis*: an acute inflammatory process of the kidney presenting as a clinical syndrome of chills, fever, and flank pain associated

with acute bacterial infection; usually associated with bacteriuria and pyuria and often with urinary frequency, urgency, and dysuria.

- *Chronic pyelonephritis*: a chronic inflammatory process often presenting as a shrunken, scarred kidney diagnosed by morphological, radiological, and/or functional evidence of renal disease.
- *Cystitis*: inflammation of the bladder; a clinical syndrome that is usually associated with dysuria, frequency, urgency, nocturia, and suprapubic pain.
- *Uncomplicated UTI*: infection in an otherwise healthy patient with a structurally and functionally normal urinary tract.
- *Complicated UTI*: infection in a patient with substantial comorbidity and/or a structurally or functionally abnormal urinary tract.
  - Clinical factors associated with increased risk of complications include diabetes mellitus, neurogenic bladders, pregnancy, congenital urinary tract anomalies, immunosuppression, end-stage renal disease, and advanced age.
- *Recurrent infections*: due to either reinfection or bacterial persistence.
  - *Reinfection* (~90%): each infection is a new event, with negative cultures between episodes, and bacteria entering from outside the urinary tract.
  - *Bacterial persistence*: multiple infections with same bacterial type; bacteria come from within the urinary tract.
- *Prophylactic antimicrobial therapy*: prevention of reinfection by the administration of antimicrobial drugs.
- *Suppressive antimicrobial therapy*: containment of a focus of bacterial persistence that cannot be eradicated (stone, hardware, etc.).

BASIC SCIENCE

BACTERIAL VIRULENCE FACTORS

- Adhesins – Type 1 pili and P pili – promote bacterial attachment by binding to tissue surface receptors:
  - Filamentous bacterial appendages
  - Type 1 pili bind to mannose residues on urothelia (mannose-sensitive)
  - Allow bacteria to ascend ureters and cause pyelonephritis.
- Capsules:
  - Promote evasion of host response.
- Hemolysins:
  - Toxic bacterial proteins.

HOST DEFENSE FACTORS

- Prevention of vaginal colonization:
  - Normal flora, *Lactobacillus*, suppress other bacteria
  - Acidic pH inhibits growth of *Escherichia coli* in the vagina
  - Secretory immunoglobulin A (IgA) in vaginal fluid.
- Prevention of bladder colonization:
  - Urine flow and voiding (mechanical clearance)
  - Low pH
  - Salts, urea, organic acids along with high osmolarity
  - Lactoferrin (scavenges iron needed by bacteria)

- Secretory IgA
- Low molecular weight oligosaccharides.
- Local antibacterial mechanisms:
  - Polymorphonuclear leukocytes
  - Antibodies
  - Cytokines.

ANTIMICROBIALS

PRINCIPLES OF ANTIBIOTIC THERAPY

- Obtain cultures before initiating therapy; tailor drugs to results.
- Consider local community and hospital susceptibility patterns.
- Adjust dosages based on renal or hepatic dysfunction when necessary.
- Be alert to potential drug toxicity.
- Monitor therapy and obtain follow-up cultures.
- Avoid overuse of antibiotics and reserve newer agents so as to minimize resistance.
- For surgical prophylaxis guidelines, refer to Chapter 30.

TRIMETHOPRIM/SULFAMETHOXAZOLE

- Mechanism: inhibits bacterial folic acid metabolism required for DNA synthesis.
- Spectrum: *Streptococcus*, *Staphylococcus*, Gram-negative rods (*not Pseudomonas*), and atypical *Mycobacteria*.
- Cautions:
  - Interacts with Coumadin (warfarin) to prolong (international normalized ratio) INR
  - May be associated with hematological abnormalities (especially in glucose-6-phosphate dehydrogenase (G6PD) deficiency and acquired immunodeficiency syndrome (AIDS)), nephrotoxicity, hepatotoxicity, and (rarely) Stevens–Johnson syndrome
  - Avoid in pregnancy.

NITROFURANTOIN

- Mechanism: inhibits several bacterial enzymes.
- Spectrum: effective against *E. coli* and *Staphylococcus saprophyticus*.
- Achieves high urinary levels but poor tissue penetration.
  - Therefore, has diminished efficacy for pyelonephritis and prostatitis.
- Cautions:
  - Neurotoxicity
  - Pulmonary fibrosis, interstitial pneumonitis
  - Hematological abnormalities and frequent gastrointestinal (GI) intolerance
  - Requires longer treatment course (7 days instead of 3)
  - Avoid in G6PD, renal failure.

AMPICILLIN OR AMOXICILLIN

- Mechanism: inhibits bacterial cell wall synthesis by binding beta-lactam ring.
- Spectrum: *Streptococcus*, *Staph. saprophyticus*, *Enterococcus*, *E. coli*, *Proteus*.

- Cautions:
  - Penicillin (PCN) allergy cross-reactivity
  - High prevalence of *E. coli* resistance in some regions
  - More prone to disrupt normal vaginal flora
  - Frequent GI intolerance and diarrhea
  - Associated with acute interstitial nephritis.

CEPHALOSPORINS

- Mechanism: inhibit bacterial cell wall synthesis
- Spectrum by generation:
  - 1st: *Streptococcus,* methicillin-sensitive *Staphylococcus aureus,* some Gram-negative rods
  - 2nd: *Streptococcus*, some Gram-negative rods, some anaerobes
  - 3rd: *Streptococcus*, most Gram-negative rods, including *Pseudomonas.*
- Cautions:
  - 10% cross-reactivity with PCN allergy
  - Synergistic toxicity with aminoglycosides.

AMINOGLYCOSIDES

- Mechanism: inhibit ribosomal protein synthesis
- Spectrum: most Gram-negative rods, including *Pseudomonas.*
- Cautions:
  - Ototoxicity – usually irreversible
  - Nephrotoxicity – usually reversible, non-oliguric acute renal failure (ARF) after 5–10 days
  - Avoid in pregnancy
  - Neuromuscular blockade – rare
  - Once-daily dosing has less nephrotoxicity but similar ototoxicity.

FLUOROQUINOLONES

- Mechanism: inhibit bacterial DNA gyrase.
- Spectrum: Gram positives, most Gram-negative rods, including *Pseudomonas, Neisseria gonorrhoeae.*
- Good tissue penetration, including prostate.
- Cautions:
  - Avoid during pregnancy and in children
  - May cause false-positive urine opiate test
  - Peripheral neuropathy (rare).

TETRACYCLINES

- Mechanism: inhibit protein synthesis.
- Spectrum: wide, but high prevalence of resistance.
- Good penetration into the prostate and effective against several sexually transmitted diseases.
- Cautions:
  - Photosensitivity
  - Avoid in pregnancy and children (teeth discoloration, bone development abnormalities).

VANCOMYCIN

- Mechanism: inhibits bacterial cell wall synthesis.
- Spectrum: Gram positives, including methicillin-resistant *Staphylococcus aureus* (MRSA).
- Cautions:
  - Nephrotoxicity and ototoxicity
  - 'Red-man syndrome': erythematous rash or flushing of the face, neck, or torso with pruritus and, in severe cases, hypotension or shock; attributed to histamine release caused by rapid infusion.

LINEZOLID

- Mechanism: inhibits protein synthesis.
- Spectrum: Gram positives, including most MRSA and vancomycin-resistant *Enterococcus* (VRE).
- Excellent oral bioavailability.
- Cautions:
  - Monoamine oxidase (MAO) inhibition – watch for drug interactions, including selective serotonin reuptake inhibitors (SSRIs)
  - Rare lactic acidosis
  - Bone marrow suppression
  - Avoid in pregnancy.

METRONIDAZOLE

- Mechanism: inhibits DNA synthesis.
- Spectrum: anaerobes (including *Bacteroides fragilis*), some Gram-negative rods, *Clostridium difficile*, *Trichomonas*, parasites.
- Gold standard oral and parenteral agent for anaerobes.
- Cautions:
  - GI and neurological symptoms
  - Interacts with Coumadin (warfarin) to prolong INR
  - Must avoid alcohol, because of disulfiram-like reactions.

CLINDAMYCIN

- Mechanism: inhibits bacterial protein synthesis.
- Spectrum: Gram positives and anaerobes.
- Often used for GP coverage in PCN-allergic patients.
- Cautions:
  - GI disturbances, notably *C. difficile* colitis.

SITE-SPECIFIC INFECTIONS OF THE URINARY TRACT: BLADDER

CYSTITIS

Etiology

- Bacteria ascend into urethra and bladder.
- When host defenses are ineffective (do not eliminate bacteria), cystitis develops.

Organisms

- Most common: *E. coli* (~80%).
- *Staph. saprophyticus* (~10% in young women).
- Other organisms: *Enterococcus*, *Klebsiella*, *Proteus*, and *Pseudomonas*.
  - Especially in complicated, recurrent, and nosocomial infections.

Risk factors

- Female gender.
- Altered vaginal flora.
- Coitus and spermicides.
- Instrumentation and urethral catheters.
- Menopause (increases vaginal pH).
- Epithelial cell receptivity (may be genetic).
- Antibiotics, especially beta-lactams.
- Voiding dysfunction.
- Immunosuppression.
- Diabetes mellitus.

UNCOMPLICATED CYSTITIS

- Presentation: acute onset of irritative voiding symptoms, without flank pain or systemic symptoms.
- Urinalysis (U/A):
  - Dipstick positive for nitrites or leukocyte esterase ~75% sensitive for infection
  - Bacteria convert urinary nitrates to nitrites
  - Leukocyte esterase is a neutrophil enzyme.
- Urine culture:
  - Historical definition of UTI was $>10^5$ CFU/ml
  - Now may consider $>10^2$ CFU/ml in setting of acute symptoms.
- Treatment:
  - Best options are trimethoprim/sulfamethoxazole, trimethoprim, nitrofurantoin, or fluoroquinolones
  - Duration: usually 3 days; 7 days if using nitrofurantoin, symptom duration >7 days, elderly, or recent UTI.

RECURRENT UNCOMPLICATED CYSTITIS

- Evaluation:
  - Depending upon history and clinical scenario, should consider pelvic exam, U/A, culture, cystoscopy, upper urinary tract imaging, and urodynamics.
- Treatment options include:
  - Change contraception and avoid spermicides
  - Postcoital antibiotics
  - Vaginal cream in postmenopausal women
  - Suppressive antibiotics to prevent vaginal colonization
  - Intermittent, self-start therapy: 3 days of antibiotics when symptoms arise and office visit if symptoms persist.

COMPLICATED CYSTITIS

- Evaluation:
  - Consider full genitourinary evaluation as above, particularly upper urinary tract imaging.
- Treatment:
  - Fluoroquinolones as empiric treatment
  - Antibiotic duration >7 days.

PYOCYSTITIS

- Defined as the presence of purulent material within the bladder lumen.
- May occur in dialysis patients with low urine output or in patients with an isolated bladder status post urinary diversion.
- May present with fever, suprapubic pain, and/or palpable mass.
- Diagnosis: abdominal imaging and bladder aspiration.
- Treatment:
  - Intravenous (IV) antibiotics and drainage
  - May also consider gentamicin bladder washes.

EMPHYSEMATOUS CYSTITIS

- Rare.
- Presence of gas within the bladder wall, resulting from severe infection by gas-producing organisms (*E. coli*, *Proteus*, *Pseudomonas*):
  - Kidney, ureter, and bladder/computed tomography (KUB/CT) may have pathognomonic picture, but may require cystogram
  - Must distinguish from instrumentation and colovesical fistula.
- Associated with diabetes.
- Treatment:
  - IV antibiotics and catheter drainage.

SITE-SPECIFIC INFECTIONS OF THE URINARY TRACT: KIDNEY

PYELONEPHRITIS

Etiology

- Organisms ascend ureters retrograde from bladder.
- May also have hematogenous seeding (rare).

Risk factors

- Same as for cystitis.
- Additional factors:
  - Bacterial P pili
  - Vesicoureteral reflux
  - Urinary stasis.

Evaluation

- History, exam, urinalysis, urine culture, complete blood count (CBC), blood cultures.
- Indications for imaging – CT scan/renal ultrasound (US) normal in ~75%:
  - History of stones or surgical procedures

- Suspected stones/urinary obstruction
- Severely ill or septic patient
- Persistently febrile for 72 hours despite antibiotics.

Outpatient treatment

- May be considered for community-acquired infection in an otherwise healthy patient with good compliance who is tolerating oral fluids and antibiotics.
- Fluoroquinolone × 14 days.
  - Alternative: trimethoprim/sulfamethoxazole (check sensitivity).

Inpatient treatment

- Initial IV antibiotics:
  - Fluoroquinolone
  - Aminoglycoside and ampicillin (or third-generation cephalosporin)
  - Convert to oral medications when afebrile for 48 hours
  - Total duration of treatment: 14 days (21 days if complicated).
- Maintain low threshold for upper tract imaging.

ACUTE LOBAR NEPHRONIA

- Focal acute pyelonephritis.
- On CT, may appear as either hyper- or hypoechoic lesions associated with focal parencyhmal inflammation/infection.

PYONEPHROSIS

- Acute pyelonephritis complicated by obstructed hydronephrosis.
- CT urogram shows decreased visualization of involved kidney.
- Treatment:
  - IV antibiotics and urgent relief of obstruction (ureteral stent or nephrostomy tube).

EMPHYSEMATOUS PYELONEPHRITIS

- Acute necrotizing parenchymal and perinephric infection resulting from complicated pyelonephritis by gas-producing organisms.
- Associated with pyonephrosis and diabetes mellitus.
- Poor overall prognosis.
- Treatment:
  - IV antibiotics, relief of obstruction, supportive care, and, if necessary, nephrectomy.

XANTHOGRANULOMATOUS PYELONEPHRITIS

- Uncommon, atypical chronic renal parenchymal infection associated with chronic infection, obstruction, and urinary stones.
- The involved kidney is often non-functioning.
- Patients may present with fevers, chills, flank pain, and flank mass.
- *Proteus* is the most common infecting organism.
  - *E. coli* is also common.

- Pathology:
  - Xanthomas are lipid-laden macrophages that are seen in association with other inflammatory cells surrouding parenchymal abscesses and calyces.
- CT may show a renal mass with associated calcifications/nephrolithiasis.
- Treatment: nephrectomy.

RENAL ABSCESS

- Cortical or medullary abscess, classically arising from focus of pyelonephritis, but can also occur by hematogenous seeding.
- Diagnosis: abdominal CT or magnetic resonance imaging (MRI).
- Treat with IV broad-spectrum antibiotics, percutaneous drainage, and rarely nephrectomy.

PERINEPHRIC ABSCESS

- Abscess between renal capsule and Gerota's fascia. May result from rupture of renal abscess or hematogenous seeding.
- May have high morbidity/mortality, especially in polycystic kidney disease and end-stage renal disease (ESRD).
- Diagnosis: abdominal CT or MRI.
- Treat with IV broad-spectrum antibiotics, percutaneous drainage, and rarely nephrectomy.

SITE-SPECIFIC INFECTIONS OF THE URINARY TRACT: PROSTATE

ACUTE BACTERIAL PROSTATITIS (NIH TYPE I)

Etiology

- Bacterial:
  - *E. coli* ~65–80%
  - *Enterococcus* ~5–10%
  - Other (including *Pseudomonas*, *Enterobacter*, *Klebsiella*) ~10–30%.
- Risk factors: UTI, catheter, transurethral surgery.

Presentation

- Acute-onset perineal and low back pain, lower urinary tract symptoms, fever, chills, and dysuria.
- On exam, prostate may be boggy and tender.

Evaluation

- Urinalysis and culture.

Treatment

- Fluoroquinolone (IV or PO) or aminoglycoside and ampicillin/third-generation cephalosporin.
- When afebrile, may continue fluoroquinolone or switch to trimethoprim or trimethoprim/sulfamethoxazole.
- Total duration of therapy should be 4–6 weeks.

- If not improved after 36 hours of antibiotics, consider abdominal CT to evaluate for abscess (particularly in immunosuppressed or otherwise compromised patients).
  - Treatment for abscess: transurethral unroofing.

CHRONIC BACTERIAL PROSTATITIS (TYPE II)

Presentation

- Persistent symptoms of prostatitis (lower urinary tract symptoms, pelvic pain, dysuria, +/− fevers).
- Prostate may be normal size or enlarged; may or may not be boggy or tender.

Evaluation

- Urinalysis and culture.

Prostate massage and '2-glass test'

- Traditionally has been performed to distinguish between type II, IIIA, and IIIB prostatitis.
- Protocol: two urine samples obtained, one pre- and one post-prostate massage.
- Interpretation:
  - Both specimens positive = cystitis/acute UTI
  - First culture negative but second positive = type II
  - Both cultures negative = type III.
- The value of this diagnostic test is unclear. Objective, definitive evidence from clinical trials is lacking.

Treatment

- 4–8 weeks of antibiotics as above.

CHRONIC NON-BACTERIAL PROSTATITIS/PELVIC PAIN SYNDROME (TYPES IIIA AND IIIB)

Presentation

- Usually characterized by chronic symptoms of prostatitis/pelvic pain with no identifiable etiology despite multiple tests and persisting despite multiple courses of antibiotics.
  - Multiple urine cultures are usually negative.
- IIIA versus IIIB
  - IIIA (inflammatory) = WBCs in post-massage urine
  - IIIB (non-inflammatory) = no WBCs
  - Clinical significance of this distinction is unclear.

Treatment

- The following medications have shown benefit in clinical trials:
  - Flomax (tamsulosin hydrochloride) 0.4 mg PO qd
  - Elmiron (pentosan polysulfate) 100 mg PO tid
  - Nonsteroidal anti-inflammatory medications.

- *Also consider a diagnosis of interstitial cystitis and treat accordingly (see Chapter 8).*

ASYMPTOMATIC PROSTATITIS (CATEGORY IV)

- Asymptomatic inflammation.
- Usually detected on prostate needle biopsy.
- No definitive indications for treatment.

ASYMPTOMATIC BACTERIURIA

Prevalence

- ~5% of young women.
- ~20–50% of elderly women.
- ~15–30% of elderly men.

Treatment

- Indicated for:
  - Pregnant women (see below)
  - Stones, obstruction, or GU tract abnormalities
  - Preoperative prophylaxis.
- Not indicated for (unless presence of above conditions):
  - Non-pregnant young women
  - Diabetes
  - The elderly
  - Chronic catheter.

In pregnancy

- Prevalence of asymptomatic bacteriuria (and rate of recurrent infection) in pregnant women is the same as in non-pregnant women.
  - However, in pregnant women bacteriuria progresses to pyelonephritis more frequently (up to 30% of affected women).
  - Pyelonephritis may lead to adverse fetal outcomes.
- Diagnosis.
  - Clean-catch urine culture at first prenatal visit.
- Treatment:
  - 3–10 days of antibiotics
  - Repeat culture 10 days later, repeat treatment if needed.

ATYPICAL INFECTIONS: FUNGAL

GENERAL PRINCIPLES

- Most common organism is *Candida* (~80% of infections).
- Risk factors:
  - Urinary catheters
  - Antibiotics
  - Diabetes mellitus
  - Impaired host
  - Structurally abnormal or previously reconstructed urinary tract.

TREATMENT

Nystatin

- Mechanism: disrupts fungal cell membranes by binding to sterols.
- Cautions:
  - GI side effects.

Amphotericin B

- Mechanism: disrupts fungal cell membranes by binding to sterols.
- Effective treatment for disseminated or invasive infections.
- Cautions:
  - Nephrotoxicity
  - Hepatotoxicity
  - Electrolyte abnormalities
  - Phlebitis
  - Fevers/chills
  - Infusion-related reactions (less for liposomal form).

Imidazoles and triazoles

- Mechanism: inhibit fungal P450 enzymes and synthesis of steroids for cell membrane.
- Cautions:
  - GI intolerance
  - Liver function test (LFT) elevation
  - May affect clearance of drugs metabolized by P450 system
  - Avoid in pregnancy.
- Fluconazole:
  - Oral or IV
  - Some resistant strains of *Candida.*
- Ketoconazole
  - Suboptimal for kidney and bladder infections (low urine levels).

Caspofungin

- Mechanism: inhibits cell wall synthesis.
- For invasive *Candida*, with efficacy similar to amphotericin B.
- Cautions:
  - Substantial histamine release in 2%.

ASYMPTOMATIC FUNGURIA

- Remove or change indwelling urinary hardware.
- Mitigate risk factors (stop antibiotics, improve nutrition, treat primary disease).
- Prophylaxis with fluconazole (or culture-appropriate agent) is required for GU procedures.
- Therapy should also be considered for immunocompromised, renal transplant, premature newborn, neutropenic, or hospitalized patients with comorbid conditions.

CYSTITIS

- Remove or change indwelling catheter.
- Alkalinize urine.
- Administer oral fluconazole or bladder irrigation with amphotericin B.

UPPER URINARY TRACTS

- Fluconazole, amphotericin B, or caspofungin.
- Imaging to look for fungus balls.
- May need drainage with amphotericin B irrigation via nephrostomy tube and/or endoscopic or surgical removal.

ATYPICAL INFECTIONS: TUBERCULOSIS

EPIDEMIOLOGY

- Incidence in United States is declining, but one-third of the world's population is infected with TB.
- 1.2–20% of patients with TB have genitourinary manifestations, mostly male.

PATHOGENESIS

- Almost all TB is acquired by inhalation.
- Bacteria multiply in lungs and disseminate (primarily) hematogenously.
- Most immunocompetent hosts never develop clinical disease.
- Genitourinary TB can present up to 15–20 years after initial infection.

KIDNEY

- Most common site.
- Results from hematogenous seeding.
- Inflammatory response may lead to scar tissue formation with fibrosis and obstruction of collecting system with calyceal strictures.

URETER/BLADDER

- Results from antegrade seeding from kidney.
- Most common site is at ureterovesical junction (UVJ)/ureteral orifice.
- Often results in small, contracted, fibrotic bladder.

EPIDIDYMIS

- Second-most common site.
- Results from hematogenous seeding.
- May present with acute symptoms of epididymitis.

TESTIS

- Results from testicular seeding.

PROSTATE

- Extremely rare.
- Results from hematogenous seeding.

PENIS

- Rare.
- Results from contact with infected partner, resulting in ulcerations.

PRESENTATION

- Symptoms are often minimal. History (i.e. travel) is important.
- Systemic symptoms: malaise, weight loss, lethargy, low-grade fever.
- Suprapubic and/or flank pain.
- Scrotal pain and/or swelling.

EVALUATION/DIAGNOSIS

- U/A:
  - Sterile pyuria is classic (~80%).
- Urine culture:
  - 3–5 early morning samples for acid-fast bacilli (AFB).
- KUB:
  - Often shows calcifications.
- Intravenous pyelogram (IVP)/CT urogram:
  - Findings often sufficient for diagnosis
  - Irregular calyces
  - Infundibular stenosis
  - Hydrocalyx, hydronephrosis, hydroureter
  - Superiorly displaced ureteropelvic junction (UPJ)
  - Ureteral strictures, usually distal (multiple scars is pathognomonic)
  - Small and contracted bladder ('thimble bladder').
- Endoscopy:
  - Limited value.

TREATMENT

- Antibiotics:
  - 6-month total duration: 2 months of isoniazid (INH) + rifampin + pyrazinamide + ethambutol, then 4 months of INH + rifampin
  - Second-line agents: cycloserine, ethionamide, streptomycin, kanamycin, amikacin, para-amino salicylic acid, and levofloxacin.

SURGERY

Patients should be on appropriate antibiotics prior to surgery.
- Nephrectomy – indications:
  - Non-functional kidney
  - Extensive disease involving most or all of affected kidney (investigate contralateral renal function)
  - Coexisting renal cell carcinoma.
- Epididymectomy and/or orchiectomy – indications:
  - Failed drug therapy with persistent severe symptoms
  - Suspicion for associated testis cancer.
- Ureteral strictures:
  - Initially, ureteral stent with antibiotic therapy

- If not improved after 4 weeks, add steroid therapy
- Persistent stricture: endoscopic incision, balloon dilation, ureteral reimplantation/reconstruction.

ATYPICAL INFECTIONS: HUMAN IMMUNODEFICIENCY VIRUS (HIV) AND ACQUIRED IMMUNODEFICIENCY SYNDROME (AIDS)

ASSOCIATED UROLOGICAL ISSUES

- Opportunistic infections of genitourinary tract.
- Increased incidence of malignancies.
- Renal cancer.
- Squamous cancers of the genitalia: i.e. associated human papillomavirus (HPV) infections.
- Kaposi's sarcoma of genitalia.
- Hypogonadism.

ATYPICAL INFECTIONS: PARASITIC DISEASES

SCHISTOSOMIASIS (BILHARZIASIS)

- Blood fluke (trematode) endemic in Africa and Middle East.
- Usually presents with hematuria and dysuria.
- Associated with bladder ulcers, stone formation, obstruction, and increased risk of squamous cell carcinoma.

ECHINOCOCCOSIS

- Tapeworm: endemic in Middle East, Australia, and Argentina.
- Hydatid cysts primarily invade liver, but can also involve kidneys.
- Presents as renal mass (may be calcified), often asymptomatic.
- Requires surgical resection.

FILARIASIS

- Nematodes spread by mosquitos, endemic in tropical regions.
- May cause lymphatic obstruction, which may induce epididymitis and elephantiasis of the penis/scrotum.

FURTHER READING

Boucher H, Groll AH, Chiou CC, Walsh TJ: Newer systemic antifungal agents: pharmacokinetics, safety and efficacy. Drugs 64(18):1997, 2004.

Erickson DR: Urethritis and interstitial cystitis, sexually transmitted diseases, urinary tract infections. American Urological Association Annual Review Course 2: 2005.

Gerber GS, Brendler CB: Evaluation of the urologic patient: history, physical examination, and urinalysis. In: Walsh PC, Retik AB, Vaughan ED, Wein AJ, eds. Campbell's Urology, 8th edn. Philadelphia: WB Saunders, 2002, pp 83–110.

Hooton TM: The current management strategies for community-acquired urinary tract infection. Inf Dis Clin North Am 17(2):303, 2003.

Johnson CW, Lowe FC, Johnson WD: Genitourinary tuberculosis. American Urological Association Update Series 22(38):302, 2003.

Johnson JR: Microbial virulence determinants and the pathogenesis of urinary tract infection. Inf Dis Clin North Am 17(2):261, 2003.

INFECTIONS OF THE URINARY TRACT

1

Johnson WD, Johnson CW, Lowe FC: Tuberculosis and parasitic diseases of the genitourinary system. In: Walsh PC, Retik AB, Vaughan ED, Wein AJ, eds. Campbell's Urology, 8th edn. Philadelphia: WB Saunders, 2002, pp 743–95.

Kass EH, Finland M: Asymptomatic infections of the urinary tract. J Urol 168(2):420, 2002.

Le J, Briggs GG, McKeown A, Bustillo G: Urinary tract infections during pregnancy. Ann Pharmacother 38(10):1692, 2004.

Lynch DM: Cranberry for prevention of UTIs. Am Fam Physician 70(11):2175, 2004.

Macfarlane MT: Urology, 3rd edn. Louisville: Lippincott Williams & Wilkins, 2001.

McLaughlin SP, Carson CC: Urinary tract infections in women. Med Clin North Am 88(2):417, 2004.

Nickel JC: Prostatitis and related conditions. In: Walsh PC, Retik AB, Vaughan ED, Wein AJ, eds. Campbell's Urology, 8th edn. Philadelphia: WB Saunders, 2002, pp 603–30.

Nickel JC: Recommendations for the evaluation of patients with prostatitis. World J Urol 21(2):75, 2003.

Physicians' Desk Reference, 59th edn., 2005.

Pohl HG, Rushton HG: The diagnosis and management of urinary tract infection in children. American Urological Association Update Series 17(31):242, 1998.

Safir MH, Schaeffer AJ: Urinary tract infection: simple and complicated. American Urological Association Update Series 16(10):74, 1997.

Salyers AA, Whitt DD: Bacterial Pathogenesis: A Molecular Approach. Washington, DC: American Society for Microbiology Press, 1994.

Schaeffer AJ: Infections of the urinary tract. In: Walsh PC, Retik AB, Vaughan ED, Wein AJ, eds. Campbell's Urology, 8th edn. Philadelphia: WB Saunders, 2002, pp 515–602.

Stapleton A: Novel approaches to prevention of urinary tract infections. Inf Dis Clin North Am 17(2):457, 2003.

Wang LJ, Wu CF, Wong YC et al: Imaging findings of urinary tuberculosis on excretory urography and computerized tomography. J Urol 169(2):524, 2003.

Wise GJ: Fungal and actinomycotic infections of the genitourinary system. In: Walsh PC, Retik AB, Vaughan ED, Wein AJ, eds. Campbell's Urology, 8th edn. Philadelphia: WB Saunders, 2002, pp 797–827.

Nephrolithiasis: etiology, stone composition, medical management, and prevention

Andrew A Wagner

SUMMARY

- The most common type of urinary stone is calcium oxalate. Treatment is typically surgery.
- Uric acid stones form at pH <5.5. Primary treatment and prevention is to alkalinize the urine; surgery is also an option.
- Struvite stones are composed of magnesium ammonium phosphate crystals. They are classically caused by infection with a urease-producing bacterium. Urinary pH is >7.2. Treatment is surgery and antibiotics.
- Cystine stones are caused by a congenital autosomal recessive disorder. Treatment is urinary alkalinization and cystine chelating agents.
- Calcium phosphate stones are associated with Type 1 renal tubular acidosis (RTA).
- Dietary interventions to prevent stones include increased fluid intake, decreased protein intake, and decreased sodium intake.
- Pharmacological interventions to prevent stones include thiazides, citrate, allopurinol, sodium cellulose phosphate, and chelating agents.

GENERAL PRINCIPLES

EPIDEMIOLOGY[1]

- Prevalence is generally 2–3%; may be increased in mountainous, desert, and tropical areas.
- Men affected more than women by a ratio of 3:1.
- White men are at greatest risk:
  - 1 in 8 will have at least one stone episode by age 70 years.
- 25% of stone formers have a family history of stone disease.
- Anatomic abnormalities, including medullary sponge kidney, ureteropelvic junction (UPJ) obstruction, and congenital abnormalities, may increase stone risk.
- The four most common kinds of stones are calcium oxalate, uric acid, struvite, and cysteine.

STONE FORMATION

- Crystallization:
  - Stones are essentially salts that precipitate out of urine
  - The point of saturation of a salt in solution is called the solubility product (K_{sp})
  - When the product of the components of a salt (e.g. calcium and oxalate) exceeds K_{sp}, salt crystals will precipitate out of solution
  - Crystallization is based on K_{sp}, pH, and the presence of stone inhibitors and promoters

- Some stone inhibitors increase the concentration of stone components required for the crystals to precipitate out of solution (i.e. for the stone crystals to form).
- Nucleation:
  - Nucleation is the process by which stones form around a core, or nucleus
  - Homogeneous stone nuclei form in solution
  - Heterogeneous stone nuclei form around existing structures, such as cellular debris.
- Aggregation:
  - Crystals join together to form larger clumps.

TYPES OF STONES

CALCIUM OXALATE

- The most common type of stone.

CALCIUM AND PHOSPHATE METABOLISM

- Calcium is absorbed in the intestinal tract.
  - Vitamin D stimulates absorption.
  - Calcium may complex in the intestinal lumen with oxalate, citrate, phosphate, or fatty acids; complexing decreases the amount available for absorption.
- Vitamin D (1,25-dihydroxyvitamin D_3 or 1,25 D_3):
  - Increases calcium and phosphate absorption in the intestine
  - Increases bone resorption
  - Precursors synthesized in skin and liver, active form synthesized in kidney (25-hydroxyvitamin $D_3 \rightarrow$ 1,25 D_3)
  - Synthesis stimulated by parathyroid hormone (PTH).
- PTH:
  - Stimulated by decreased serum calcium
  - Directly stimulates osteoclasts and the release of calcium and phosphate
  - Increases renal reabsorption of calcium
  - Decreases renal reabsorption of phosphate
  - Increases 1,25 D_3 production in kidney.

OXALATE METABOLISM

- Oxalate is absorbed in the intestinal tract.
  - Absorption may be increased after small bowel resection or inflammatory bowel disease.
- Fecal bacteria degrade oxalate (*Oxalobacter formigenes*, *Pseudomonas oxalaticus*).
- Filtered and secreted by kidney.
- Ascorbic acid (vitamin C) is metabolized to oxalate.

INHIBITORS[2]

- Citrate:
  - Only inhibitor with proven clinical applications
  - Metabolic acidosis can decrease urinary citrate excretion.

- Pyrophosphate.
- Glycosaminoglycans.
- Prothrombin fragment 1.
- Nephrocalcin.
- Tamm–Horsfall glycoprotein.
- RNA fragments.
- Complexors:
  - Bind with components and decrease saturation of ions
  - Citrate complexes with phosphate
  - Calcium, magnesium, and sodium may complex with oxalate.

METABOLIC ABNORMALITIES CONTRIBUTING TO CALCIUM OXALATE NEPHROLITHIASIS

HYPERCALCIURIA

- Idiopathic: ↑ urine calcium, normal serum calcium.
- Absorptive hypercalciuria:
  - ↑ intestinal absorption
  - Could be secondary to ↑ vitamin D
  - ↓ PTH
  - Normal fasting urine calcium.
- Renal hypercalciuria:
  - Renal wasting causes ↓ serum calcium
  - ↑ PTH
  - elevated fasting urine calcium.
- Resorptive hypercalciuria:
  - Primary hyperparathyroidism
  - Excess PTH-dependent bone resorption.
- Recommended treatment:
  - Absorptive: calcium restriction, sodium cellulose phosphate, thiazides, and increased fluid intake
  - Other types: thiazide and increased fluid intake.

HYPERCALCEMIA

- Primary hyperparathyroidism:
  - Most common cause of outpatient hypercalcemia
  - Prevalence of stone disease only 1%
  - Suspect when serum calcium >10.1 mg/dl
  - Diagnosis: serum PTH
  - Treatment: remove the adenoma (if stones are symptomatic, then treat them first).
- Malignancy:
  - The most common cause of inpatient hypercalcemia but a very rare cause of stones
  - PTH-like polypeptide causes increased bone resortion.
- Sarcoidosis:
  - Granuloma produces 1,25 D_3
  - Low/absent PTH levels.

NEPHROLITHIASIS: ETIOLOGY, COMPOSITION, MANAGEMENT, AND PREVENTION

2

- Other causes:
  - Hyperthyroidism and cortisol excess (Cushing's syndrome).

HYPEROXALURIA

- Mild hyperoxaluria:
  - Causes: ↑ dietary oxalate/↑ absorption/↑ vitamin C
  - Treatment: oxalate restriction, pyridoxine, thiazides, ↑ fluids.
- Primary hyperoxaluria:
  - Deficiency of alanine–glycoxylate aminotransferase (AGT) in liver results in ↑ oxalate
  - Nephrocalcinosis, renal failure, death before 20 years old
  - Treatment: pyridoxine, liver/kidney transplant.
- Enteric hyperoxaluria:
  - Etiology
    - Small bowel resection, inflammatory bowel disease (IBD), other causes of malabsorption
  - Pathophysiology
    - Colonic permeability from ↑ bile salt exposure
    - ↓ Calcium in colon from saponification with fat allows ↑ oxalate reabsorption
  - Treatment: low oxalate/fat diet, calcium supplements, cholestyramine, ↑ fluids.

HYPERURICOSURIA

- Facilitates calcium oxalate crystallization:
  - Etiology
    - ↑ Dietary purines
    - ↑ Endogenous purine production
  - Most hyperuricosuric calcium oxalate stone patients have normal serum uric acid
  - Treatment: purine restriction, allopurinol, ↑ fluids.

HYPOCITRATURIA

- Citrate is a stone inhibitor:
  - Complexes with calcium
  - Inhibits crystallization and aggregation.
- 15–63% stone patients.
- Etiology:
  - Metabolic acidosis, UTIs.
- Treatment:
  - Citrate supplementation
  - ↑ fluids.

HYPOMAGNESURIA

- Magnesium is a stone inhibitor.
- Etiology:
  - IBD
  - Deficient diet.

OTHER TYPES OF URINARY STONES

URIC ACID STONES

- Comprise 5–10% of all stones.
- There is no known inhibitor of crystallization, which occurs at low pH.
- Urine pH <5.5.
- Associated with ↑ uric acid in urine.
  - Not necessarily associated with hyperuricemia.
- Secondary causes:
  - Gout – affects up to 20% of patients
  - Chemotherapy for myeloproliferative cancer.
- Most common radiolucent stone.
- Treatment: dissolve:
  - ↑ fluids, alkali (citrate therapy), allopurinol, protein restriction
  - Aim urine output >2500 ml per day:
  - Potassium citrate or sodium bicarbonate
    - Achieve urine pH 6.5–7.0
    - Avoid pH>7.0 as it can precipitate calcium phosphate
  - If hyperuricemic or hyperuricosuric, then allopurinol.

STRUVITE STONES

- Composed of magnesium ammonium phosphate crystals (MAP).
- Also known as infection stones or triple phosphate stones.
- Staghorn calculi are typically struvite stones.
- Caused by infection with urease-producing bacteria:
  - *Proteus* is the most common
  - Urease hydrolyzes urea to form ammonia, which alkalinizes the urine, raises the pH, and allows crystals to form.
- Urine pH will be >7.2.
- Stones may harbor organisms different than those in the urine.[3]
  - Therefore, culture stone fragments separately if possible.
- Treatment:
  - Surgery (see Chapter 3)
  - Antibiotics to prevent infection/stone recurrence
  - Irrigation with acidic solution (hemiacidrin, Suby G).
    - Successful but requires lengthy, complicated treatment and ↑ costs.[4–6]
    - Dangers:
      - Risk of sepsis; therefore, urine must be sterile
      - Hypermagnesemia.
- Acetohydroxamic acid:
  - Inhibits urease
  - 20–70% severe side effects.

CYSTINE STONES

- 1% of all stones.
- Congenital disorder that is autosomal recessive.
- Caused by a defect in cystine reabsorption in the proximal tubule.
- Cystine poorly soluble at normal pH (pKa 8.3).

2

NEPHROLITHIASIS: ETIOLOGY, COMPOSITION, MANAGEMENT, AND PREVENTION

- Crystals form characteristic benzene rings on microscopy.
- Cyanide–nitroprusside screening test shows magenta ring.
- Treatment:
  - Low methionine/sodium diet
  - Hydrate to 3 L urine output/day
  - Alkalinize urine
    - Potassium citrate
    - Complex cystine
      - D-penicillamine (high side effects) or MPG (mercaptopropionylglycine).
        - Pyridoxine to prevent vitamin B_6 deficiency.
- Extracorporeal shock wave lithotripsy (ESWL) not effective.

CALCIUM PHOSPHATE STONES

- Associated with type 1 RTA:
  - Also known as distal RTA
  - Inability of distal nephron to acidify urine, with characteristic hypokalemic, hyperchloremic, non-anion gap metabolic acidosis
  - Urine pH >5.5
  - Hypocitraturia
  - 70% of adults with type I RTA have stones
  - 80% are women
  - Associated with renal cysts.
- Inhibitors of calcium phosphate crystallization:
  - Magnesium
  - Citrate
  - Pyrophosphate
  - Nephrocalcin.
- Treatment:
  - Potassium bicarbonate or potassium citrate, corrects acidosis and ↑ urine citrate
  - ↑ fluids
  - Thiazides if hypercalciuric.

OTHER STONES

- Dihydroxyadenine:
  - Radiolucent.
- Xanthine:
  - Deficiency of xanthine oxidase
  - Also seen in Lesch–Nyhan syndrome patients on allopurinol
  - Radiolucent.
- Matrix:
  - Ureolytic urinary tract infection (UTI)
  - *Alkaline* urine
  - Radiolucent.
- Ammonium acid urate:
  - Ureolytic UTI
  - Children of developing countries and laxative-abusing women.
- Triamterene.

- Indinavir:
  - Radiolucent on kidney, ureter, and bladder (KUB) and computed tomography (CT) scanning.

MEDICAL MANAGEMENT

DIETARY PREVENTION[7,8]

- Fluids:
  - Increased urine output will decrease stone formation[9]
  - If possible, maintain >2.5 L urine output/day.
- Coffee/tea, beer, and wine decrease stone risk.[10]
- Fruit juice has an unclear effect.
  - Lemon juice increases urinary citrate, which decreases risk.
  - Grapefruit juice increases stone risk.

PROTEIN

- Decreasing dietary protein will decrease urine calcium/uric acid/oxalate and increase urine citrate – low/moderate protein intake is desirable.[11]

CALCIURIA

- Except in cases of absorptive hypercalciuria, increased calcium intake may *decrease* stone risk.[12]
  - Calcium binds intestinal oxalate and prevents its absorption.
- Therefore, unless patients have absorptive hypercalciuria, they should maintain adequate calcium intake.

SODIUM

- Increased dietary sodium will increase urinary sodium.
  - However, increased dietary sodium has not been proven to increase stone risk.
- Advise: sodium in moderation.

ASCORBIC ACID (VITAMIN C)

- Metabolized to oxalate.
- Increased vitamin C intake may increase urinary oxalate.[13]
- Advise: vitamin C in moderation.

OXALATE

- Tea, instant coffee, spinach, chocolate, nuts, and rhubarb contain oxalate and may increase urinary oxalate.
- Advise: high-oxalate foods in moderation for calcium oxalate stone formers.

PHARMACOLOGICAL PREVENTION[7]

Thiazides

- Increase calcium resorption and sodium excretion in distal nephron.
- Effective in hypercalciuric and non-hypercalciuric patients.[14]
- Excess urinary sodium may block thiazide-induced calcium reabsorption.

2

NEPHROLITHIASIS: ETIOLOGY, COMPOSITION, MANAGEMENT, AND PREVENTION

- HCTZ 25–50 mg qd-bid or chlorthalidone 12.5–25 mg (up to 100 mg) qd:
  - Start with small dose, titrate as needed
  - Administer concomitant potassium citrate
  - May need ≥2 years for effect.
- Long-term effects:
  - Volume depletion
  - Hypokalemia (correct with potassium-citrate or K-sparing diuretic)
  - Acidosis
  - Hypocitraturia.
- Side effects (30%):
  - Sleepiness
  - ↓ Libido.

Citrate

- Inhibits calcium oxalate crystallization.
- Effective for hypocitraturic stone disease.[15]
- Potassium citrate 10–20 mEq tid w/meals.
- Side effects:
  - Gastrointestinal (GI) intolerance.
- Give liquid prep in diarrhea conditions.

Allopurinol

- Inhibits xanthine oxidase and decreases uric acid production.
- Use in uric acid and hyperuricosuric calcium oxalate stone formers.[16]
- 300 mg PO qd, max 800 mg qd.
- ↓ Dose in renal failure.
- Side effects (rare):
  - Rash
  - LFT abnormalities.

Phosphate (orthophosphate)

- Decreased vitamin D levels, therefore decreased urinary calcium excretion.
- Also increases urine pyrophosphate and citrate.
- However, clinical benefits are uncertain.

Magnesium

- Increases urinary citrate.
- May cause diarrhea.
- Clinical benefits uncertain, but randomized study using potassium magnesium citrate showed potential benefit.[17]

Sodium cellulose phosphate

- Binds calcium in the gut and inhibits absorption.
- Indicated for use in absorptive hypercalciuria.
- 5 g qd–tid with meals.
- Side effects:
  - Diarrhea
  - Hypomagnesemia.

Antibiotics

- Long-term prophylaxis for struvite stone formers after surgical treatment.
- Drug should be culture-specific.

Acetohydroxamic acid

- Urease inhibitor for infection stones.
- 250 mg PO q 8 h bid–qid.
- 20–70% have severe side effects.

Chelating agents

- Indicated for cystinuria (i.e. cystein stone formers).
- D-penicillamine:
  - 250 mg qd to 750 mg tid before meals
  - Side effects occur in 70% of patients.
- MPG (or Thiola):
  - Side effects 40%
  - Pyridoxine 50 mg bid to prevent vitamin B_6 deficiency.

REFERENCES

1. Menon M, Resnick MI: Urinary lithiasis: etiology, diagnosis, and medical management. In: Walsh PC, Retik AB, Vaughan ED, Wein AJ, eds. Campbell's Urology, 8th edn. Philadelphia: WB Saunders, 2002.
2. Marangella M, Bagnis C, Bruno M et al: Crystallization inhibitors in the pathophysiology and treatment of nephrolithiasis. Urol Int 72 (Suppl 1):6, 2004.
3. Rodman JS: Struvite stones. Nephron 81 (Suppl 1):50, 1999.
4. Streem SB, Lammert G: Long-term efficacy of combination therapy for struvite staghorn calculi. J Urol 147:563, 1992.
5. Tiselius HG, Hellgren E, Andersson A, Borrud-Ohlsson A, Eriksson I. Minimally invasive treatment of infection staghorn stones with shock wave lithotripsy and chemolysis. Scand J Urol Nephrol 33:286, 1999.
6. Wall I, Tiselius H, Hellgren E: Minimally invasive treatment of hemiacidrin soluble staghorn renal stones. J Lithotr Stone Dis 3:31, 1991.
7. Pearle MS: Prevention of nephrolithiasis. Curr Opin Nephrol Hypertens 10:203, 2001.
8. Assimos DG, Holmes RP: Role of diet in the therapy of urolithiasis. Urol Clin North Am 27:255, 2000.
9. Borghi L, Meschi T, Schianchi T et al: Urine volume: stone risk factor and preventive measure. Nephron 81 (Suppl 1):31, 1999.
10. Curhan GC, Willett WC, Speizer FE, Stampfer MJ: Beverage use and risk for kidney stones in women. Ann Intern Med 128:534, 1998.
11. Giannini S, Nobile M, Sartori L et al: Acute effects of moderate dietary protein restriction in patients with idiopathic hypercalciuria and calcium nephrolithiasis. Am J Clin Nutr 69:267, 1999.
12. Curhan GC, Willett WC, Rimm EB, Stampfer MJ: A prospective study of dietary calcium and other nutrients and the risk of symptomatic kidney stones. New Engl J Med 328:833, 1993.
13. Traxer O, Huet B, Poindexter J, Pak CY, Pearle MS: Effect of ascorbic acid consumption on urinary stone risk factors. J Urol 170:397, 2003.
14. Pearle MS, Roehrborn CG, Pak CY: Meta-analysis of randomized trials for medical prevention of calcium oxalate nephrolithiasis. J Endourol 13:679, 1999.
15. Barcelo P, Wuhl O, Servitge E, Rousaud A, Pak CY: Randomized double-blind study of potassium citrate in idiopathic hypocitraturic calcium nephrolithiasis. J Urol 150:1761, 1993.

2

NEPHROLITHIASIS: ETIOLOGY, COMPOSITION, MANAGEMENT, AND PREVENTION

16. Ettinger B, Tang A, Citron JT, Livermore B, Williams T: Randomized trial of allopurinol in the prevention of calcium oxalate calculi. New Engl J Med 315:1386, 1986.
17. Ettinger B, Pak CY, Citron JT et al: Potassium-magnesium citrate is an effective prophylaxis against recurrent calcium oxalate nephrolithiasis. J Urol 158:2069, 1997.

Nephrolithiasis: surgical treatment and metabolic evaluation

Andrew A Wagner

SUMMARY

- Acute stones present as flank pain radiating to the contralateral lower abdomen and groin, nausea/vomiting, hematuria, irritative voiding symptoms, and fevers.
- Urinalysis (U/A) typically shows red cells and white cells, with bacteria if there is a concomitant infection.
- Treatment of acute stone episodes includes IV fluids, pain control, antibiotics if urine infection is present, and, if necessary, decompression of the urinary tract with a ureteral stent or nephrostomy tube.
- Treatment of stones includes expectant management, extracorporeal shock wave lithotripsy (ESWL), ureteroscopy, and percutaneous nephrolithotomy (PCNL).
- Type of treatment depends upon stone size and location.

PRESENTATION AND HISTORY

PRESENTATION

- Renal colic:
  - Classically described as flank pain, often acute in onset, radiating to the ispilateral abdomen
  - Distal ureteral stones may be associated with ipsilateral groin, testicular (in men – can mimic torsion or epididymitis), and vulvar (in women) pain
  - Usually waxes and wanes; continuous pain may indicate pyelonephritis
  - In contrast to patients with peritonitis, patients with renal colic will frequently move about to find a more comfortable position.
- Nausea and vomiting.
- Irritative voiding symptoms.
- Hematuria (gross or microscopic).
- Urinary infection.
- Fever, especially if infection is present.
- Occasionally asymptomatic, with stones detected incidentally.

PAST MEDICAL HISTORY

- Decreased fluid intake.
- Urinary tract infections.
- High-protein diet (associated with acidosis, hypocitraturia, hypercalciuria, hyperuricosuria, and hyperoxaluria).
- Inflammatory bowel disease, small bowel resection, or jejunoileal bypass (hyperoxaluria and calcium oxalate stones).
- Primary hyperparathyroidism (hypercalciuria and calcium oxalate stones).
- Gout (uric acid stones).
- Total colectomy (uric acid stones).

- Renal tubular acidosis (calcium phosphate stones).
- Medications:
  - Steroids (hypercalciuria)
  - Loop diuretics (hypercalciuria)
  - Colchicine (hyperuricosuria)
  - Vitamin D
  - Antacids
  - Triamterene
  - Indinavir.
- Associated genitourinary diseases:
  - Ureteropelvic junction (UPJ) obstruction
  - Bladder reconstruction
  - Benign prostatic hyperplasia (BPH)
  - Medullary sponge kidney.
- Family history of stones.[1]
- Social history:
  - Immobility and sedentary lifestyle increase risk
  - Wine/beer decrease risk.

EVALUATION IN THE ACUTE SETTING

PHYSICAL EXAM

- Evaluate for fever.
  - Concomitant infection may be associated with tachycardia and/or hypotension.
- Abdominal exam to evaluate for flank tenderness/peritonitis.

URINALYSIS AND URINE CULTURE

- Red blood cells (RBCs) are usually present, although up to 15% may have none.[1]
- White blood cells (WBCs) may be present.
- pH:
  - <5.5 and radiolucent stone: consider uric acid
  - >5.5 with metabolic acidosis, hypokalemia, and hyperchloremia: consider renal tubular acidosis (RTA)
  - >6.0: consider struvite.
- Crystals:
  - Calcium oxalate: dumbbell/hourglass/bipyramidal
  - Calcium phosphate: needle-shaped/amorphous
  - Uric acid: amorphous/rosettes
  - Struvite: coffin lid
  - Cystine: benzene ring/hexagonal.

SERUM STUDIES

- Complete blood count (CBC).
- Electrolytes.
- Calcium.
- Phosphate.
- Uric acid.

IMAGING

KUB

- Pelvic phleboliths tend to be round, while stones are irregular.
- 5 typical locations of stone impaction:
  - Calyx
  - Ureteropelvic junction (UPJ)
  - Pelvic brim (iliacs)
  - Posterior pelvis (broad ligament, females)
  - Ureterovesical junction (UVJ).

Intravenous pyelogram (IVP)

- Nowadays, rarely used in the acute setting.
- Occasionally useful for preoperative planning for PCNL or to identify a level of obstruction when computed tomography (CT) is equivocal.

Ultrasound

- Pregnancy and pediatrics: avoids radiation.
- Poor visualization of small renal and ureteral stones.

Non-contrast computed tomography

- 97% sensitive and 97% spccific for stone disease.
- 4 signs of obstruction:
  - *I lydroureter*
  - *Perinephric stranding*
  - Hydonephrosis
  - Nephromegaly.

MANAGEMENT

ACUTE MANAGEMENT

- Pain control:
  - Narcotics
  - NSAIDs: may consider ketorolac if no history of renal disease, bleeding diathesis, peptic ulcer disease, or gastroesophageal reflux disease.
- IV fluids.
- Antibiotics if urinary infection is present.
- Strain urine.
- Recommended indications for admission:
  - Uncontrolled pain
  - Unremitting nausea/vomiting with inability to tolerate PO
  - Obstructed, infected renal unit
  - Obstructed, solitary renal unit
  - Bilateral obstruction
  - Anuria.
- Recommended indications for acute intervention (ureteral stent, percutaneous nephrostomy, or stone removal):
  - Obstructed infected system (drainage only! Definitive stone treatment is not recommended due to risk of sepsis)
  - Obstructed solitary kidney

- Stone unlikely to pass (>5 mm)
- Intolerable symptoms
- Symptom duration >2 weeks.
- Recommended indications for watchful waiting:
  - No evidence of infection
  - Pain well-controlled with oral medications
  - Stone <5 mm
  - No obstruction.
- Overall spontaneous stone passage rates are shown in Table 3.1.
- Spontaneous stone passage rates based on location:
  - Proximal: 20%
  - Distal: 70%.

MEDICAL OPTIONS DURING EXPECTANT MANAGEMENT[2-7]

- Pain control.
- Antibiotic prophylaxis:
  - Reasonable to start, especially in high-risk patients (i.e. diabetics, elderly)
  - UTI occurs in up to 3% of patients during watchful waiting
  - Potential options: Macrodantin (nitrofurantoin) 100 mg PO qd or Bactrim DS (trimethoprim/sulfamethoxazole) 1 tab PO qd or Levaquin (levofloxacin) 250 mg PO qd.
- Alpha-blockers:
  - α-1 receptors located on terminal ureter
  - α-1 antagonists may decrease ureteral tone
  - A few small clinical trials suggest that Flomax (tamsulosin) 0.4 mg PO qd or other alpha-blockers facilitate passage of distal stones, especially when combined with steroids.[3,4]
- Calcium channel blockers:[5,6]
  - Decrease ureteral muscle spasm
  - Speeds passage when used with steroids
  - A few small clinical trials suggest that nifedipine XL 30 mg PO qd × 7 days facilitates passage of ureteral stones.
- Steroids:[5-7]
  - May decrease local inflammation and/or ureteral spasm
  - Typical dose: prednisone 10 mg PO bid × 5 days; may need to consider tapered dose.

TABLE 3.1

STONE PASSAGE RATES

	Stone size		
	<4 mm	4–6 mm	>6 mm
Spontaneous passage within 1 year	90%	60%	20%

SURGERY

PREOPERATIVE CHECK LIST

- KUB (same day) and other appropriate imaging.
- Urinalysis and urine culture.
- Appropriate prophylactic and perioperative antibiotics.[8]

PROCEDURES

Extracorporeal shock wave lithotripsy

- Imaging: fluoroscopy (most common) or ultrasound (less common; difficult visualization).
- Anesthesia: sedation or general; consider EMLA cream at skin site.
- Associated with transient decreases in renal blood flow.
- Potential long-term renal effects:[9]
  - Renal injury/scar
  - Hypertension especially if kidney small or impaired.
- Complications:
  - Hematoma (<1%)
  - UTI/sepsis
  - Obstruction (*Steinstrasse*)
  - Injury to nearby organs (bowel, lung, pancreas, spleen, liver) – very rare!
- Contraindications:
  - Pregnancy
  - Calcified aneurysm
  - Morbid obesity
  - Bleeding diathesis.
- Postoperative follow-up should include:
  - KUB in 2–4 weeks to document stone fragment passage
  - Monitor blood pressure.

Ureteroscopy

- Rigid scope useful for:
  - Distal ureteral stones in men
  - Distal and proximal ureteral stones in women.
- Flexible scope useful for:
  - Proximal ureteral and renal stones.

Percutaneous nephrolithotomy

- Major complications (1–7%):[10]
  - Bleeding, sepsis, organ injury, perforation, hydrothorax, or pneumothorax (from supracostal percutaneous access tract).
- Minor (11–25%).[10]
- Consider non-contrast CT on postoperative day 1 to evaluate for residual stones.

3

NEPHROLITHIASIS: SURGICAL TREATMENT AND METABOLIC EVALUATION

TREATMENT OF RENAL STONES (BY SIZE)

RENAL STONES <2.0 CM

Expectant management

- Consider if asymptomatic and <5 mm.
- Most stones will increase in size.
- Up to 50% will become symptomatic (i.e. pain/infection) within 5 years.
- If UA stone, consider trial of dissolution with potassium citrate.

ESWL

- Typically, first-line therapy.
- Success rates by size:[10]
  - <10 mm: 80%
  - 11–20 mm: 65%
  - >20 mm: 50%.
- Consider placement of ureteral stent for stone >1.0 cm to prevent *Steinstrasse* (symptomatic obstruction of ureter by stone fragments).
- Situations where ESWL may have more limited success:
  - Larger stone
  - Harder stones: cystine, calcium phosphate, and calcium oxalate monohydrate
  - Obese patient
  - UPJ obstruction
  - Calyceal diverticulum
  - Lower pole location.

Ureteroscopy

- Up to 90% success rate in expert hands.[11]
- Ureteral access sheath can facilitate fragment removal.
- Should reposition lower pole stones to upper pole for easier fragmentation and passage.

Approach to lower pole stones: ESWL vs PCNL

- <10 mm – ESWL first-line therapy:
  - ~70% stone-free with ESWL[12,13]
  - 100% stone-free with PCNL.
- >20 mm – PCNL first-line therapy:
  - ~90% stone-free with PCNL[12,13]
  - ~30% stone-free with ESWL.
- 10–20 mm – the controversy!
  - ~90% stone-free with PCNL[12,13]
  - ~50% stone-free with ESWL
  - Also take into account: stone composition, renal anatomy, and patient preference.
- PCNL may be superior for:
  - Stone >1.5 cm
  - Acute infundibular-pelvic angle (<90°)
  - Narrow infundibulum (<4 mm)
  - Previous failed ESWL.

RENAL STONES >2.0 CM

PCNL

- Typically is first-line therapy.

Ureteroscopy

- Consider if patient is morbidly obese, is coagulopathic, or has other clinical conditions/comorbidities that would render PCNL problematic.
- Note that, depending on stone size, compared with ESWL, may be more tedious and more difficult to remove all stone fragments.

ESWL

- Consider if patient is morbidly obese, is coagulopathic, or has other clinical conditions/comorbidities that would render PCNL problematic.
- Will likely require multiple sessions.
- Ureteral stent should be placed to prevent Steinstrasse.

Open surgery

- Rarely performed nowadays.
- Approach: pyelolithotomy.

Approach to staghorn calculi[14]

- Most commonly struvite.
- Definitions:
  - Partial: extends into $\geq$2 calyces
  - Complete: extends into all calyces.
- PCNL:
  - First line therapy and mainstay of treatment.
- PCNL/ESWL combination therapy:
  - 'Sandwich therapy'
  - Three stages: PCNL, followed by ESWL, followed by PCNL
  - Stages separated by 1–2 days
  - CT imaging should be performed after each stage to assess for residual stones
  - Flexible nephroscopy at the final stage can assess and treat residual stone fragments.
- ESWL monotherapy:
  - Typically not recommended
  - May be useful in young children/infants
  - Percutaneous nephrostomy tube or ureteral stent mandatory in adults.

STONE-FREE RATES[14]

- PCNL: 78%.
- Combo PCNL/ESWL: 66%.
- ESWL: 54%.
- Open surgery: 71%.

SIGNIFICANT COMPLICATIONS[14]

- PCNL: 15%.
- Combo PCNL/ESWL: 14%.
- ESWL: 19%.
- Open surgery: 13%.

TREATMENT OF RENAL STONES: ANATOMIC VARIANTS

URETEROPELVIC JUNCTION OBSTRUCTION

- PCNL combined with direct vision endopyelotomy:
  - 80% successful.
- Laparoscopic pyeloplasty with pyelolithotomy.

CALYCEAL DIVERTICULUM

- PCNL:
  - >90% successful
  - Allows ablation of diverticulum/incision of calyceal neck.
- Ureteroscopy with ablation and/or dilation of calyceal neck:
  - Technically difficult
  - Use only for small stones (<1 cm).

HORESHOE KIDNEYS

- ESWL:[10]
  - For small stones (<1.5 cm)
  - Overall treatment success rate tends to be lower (28–78%)
  - Use prone position for anteromedial calyces.
- PCNL:
  - For larger stones (≥ 1.5 cm) and/or other conditions rendering ESWL problematic (i.e. morbid obesity)
  - Upper poles tend to be best for percutaneous access since they are oriented posterolaterally.
- May also consider ureteroscopy.

TREATMENT OF URETERAL STONES (BY SIZE AND LOCATION)[15]

UETERAL STONES <5 MM: ANY LOCATION

Expectant management

- Stone has a >50% chance of spontaneous passage, slightly increased if in the distal ureter.
- Some medications may abet passage (see above).

ESWL (proximal)

Ureteroscopy (distal)

URETERAL STONES <1.0 CM: PROXIMAL

ESWL

- First-line therapy.
- Ureteral stent:
  - Will not improve fragmentation
  - Used for relief of symptoms/obstruction
  - Displacement of stone into renal pelvis may potentially improve results.

Ureteroscopy or PCNL

- For ESWL failure.

URETERAL STONES >1.0 CM: PROXIMAL

- ESWL, ureteroscopy, and PCNL are all acceptable alternatives.

URETERAL STONES <1.0 CM: DISTAL

- ESWL and ureteroscopy are acceptable alternatives.

URETERAL STONES >1.0 CM: DISTAL

- ESWL and ureteroscopy are acceptable alternatives.
- Blind basketing of stone should not be performed.

STONE-FREE RATES[15]

- Stone-free rates are shown in Table 3.2.

TABLE 3.2		
STONE-FREE RATES		
	Proximal ureter	Distal ureter
<1.0 cm		
ESWL	84%	85%
Ureteroscopy	56%	89%
PCNL	76%	–
≥1.0 cm		
ESWL	72%	74%
Ureteroscopy	44%	73%
PCNL	74%	–

NEPHROLITHIASIS: SURGICAL TREATMENT AND METABOLIC EVALUATION

3

STONE FRAGMENTATION TECHNOLOGIES

ELECTROHYDRAULIC LITHOTRIPSY (EHL)

- Spark creates hydraulic shock wave.
- Probe placed 1 mm from stone.
- Use normal saline for irrigation.
- Start with 50 V and gradually increase as needed.
- Perforation of urinary tract is possible without contact between probe tip and urothelium.
- 1.6F probe for flexible ureteroscopy.
- May allow more rapid fragmentation than holmium laser although smallest probes are fragile.

HOLMIUM:YAG LASER

- Generally safer than EHL.
- Can fragment all stone types.
- 200 μm or 365 μm fibers for ureteroscopy.
- 550 μm or 1000 μm fiber for bladder stones.
- Probe must touch stone.
- Keep probe 1 mm from urothelium.
- Beginning settings:
  - Power 0.5 J; frequency 5 Hz
  - ↑ frequency (up to 15 Hz), then energy (up to 1.0 J), as needed, to speed lithotripsy.[16]

BALLISTIC LITHOTRIPSY (PNEUMATIC)

- Instrument acts like jackhammer.
- More efficient fragmentation of larger/hard stones.
- Lowest risk of perforation compared with laser, EHL, or U/S lithotripsy.
- Small probes available for rigid ureteroscopy.

ULTRASONIC LITHOTRIPSY

- Ultrasonic waves vibrate probe, transmitting energy to the stone:[10]
- Simultaneous suction of fragments through probe.
- Mostly used in PCNL.
- *Gentle* pressure on stone to avoid perforation.

METABOLIC STONE EVALUATION[17,18]

- All stone patients should have work-up as defined under 'Evaluation in the Acute Setting' above.
  - In addition, if stones are recovered during treatment/follow-up, they should be sent for chemical analysis.
- High-risk patients should have a full metabolic evaluation.
- Wait at least 4 weeks after resolution of acute stone episode or stone procedures prior to initiating evaluation.
- Definition of high-risk patients:[17,18]
  - Stones during childhood

- Cystine, uric acid, or struvite stones
- Concomitant intestinal diseases
- Multiple/recurrent stones
- Family history
- Osteoporosis
- Nephrocalcinosis.
- Evaluation in high-risk patients:
  - 24 h urine stone risk analysis × 2.
- Patient should stop stone-prevention medications for 5 days prior to study.

EVALUATION

- Volume.
- pH.
- Creatinine.
- Calcium.
- Phosphate.
- Potassium.
- Sodium.
- Uric acid.
- Oxalate.
- Citrate.
- Magnesium:
  - Specific treatments based on results: see Chapter 2 for details.
  - Follow-up urine stone risk analysis to monitor treatment efficacy.

URINARY STONES DURING PREGNANCY[19]

URINARY TRACT CHANGES DURING PREGNANCY

- Bilateral hydronephrosis:
  - Classically associated with the right renal unit
  - Associated with increased progesterone and ureteral compression by gravid uterus.
- Absorptive hypercalciuria and hyperuricosuria.
- Increased urinary excretion of citrate and magnesium.
- Decreased serum creatinine.

DIAGNOSIS

- Radiation issues:
  - Exposure hazardous during first trimester
  - Risk of congenital anomaly doubles at 25–80 cGy[20]
  - KUB: 0.14 cGy; IVP: 0.17 cGy; CT: 2.5 cGy
  - KUB or limited IVP have <1% of critical dose of radiation and are safe if medically necessary.
- Ultrasound:
  - First-line modality for diagnosis
  - Unreliable for ureteral stones; vaginal ultrasound may aid diagnosis of distal ureteral stones
  - Resistive index may be helpful.[21]

- IVP:
  - Second-line modality for diagnosis: not recommend as first-line diagnostic test because of potential radiation exposure
  - 3 film limited study may be considered: scout, 30 seconds after injection, and 20 minutes after injection.
- MRI or nuclear scan:
  - Third-line modalities for diagnosis.

TREATMENT

- 75% will pass spontaneously with hydration, pain medications, and antibiotics.
- For intractable pain and/or obstruction, obtain drainage with ureteral stent or percutaneous nephrostomy tube utilizing ultrasound guidance.
- Note that ureteral stents will tend to calcify early in pregnant women and require changing every 4–8 weeks.
- Ureteroscopy with basketing or holmium laser lithotripsy is safe in experienced hands.[22,23]
- ESWL, EHL, and ultrasonic lithotripsy are contraindicated.

REFERENCES

1. Menon M, Resnick MI: Urinary lithiasis: etiology, diagnosis, and medical management. In: Walsh PC, Retik AB, Vaughan ED, Wein AJ, eds. Campbell's Urology, 8th Edn. Philadelphia: WB Saunders, 2002.
2. Porena M, Guiggi P, Balestra A, Micheli C: Pain killers and antibacterial therapy for kidney colic and stones. Urol Int 72 (Suppl 1):34, 2004.
3. Dellabella M, Milanese G, Muzzonigro G: Efficacy of tamsulosin in the medical management of juxtavesical ureteral stones. J Urol 170:2202, 2003.
4. Porpiglia F, Ghignone G, Fiori C, Fontana D, Scarpa RM: Nifedipine versus tamsulosin for the management of lower ureteral stones. J Urol 172:568, 2004.
5. Borghi L, Meschi T, Amato F et al: Nifedipine and methylprednisolone in facilitating ureteral stone passage: a randomized, double-blind, placebo-controlled study. J Urol 152:1095, 1994.
6. Porpiglia F, Destefanis P, Fiori C, Fontana D: Effectiveness of nifedipine and deflazacort in the management of distal ureter stones. Urology 56:579, 2000.
7. Cooper JT, Stack GM, Cooper TP: Intensive medical management of ureteral calculi. Urology 56:575, 2000.
8. Pearle MS: Prevention of nephrolithiasis. Curr Opin Nephrol Hypertens 10:203, 2001.
9. Bataille P, Cardon G, Bouzernidj M et al: Renal and hypertensive complications of extracorporeal shock wave lithotripsy: who is at risk? Urol Int 62:195, 1999.
10. Lingeman JE, Lifshitz DA, Evan AP: Surgical management of urinary lithiasis. Campbell's Urology, 4: 2003.
11. Fabrizio MD, Behari A, Bagley DH: Ureteroscopic management of intrarenal calculi. J Urol 159:1139, 1998.
12. Lingeman JE, Siegel YI, Steele B, Nyhuis AW, Woods JR: Management of lower pole nephrolithiasis: a critical analysis. J Urol 151:663, 1994.
13. Albala DM, Assimos DG, Clayman RV et al: Lower pole I: a prospective randomized trial of extracorporeal shock wave lithotripsy and percutaneous nephrostolithotomy for lower pole nephrolithiasis – initial results. J Urol 166:2072, 2001.
14. Preminger GM, Assimos DG, Lingeman JE et al: AUA guideline: report on the management of staghorn calculi. AUA, Office of Education and Research 1:1, 2005.

15. Segura JW, Preminger GM, Assimos DG et al: Ureteral Stones Clinical Guidelines Panel summary report on the management of ureteral calculi. The American Urological Association. J Urol 158:1915, 1997.
16. Spore SS, Teichman J, Corbin NS et al: Holmium:YAG lithotripsy: optimal power settings. J Endourol 13:559, 1999.
17. Consensus conference. Prevention and treatment of kidney stones. JAMA 260:977, 1988.
18. Lifshitz DA, Shalhav AL, Lingeman JE, Evan AP: Metabolic evaluation of stone disease patients: a practical approach. J Endourol 13:669, 1999.
19. McAleer SJ, Loughlin KR: Nephrolithiasis and pregnancy. Curr Opin Urol 14:123, 2004.
20. Swartz HM, Reichling BA: Hazards of radiation exposure for pregnant women. JAMA 239:1907, 1978.
21. Shokeir AA, Mahran MR, Abdulmaaboud M: Renal colic in pregnant women: role of renal resistive index. Urology 55:344, 2000.
22. Watterson JD, Girvan AR, Beiko DT et al: Ureteroscopy and holmium:YAG laser lithotripsy: an emerging definitive management strategy for symptomatic ureteral calculi in pregnancy. Urology 60:383, 2002.
23. Kavoussi LR, Jackman SV, Bishoff JT: Re: renal colic during pregnancy: a case for conservative treatment. J Urol 160:837, 1998.

3

NEPHROLITHIASIS: SURGICAL TREATMENT AND METABOLIC EVALUATION

Infertility

Wilmer B Roberts

SUMMARY

- Infertility is the inability of a couple to become pregnant after 1 year of frequent, unprotected intercourse.
- Among couples with normal fertility parameters, 20–25% will typically conceive within 1 month, 75% within 6 months, and 90% within 1 year.
- 15% of US couples are infertile: 40% female factors, 20% male factors, 30% both male and female factors, and 10% untraceable.
- Initial evaluation of male factor infertility includes history, physical exam, and semen analysis.
- Further evaluation and treatment depends upon semen analysis results. Patients may have low volume or absent ejaculate, azoospermia, oligospermia, asthenospermia (abnormalities of sperm movement), sperm morphological defects, and/or combinations of these abnormalities.
- Of infertile couples, 25–35% will conceive by intercourse alone without treatment.
- Intracytoplasmic sperm injection is an efficacious modality.

GENERAL INFORMATION

DEFINITION[1]

- The inability of a couple to become pregnant after 1 year of frequent, unprotected intercourse.
- Among couples with normal fertility parameters, 20–25% will typically conceive within 1 month, 75% within 6 months, and 90% within 1 year.

EPIDEMIOLOGY[2–4]

- 15% of US couples are infertile:
  - 40% involve primarily female factors
  - 20% primarily male factors
  - 30% both male and female factors
  - 10% untraceable.

PHYSIOLOGY AND PATHOPHYSIOLOGY OF MALE REPRODUCTION

HYPOTHALAMUS–PITUITARY–TESTICULAR AXIS

- Controls normal spermatogenesis.
- Hypothalamus: secretes gonadotropin-releasing hormone (GnRH).
  - GnRH-secreting neurons receive signals from multiple sites in the brain, including the amygdala, olfactory, and visual cortex
  - GnRH secreted in pulsatile fashion, every 90–120 minutes, highest in a.m. and seasonally in the spring.

- Failure of GnRH-secreting cells to migrate properly during embryogenesis results in Kallmann's syndrome (congenital hypogonadotropic hypogonadism, which is associated with anosmia and midline defects).
- Anterior pituitary:
  - Secretes luteinizing hormone (LH) and follicle-stimulating hormone (FSH) in response to GnRH.
- Testes:
  - Leydig cells, stimulated by LH, produce testosterone
  - Testosterone feeds back on hypothalamus to inhibit GnRH secretion
  - Sertoli cells, stimulated by FSH, produce inhibin
  - Inhibin feeds back on anterior pituitary and inhibits FSH secretion.

SEMINIFEROUS TUBULES

- Site of spermatogenesis.
- Sertoli cells (non-dividing):
  - Stimulated by FSH
  - Support spermatogenesis in the seminiferous epithelium
  - Form the 'blood–testis barrier' with tight junctions between adjacent cells.[5,6]
- Germinal cells (dividing):
  - Develop into sperm cells: one primary spermatocyte (46N) undergoes meiosis to form two secondary spermatocytes (23N), which divide to form four spermatids (23N), which undergo spermiogenesis to form four mature sperm cells (23N)
  - Renew epithelial stem cells (likely a c-kit mediated process).[7]
- Spermatogenesis takes 74 days.
- Azoospermia linked in 12 men to deletions of the azoospermic factor region on the Y-chromosome involving the *DAZ* (deleted in azoospermia) gene.[8]

SPERM MATURATION

- Sperms mature as they progress from seminiferous tubules to vas (also called ductus) deferens.
- Normal sperm transport and maturation:
  - Seminiferous tubules → rete testis → ductuli efferentes → caput epididymis (in which sperm develop motility through unknown mechanism) → vas (ductus) deferens.
- Intermesenteric nerves and renal plexus provide autonomic innervation (no somatic) to Leydig cell clusters (neural modulation of testosterone production implicated).
- Epididymal innervation arises from intermediate spermatic nerves (superior hypogastric plexus) and inferior spermatic nerves (pelvic plexus).
- Epididymal transport requires 2–12 days (5α-reductase important).[9,10]
- Vas (ductus) deferens:
  - Arterial supply = deferential artery from inferior vesicular
  - Nerve supply = sympathetic and parasympathetic from hypogastric plexus via presacral nerve.[11,12]

TESTICULAR ANATOMY

- Embryology:
  - Testicle: formed from coelomic epithelium of the genital ridge and underlying mesenchyme and migration of primordial germ cells
  - Epididymis and vas deferens: from Wolffian (mesonephric) duct.
- Typical volume: 15–25 ml.
- Typical longitudinal length: 4.5–5.1 cm.
- Arterial supply:
  - Internal spermatic artery
  - Deferential artery
  - Cremasteric artery.
- Venous drainage:
  - Via the pampiniform plexus
  - Countercurrent exchange of heat lowers testicular temperature by 2–4°C, which is important for normal spermatogenesis.

SEMINAL FLUID

Composition

- Secretions from the testis, epididymis, Cowper's bulbourethral glands, periurethral glands of Littre, prostate (acidic) and seminal vesicles (alkaline).
- Initially a coagulum due to seminal vesicle fluid, which is high in fructose.
  - Liquefaction occurs secondary to prostate-derived proteases [prostate-specific antigen (PSA) and plasminogen activator].

Volume

- Normal volume is ≥2.0 ml.
- Abnormal/small volume ejaculate caused by:
  - Ejaculatory duct obstruction (acidic pH, low fructose)
  - Androgen deficiency (acidic pH, low fructose)
  - Retrograde ejaculation
  - Sympathetic denervation
  - Agenesis of the vas deferens/seminal vesicles (acidic pH, low fructose, lack of coagulation)
  - Drug therapy
  - Bladder neck surgery.

Sperm count

- Median 70–100 million/ml.

Sperm motility

- Zero-to-Four Scale:[13]
  - 0 = no motility (alive, but flagellar defects vs dead sperm)
  - 1 = sluggish/non-progressive movement
  - 2 = slow/meandering forward progression
  - 3 = relatively straight movement with moderate speed
  - 4 = straight movement with high speed.
- WHO scale (1999):[14]
  - A = rapid-progressive motility

4

INFERTILITY

- B = slow/sluggish progressive motility
- C = non-progressive motility
- D = no motility (ultrastructural defects vs necrospermia).

Morphology

- Head:
  - Oval-shaped
  - 5.0–6.0 × 2.5–3.5 µm.
- Acrosome:
  - Comprises 40–70% of head.
- Midpiece:
  - 1.5 × head length
  - <1.0 µm wide.
- Tail:
  - Uncoiled, free from kinks
  - ~45 µm long.
- Cytoplasmic droplets:
  - In midpiece *only* and <50% of the head area.
- Normal semen:
  - >60% normal forms *and* <3% immature forms with equivalent sperm densities (i.e. >20 million/ml)
  - In vitro fertilization (IVF) rates 37% with <14% normal sperm and 91% with >14% normal sperm.

QUICK NORMAL REFERENCE VALUES[14]

- Volume ≥2.0 ml.
- pH ≥7.2.
- Number >20 million/ml or >40 million/ejaculate.
- Motility >50% grade A + B or >25% grade A.
- Normal morphology >15%.
- Viability >75%.
- White blood cells (WBCs) <1 million/ml.

EVALUATION

HISTORY

- Developmental:
  - Testicular descent, delayed pubertal development, decreased sexual function/libido, loss of body hair or decrease in frequency of shaving.
- Sexual:
  - Libido, intercourse frequency, prior fertility assessments.
- School performance:
  - Learning disabilities suggestive of Klinefelter's syndrome.
- Chronic medical illnesses and infections:
  - Mumps, sinopulmonary symptoms, sexually transmitted diseases (STDs), genitourinary infections.
- Surgical procedures involving the inguinal and scrotal regions:
  - Vasectomy, orchiectomy, herniorraphy.

- Drugs/environmental exposures:
  - Ethanol (alcohol) frequency, anabolic steroids, chemo/radiation therapy, drugs causing hyperprolactinemia, pesticides, hormonal disrupters.

PHYSICAL EXAMINATION

- External genitalia:
  - Measure testicular size
  - Assess for vasal and/or epididymal thickening, varicocele, hernia
  - Assess for ambiguous genitalia, micropenis, and hypospadias.
- General:
  - Assess for eunuchoidal proportions: arm span >2 cm more than height, heel-to-pubis >2 cm more than pubis-to-crown
  - Assess for loss of pubic, axillary, and facial hair; decreased oiliness of the skin and fine facial wrinkling; and gynecomastia (suggests decreased androgen-to-estrogen ratio).

SEMEN ANALYSIS

- Collect at least two samples, at least 1–2 weeks apart, each after at least 2–7 days of abstinence.
- Assess volume and pH (see normal criteria above).
- Microscopy:
  - Debris and agglutination
  - Sperm concentration/motility/morphology
  - Leukocyte count
  - Look for immature germ cells.

LABORATORY ANALYSIS

Postcoital test

- In vivo assessment of sperm–cervical mucus interaction.
- Woman in preovulatory phase.
- Number and motility of sperm in cervical mucus assessed 9–24 hours after vaginal intercourse.

Slide/capillary test

- In vitro assessment of sperm–cervical mucus interaction.

Advanced testing

- Computer-aided sperm analysis.
- Acrosome reaction.
- Zona-free hamster oocyte penetration test.
- Human zona pellucida binding test.
- Sperm biochemistry.
- Sperm chromatin and DNA assays.

4

INFERTILITY

EVALUATION AND TREATMENT BASED ON SEMEN ANALYSIS RESULTS[15]

LOW VOLUME/ABSENT EJACULATE

- Rule out incomplete specimen collection and short abstinence period.
- Differential diagnosis includes medications, history of retroperitoneal or bladder neck surgery, ejaculatory duct obstruction, diabetes, and spinal cord injury.
- *Perform postejaculatory urinalysis to evaluate for retrograde ejaculation:*
  - If positive (i.e. high sperm counts), treat with sympathomimetics vs bladder wash with artificial insemination
  - If negative, obtain transrectal ultrasound.
- *Transrectal ultrasound to evaluate for ejaculatory duct obstruction:*
  - If abnormal, aspirate seminal vesicles
  - If normal, treat with sympathomimetics and/or electroejaculation.
- *Transrectal aspiration of seminal vesicles to evaluate for ejaculatory duct and epididymal obstruction:*
  - If positive, perform transurethral resection of the ejaculatory ducts (TURED)
  - If negative, perform TURED and epididymovasostomy.

AZOOSPERMIA

- Absence of sperm in the ejaculate.
- Differential diagnosis (decreased spermatogenesis vs obstruction):
  - Failure of hypothalamic–pituitary function: hypogonadotropic hypogonadism (Kallmann's syndrome) or pituitary tumor
  - Primary failure of spermatogenesis: spermatogenic abnormalities, congenital chromosomal abnormalities, Y-chromosome microdeletions, gonadotoxins, varicocele, idiopathic
  - Ductal obstruction: congenital bilateral absence of the vas deferens (CBAVD, caused by deficiency of the *CFTR* gene), vasal obstruction, epididymal obstruction, ejaculatory duct obstruction.
- *Evaluate for presence of vasa on exam:*
  - Vasa not present: assume CBAVD is present – perform *CFTR* testing and consider assisted reproduction vs adoption
  - Vasa present: check testicular size.
- *Evaluate testicular size:*
  - Bilateral normal testicles or unilateral testicular atrophy: check serum FSH
  - Bilateral testicular atrophy: check serum FSH.
- *Bilateral normal testicles or unilateral testicular atrophy:*
  - Normal FSH: perform testicular biopsy – abnormal biopsy means primary testicular failure (treatment options: testicular sperm extraction and IVF, artificial insemination with donor sperm, adoption); normal biopsy means obstruction (treat with epididymovasostomy vs vasovasostomy)
  - Elevated FSH: primary testicular failure.
- *Bilateral testicular atrophy:*
  - Low FSH: hypogonadotropic hypogonadism – check LH and prolactin levels and obtain head computed tomography (CT) or magnetic resonance imaging (MRI) scan to evaluate for pituitary adenoma
  - High FSH: primary testicular failure.

- Treatment for hypogonadotropic hypogonadism:
  - Hyperprolactinemia: lower the serum prolactin concentration through discontinuation of offending medications or, if a lactotroph adenoma is present, administration of dopamine agonists and/or tumor resection
  - Hypothalamic disease: administer GnRH analogue.

OLIGOSPERMIA

- Sperm densities <20 million/ml.
- Rarely an isolated finding.
- Differential diagnosis includes varicocele, cryptorchidism, idiopathic, drugs/heat/toxins, systemic infection, endocrinopathy.
- If <10 million/ml sperm present:
  - Send testosterone and FSH.
- If testosterone and/or FSH are abnormal, consider additional hormonal evaluation, including LH, prolactin, and free testosterone.

ASTHENOSPERMIA

- Defects in sperm movement.
- Differential diagnosis includes spermatozoal structural defects, prolonged abstinence, idiopathic, genital tract infection, antisperm antibodies, varicocele, partial obstruction, and Kartagener's syndrome (immotile cilia syndrome, situs inversus, and chronic respiratory infections).
- *Send antisperm antibody assay:*
  - If positive, consider corticosteroids vs intracytoplasmic sperm injection (ICSI)
  - If negative, assess motility.
- *Sperm motility:*
  - ≥5%: evaluate for varicocele, increased scrotal temperatures (i.e. restrictive clothing), systemic illness, pyospermia
  - <5%: perform viability assay.
- *Viability assay:*
  - High: perform electron microscopy; if ultrastructural defect present, consider IVF vs ICSI
  - Low: perform transrectal ultrasound.
- *Transrectal ultrasound:*
  - Normal: evaluate for varicocele, increased scrotal temperatures (i.e. restrictive clothing), systemic illness, pyospermia
  - Abnormal: aspirate seminal vesicles as per evaluation above.

MISCELLANEOUS CAUSES OF MALE INFERTILITY

- Hemochromatosis.
- Estrogen-producing tumors.
- Exogenous androgens/glucocorticoids.
- Noonan's syndrome.
- Myotonic dystrophy.
- Drugs:
  - Chemotherapy (cyclophosphamide, chlorambucil), flutamide, cyproterone, ketoconazole, spironolactone, ethanol, cimetidine, marijuana, heroin, methadone, pesticides (dibromochloropropane), lead, cadmium, mercury.

4

INFERTILITY

- Radiation:
  - Potentially reversible damage with a single exposure of <600 rad.
- Renal failure/uremia.
- Hepatic cirrhosis.
- Sickle-cell disease.

PROGNOSIS

- Of infertile couples, 25–35% will conceive by intercourse alone without treatment.[16]
- Intrauterine insemination:
  - Limited efficacy with male factor infertility.
- In vitro fertilization:
  - With sperm concentration <5 million/ml and poor motility, pregnancy rate is <10%.
- ICSI:
  - ICSI has revolutionized treatment and improved the prognosis for fertility in men with many conditions, including maturation arrest, defective spermiogenesis, deletion of the *DAZ* gene, Klinefelter's syndrome, and long-standing azoospermia following chemotherapy
  - Fertilization rate ~60%
  - Pregnancy rate ~20% (pregnancy rates with multiple attempts: 29–38%).[17–19]
- Artificial insemination with donor semen:
  - ~50% pregnancy rate with six cycles of insemination.[20]
- Approximately 70% of men will have improvement in semen parameters (motility, then count and morphology) after varicocelectomy.[15]

REFERENCES

1. Spira A: Epidemiology of human reproduction. Hum Reprod 1(2):111–15, 1986.
2. Hull MG, Glazener CM, Kelly NJ et al: Population study of causes, treatment, and outcome of infertility. Br Med J (Clin Res Ed) 291(6510):1693–7, 1985.
3. Greenhall E, Vessey M: The prevalence of subfertility: a review of the current confusion and a report of two new studies. Fertil Steril 54(6):978–83, 1990.
4. Thonneau P, Marchand S, Tallec A et al: Incidence and main causes of infertility in a resident population (1,850,000) of three French regions (1988–1989). Hum Reprod 6(6):811–16, 1991.
5. Dym M: The fine structure of the monkey (Macaca) Sertoli cell and its role in maintaining the blood–testis barrier. Anat Rec 175(4):639–56, 1973.
6. Dym M, Fawcett DW: The blood–testis barrier in the rat and the physiological compartmentation of the seminiferous epithelium. Biol Reprod 3(3):308–26, 1970.
7. Yoshinaga K, Nishikawa S, Ogawa M et al: Role of c-kit in mouse spermatogenesis: identification of spermatogonia as a specific site of c-kit expression and function. Development 113(2):689–99, 1991.
8. Reijo R, Lee TY, Salo P et al: Diverse spermatogenic defects in humans caused by Y chromosome deletions encompassing a novel RNA-binding protein gene. Nat Genet 10(4):383–93, 1995.
9. Turner TT: On the epididymis and its function. Invest Urol 16(5):311–21, 1979.
10. Brooks DE: Epididymal functions and their hormonal regulation. Aust J Biol Sci 36(3):205–21, 1983.
11. Harrison RG, Weiner JS: Vascular patterns of the mammalian testis and their functional significance. J Exp Biol 26(3):304–16, 1949.
12. Kormano M, Reijonen K: Microvascular structure of the human epididymis. Am J Anat 145(1):23–7, 1976.

13. Amelar RD, Dubin L, Schoenfeld C: Semen analysis. an office technique. Urology 2(6):605–11, 1973.
14. World Health Organization. WHO Laboratory Manual for the Examination of Human Semen and Sperm–Cervical Mucus Interaction. 1999.
15. Sigman M, Jarow, JP: Male infertility. In: Walsh PC, Retik AB, Vaughan ED, Wein AJ, eds. Campbell's Urology, 8th edn. Philadelphia: WB Saunders, 2002.
16. Collins JA, Wrixon W, Janes LB, Wilson EH: Treatment-independent pregnancy among infertile couples. New Engl J Med 309(20):1201–6, 1983.
17. Schlegel PN, Girardi SK: Clinical review 87: In vitro fertilization for male factor infertility. J Clin Endocrinol Metab 82(3):709–16, 1997.
18. Palermo GD, Cohen J, Alikani M, Adler A, Rosenwaks Z: Intracytoplasmic sperm injection: a novel treatment for all forms of male factor infertility. Fertil Steril 63(6):1231–40, 1995.
19. Tarlatzis BC, Bili H: Intracytoplasmic sperm injection. Survey of world results. Ann NY Acad Sci 900:336–44, 2000.
20. Wang C, Swerdloff RS: Treatment of male infertility. UpToDate 13:3, 2005.

4

INFERTILITY

Erectile dysfunction and Peyronie's disease

Trinity J Bivalacqua and Mohamad E Allaf

5

SUMMARY

- Erectile dysfunction (ED) is defined as the consistent or recurrent inability of a man to attain and/or maintain a penile erection sufficient for sexual activity.
- It is present in more than 50% of men between ages 40 and 70 years and is associated with cardiovascular disease, smoking and peripheral vascular disease.
- Evaluation is primarily based upon history and physical exam.
- Oral type 5 phosphodiesterase inhibitors are a highly efficacious and safe form of treatment. They should be considered as first-line therapy.
- Other types of treatment include intracavernous injection of vasoactive agents (alprostadil, papaverine, phentolamine, or a combination of all three known as tri-mix), intraurethral injection of alprostadil, vacuum constriction devices, and penile prostheses.
- Peyronie's disease is a localized connective tissue disorder of the penis characterized by changes in the collagen composition of the tunica albuginea.
- Peyronie's disease typically presents as a palpable penile plaque, penile pain, penile curvature and erectile dysfunction. Treatment includes medical therapy (efficacy uncertain) and surgery.

ERECTILE DYSFUNCTION

DEFINITION

- Erectile dysfunction (ED) is defined as the consistent or recurrent inability of a man to attain and/or maintain a penile erection sufficient for sexual activity.[1]
- Recent data demonstrate identifiable organic causes in the majority of men.[2,3]
- Only about 10% of men with ED are found to have a psychological problem as the primary cause of their dysfunction.
- In men aged 35 years old or less, psychogenic ED is more common than organic ED.
- Psychogenic ED is a result of performance anxiety, antecedent life changes (divorce, bereavement, or vocational failure) and developmental vulnerabilities.[4]
- There is a clear association between depression and ED.[5]

EPIDEMIOLOGY

- Incidence of ED increases with age, affecting <3% of men younger than 45 years old and nearly 75% of men older than 75 years old.[6]
- Data from the Massachusetts Male Aging Study (MMAS) illustrated that 52% of men between the ages of 40 and 70 report some degree of ED.

- Based on data from the MMAS, more than 30 million men in the United States may have some degree of ED.
  - Within the studied age group, the probability of ED increased from 40% at the age of 40 to 67% at 70 years of age.
- In 1995, it was estimated that approximately 152 million men worldwide suffered from ED, with projections of 322 million affected men by 2025.[7]
- The National Ambulatory Medical Care Survey reported 525 000 physician visits in 1985 due to ED, resulting in 30 000 hospital admissions and costing a total of $146 000 000.[8]

PHYSIOLOGY OF ERECTION

- The process of penile erection is dependent on an intact central and peripheral nervous system and stable hormonal status.[9,10]
- Normal erectile function involves three synergistic and simultaneous processes:
  - Neurologically mediated increase in penile arterial inflow
  - Relaxation of cavernosal smooth muscle
  - Restriction of venous outflow from the penis.
- The penis is composed of three bodies of tissue:
  - Corpus spongiosum supports and protects the urethra on the ventral surface
  - Paired corpora cavernosa, which lie dorsally and adjacent to each other, function as blood-filling reservoirs and provide structure to the penis.
- The cavernosal bodies are composed of a network of vascular sinuses supplied by the helicine arteries (terminal branches of the cavernosal arteries).
- In the flaccid state, smooth muscle trabeculae are tonically contracted and permit only a small amount of arterial inflow. The release of neurotransmitters from cavernous nerve terminals and vascular endothelium lining the corporal smooth muscle in response to sexual stimulation results in corporal smooth muscle relaxation and erection.[11]
- The balance between contractile systems (RhoA/Rho-kinase, alpha-adrenergic, endothelin, angiotensin, thromboxane A_2) and vasodilatory second-messenger systems (nitric oxide (NO), adenylate cyclase-cyclic AMP and guanylyl cyclase-cyclic GMP) determines the tone of corpora cavernosa smooth muscle of the penis.[12,13]
- Cholinergic nerves, nonadrenergic/noncholinergic nerves (NANC; nitrergic), and other factors such as vasoactive intestinal peptide (VIP) and calcitonin gene related peptide (CGRP) mediate corporal smooth muscle relaxation (Figure 5.1).[13]
- Shear stress and muscarinic receptors on trabecular endothelium stimulate the production of NO.
- NO originating from nitrergic nerves and penile endothelium diffuses into smooth muscle cells where it directly interacts with the soluble form of guanylate cyclase to increase intracellular levels of cyclic GMP (cGMP).
- The increase in cGMP results in smooth muscle relaxation, primarily through activation of the cGMP-dependent protein kinases (PKGs) and ion channels. This mechanism reduces intracellular Ca^{2+} via Ca^{2+} sequestration/extrusion and opens potassium channels, causing hyperpolarization.[14]

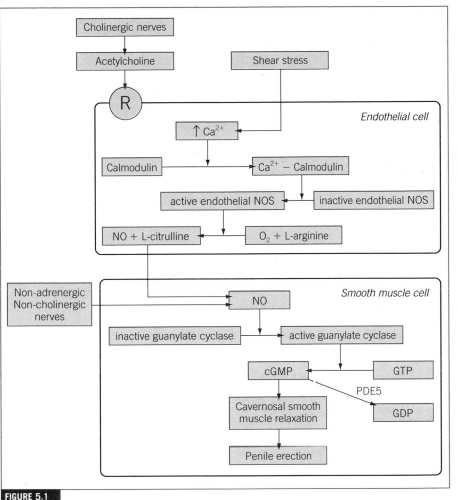

FIGURE 5.1

Overview of the nitric oxide (NO) and guanylyl cyclase pathways. Agonists acting at a receptor (R), or shear stress induce an increase in intracellular calcium concentration, leading to activation of nitric oxide synthase (NOS). NO produced by NOS diffuses to the underlying smooth muscle, where it stimulates production of cyclic GMP (cGMP), ultimately leading to vasorelaxation and penile erection.

- cGMP activity is terminated by hydrolysis of the 3′5′ bond by the type 5 phosphodiesterase (PDE5).[15]
- The increased corporal arterial inflow results in an increase in intracavernosal pressure and volume. The penis expands in length and girth, thereby compressing it between the tunica albuginea and the peripheral sinusoids. This process of veno-occlusion traps blood in the corporal bodies causing penile tumescence and rigidity.

EVALUATION

Etiology

- The relationship between vascular disease and ED is well established, both for arterial insufficiency and corporo-veno-occlusive dysfunction (venous leak).

ERECTILE DYSFUNCTION AND PEYRONIE'S DISEASE 5

- Arteriogenic ED results from poor blood flow into the penis. This can be due to traumatic occlusive disease of the hypogastric-cavernous-helicine tree or various systemic diseases (diabetes, atherosclerosis).[4]
- Veno-occlusive ED results from the inability to hold blood in the penis. This may be due to the presence of abnormally large venous channels draining the corpora cavernosa, degenerative changes (Peyronie's disease, aging, diabetes), trauma to the tunica albuginea (penile fracture), or priapism.[4]
- Neurogenic ED can be caused by disease (Alzheimer's disease, multiple sclerosis) or traumatic injury to the brain, spinal cord, or bony pelvis.
- Direct injury to the pudendal or cavernous nerves from trauma or surgery (pelvic surgery) can result in ED.
- Patients with a history of myocardial infarction, hypertension, elevated cholesterol, atherosclerosis, chronic renal failure, and peripheral vascular disease all have a higher incidence of ED when compared to the general population.[2]
- Diabetes mellitus is also associated with a higher incidence of ED at all ages. Between 35 and 75% of all men with diabetes experience some degree of ED.[16]
- The probability of ED increases with each vascular risk factor, including cigarette smoking, obesity, elevated cholesterol, diabetes and hypertension.[17]
- Approximately 5–10% of all organic ED is secondary to endocrinopathy, including hyperprolactinemia (suppression of LH secretion), hypogonadism (decreased testosterone), hyper- and hypothyroidism, and adrenal disorders involving alterations in androgen secretion.[18]
- Medications have been shown to cause ED. The most common implicated medications are antihypertensives (beta-blockers, calcium-channel blockers, diuretics, spironolactone), antihistamines, and H_2-blockers.
- Drugs with antiandrogen effects may cause ED, including luteinizing hormone-releasing hormone (LHRH) agonists, 5-alpha reductase inhibitors, and estrogens.
- Psychotropic medications, including selective serotonin reuptake inhibitors (SSRIs), lithium, monoamine oxidase inhibitors, and phenothiazines cause ED.
- Recreational illicit drugs which contribute to ED are tobacco, alcohol, heroin, cocaine, and ecstasy (MDMA).

History and physical examination

- A detailed medical and sexual history and a thorough physical examination is the most essential step in diagnosing and determining the etiology of ED.
- A psychosexual history should include the level of libido, duration of ED, the onset of dysfunction, presence of morning erections, quality of erection, and presence of any psychological conflict.
- All medical illnesses, past surgical history including radical pelvic surgery (abdominoperineal resection, radical prostatectomy), pelvic trauma, pelvic irradiation, priapism, and drug history (including alcohol and tobacco) should be documented.
- Physical examination:
  - Ascertain signs of androgen deficiency such as loss of secondary sex characteristics, eunuchoidal proportions, small testicular volume, or breast enlargement

- Neurologic findings of spinal cord lesion, previous stroke, or peripheral neuropathy; genital and perineal sensation
- Palpation of femoral and pedal pulses, and evidence of lower extremity ischemia
- Penile examination to exclude Peyronie's disease.

Laboratory assessment

- Free and total testosterone, TSH, prolactin, gonadotropins, fasting glucose, and lipid profile.
- Specialized tests are usually performed only after a trial of oral pharmacotherapy has failed.
  - Brachial penile blood pressure index
  - Intracavernosal injection of vasodilator
  - Duplex ultrasonography
  - Pelvic arteriography
  - Cavernosography.

Assessment of other patient factors

- Coexisting coronary artery disease and its symptoms and severity.
- The use of nitrates for angina.
- Exercise tolerance.
- The use of vasodilators for hypertension or congestive heart failure.

THERAPY (TABLE 5.1)

TABLE 5.1

APPROACH TO TREATMENT OF ERECTILE DYSFUNCTION

1. Psychosexual counseling if applicable.
2. First-line therapies:
   - PDE5 inhibitors
   - Vacuum constriction devices
3. Second-line therapies:
   - Intracavernosal injection therapy (PGE_1, papaverine, phentolamine)
   - Intraurethral injection therapy (PGE_1)
4. Third-line therapies:
   - Penile prosthesis

TYPE 5 PHOSPHODIESTERASE INHIBITORS

- Phosphodiesterase type 5 (PDE5) is responsible for the degradation and inactivation of cGMP. Inhibition of this enzyme increases corporal cGMP and thus promotes smooth muscle relaxation (see Figure 5.1).
- Sildenafil (Viagra), vardenafil (Levitra), and tadalafil (Cialis) selectively inhibit PDE5 and enhance NO-dependent corporal vasorelaxation by increasing vascular smooth muscle cGMP.[19–21]
- PDE5 inhibitor therapy is highly efficacious and improves erectile function in a broad population of men with ED, including hard-to-treat patients with severe diabetes mellitus and following radical retropubic prostatectomy.[22]
- Patients using PDE5 inhibitors perform better in terms of increased rigidity, frequency of vaginal penetration and maintenance of erection.

- Side effects:
  - Common adverse events for all PDE5 inhibitors include headache, flushing, rhinitis, and dyspepsia
  - Sildenafil – visual disturbances related to inhibition of PDE6
  - Tadalafil – myalgia and back pain thought to be associated with inhibition of PDE11.
- Contraindications:
  - *Absolute contraindication: concomitant use of organic nitrates such as nitroglycerin*
  - American College of Cardiology and American Heart Association recommend a minimum of 24 hours before administration of nitrates after sildenafil and vardenafil usage and 48 hours after tadalafil if patients are willing to accept the risk of severe hypotension with combination of nitrates and PDE5 inhibitors
  - Relative contraindication for the use of sildenafil, vardenafil and tadalafil with alpha-adrenergic antagonists due to possible occurrence of symptomatic hypotension
  - Sildenafil administration in doses greater than 25 mg should be postponed for at least 4 hours after taking alpha-adrenergic antagonists.
- Drug interactions:
  - Erythromycin, cimetidine, protease inhibitors, ketoconazole, rifampin.
- A delay in systemic absorption and decrease in plasma C_{max} occurs when sildenafil and vardenafil are adminstered after a high-fat meal. The pharmacokinetics of tadalafil are not affected by food.
- Pharmacokinetics:
  - Sildenafil – T_{max} = 1 hour, $T_{1/2}$ = 4 hours, duration of action = 4 hours
  - Vardenafil – T_{max} = 0.7–1 hour, $T_{1/2}$ = 4–5 hours, duration of action = 2–8 hours
  - Tadalafil – T_{max} 2 hours, $T_{1/2}$ = 17.5 hours, duration of action = 24–36 hours.

Intracavernous injection therapy

- Patients are taught how to self-inject a vasoactive agent into their corpora cavernosa with a 27- or 30-gauge needle.
- Erections occur typically 15 minutes after intracorporal injection and last 45–90 minutes.[23]
- When appropriately titrated, the success rate of this therapy in producing a rigid erection is 80–90% in a wide range of ED patients.[23]
- Side effects – penile pain, occurrence of hematoma, formation of corporal nodules, and priapism.
- Alprostadil:
  - Alprostadil (PGE_1; CAVERJECT, Pharmacia; Prostin VR, Pharmacia; Edex, Schwarz Pharma) is a cAMP-dependent corporal smooth muscle relaxing agent and induces increases in corporal blood flow and penile erection
  - Dose: 5–20 µg
  - Common side effects of intracavernosal PGE_1 injections include penile pain, fibrosis, and prolonged erections
  - Priapism occurs less commonly compared with other vasoactive agents.

- Papaverine:
  - Non-selective phosphodiesterase inhibitor which intracellularly increases both cAMP and cGMP and promotes corporal smooth muscle relaxation and erection
  - Papaverine is derived from the poppy seed
  - Dose: 5–20 mg
  - As a single agent it is efficacious, inexpensive, and does not need to be refrigerated
  - Less penile pain but is more prone to priapism and fibrosis with long-term use.
- Phentolamine:
  - Competitive alpha-1 and alpha-2 adrenergic antagonist that reduces penile vascular tone and contributes to corporal smooth muscle relaxation
  - Dose: 1 mg
  - As a single agent it is minimally efficacious but is commonly used in combination to potentiate papaverine and/or PGE_1.
- Tri-mix:
  - In an attempt to maximize efficacy and minimize side effects, a combination of PGE_1, papaverine, and phentolamine as a tri-mix is utilized
  - A common mixture is papaverine, 120 mg (4 ml of 30 mg/ml); phentolamine, 6 mg; and PGE_1, 120 μg (6 ml of 20 mg/ml) to make a total volume of 10 ml
  - The reliable patient can titrate his intracavernosal dose from 0.2 to 0.5 ml to optimize his erectile response.

Intrauretheral injection therapy

- The only commercially available pharmacological agent for intraurethal injection is an intraurethral system for delivery of alprostadil called MUSE (medicated urethral system for erection).[24]
- Alprostadil, when applied into the urethra, must be absorbed through the ventral side of the tunica albuginea and into the corpus cavernosum to cause an erection.
- High concentrations of PGE_1 must be used to maintain efficacy.
- Doses: 250, 500, and 1000 μg.
- Side effects: penile pain and urethral burning in up to 30% of patients.

Vacuum constriction devices

- The vacuum constriction device (VCD) is noninvasive and consists of a plastic cylinder which is placed over the penis. The cylinder is then connected to a vacuum-generating source that produces negative pressure, allowing for engorgement of the penis.[25]
- A constricting ring is placed at the base of the penis to maintain tumescence. The ring should not be left in place for more than 30 minutes, as this can result in an ischemic injury.
- Adequate arterial inflow to the cavernosal tissue is required for the successful use of the VCD.
- A patient's motor skills and vision must also be taken into consideration prior to prescribing a VCD, as it does require some hand–eye coordination.[25]
- Advantages – safe and noninvasive.

- Disadvantages – pain; poor duration; high drop-out rate; impaired ejaculation, resulting in entrapment of semen.

PENILE PROSTHESIS

- Penile implants are paired supports that are placed one in each of the corpora cavernosa.[26]
- Two types:
  - *Inflatable* – hydraulic or fluid-filled, which include the 3-piece and the 2-piece models. The 3-piece model utilizes a reservoir located in the pelvis behind the rectus muscle, a pump in the scrotum, and two inflatable cylinders. The two-piece device has the reservoir and pump combined, located in the scrotum, and two cylinders
  - *Semi-rigid* – bendable and positionable, but remain firm in the penis. Semi-rigid prostheses include malleable and mechanical versions.
- Infrapubic approach:
  - Easy placement of reservoir in pelvis
  - Potential injury to dorsal penile nerve.
- Penoscrotal approach:
  - Penile nerve not in surgical field
  - Easier dissection of corporal bodies
  - Difficult placement of reservoir in pelvis.
- Complications:[27,28]
  - Mechanical malfunction (5–10%)
  - Infection (1–3%)
  - Erosion (<5%).

PEYRONIE'S DISEASE

DEFINITION

- Peyronie's disease, or induratio plastica, is a penile condition named after François Gigot de la Peyronie, who first reported a clinical series of penile curvature in 1743.
- Localized connective tissue disorder characterized by changes in the collagen composition of the tunica albuginea.[29,30]
- Fibrous plaque contains excessive amount of collagen, alterations in the elastin framework, and fibroblastic proliferation altering penile anatomy.[31]
- Classified into two phases:
  - Acute inflammatory phase, which persists for 6–18 months – pain, slight penile curvature, and nodule formation
  - Chronic phase – stable plaque size, penile curvature, and, in some instances, complete erectile dysfunction.

EPIDEMIOLOGY

- Affects males between the ages of 40 and 70 years.[32,33]
- The prevalence of Peyronie's disease is 1.5%, 3.0%, 4.0%, and 6.5% for men 30–39, 40–59, 60–69, and above 70 years old, respectively.[33]
- Approximately 10% of men with erectile dysfunction have Peyronie's disease, whereas 20–40% of men with Peyronie's disease have erectile dysfunction.[34]

PATHOPHYSIOLOGY

- Trauma is thought to be the initiating factor, with fibrosis and collagen changes of the tunica albuginea resulting from an inflammatory process triggered by vascular trauma with localized aberration of wound healing.[35]
- Elevation in inflammatory cytokines and fibrotic cytokines (i.e. TGF-β).[36,37]
- May have a genetic predisposition – associated with Dupuytren's contracture and HLA-B7 antigens.[38]
- Associated with a number of systemic disease states such as diabetes, hypertension, and elevated cholesterol.[39]

PRESENTATION AND EVALUATION

- Initial presentation:
  - Penile pain
  - Penile angulation
  - Palpable plaque
  - Erectile dysfunction.
- Medical and sexual history.
- Physical examination.
- Penile rigidity during erection, shortening, induration, hourglass constriction or pain with or without erection.
- Plaque may be located on either the dorsal or ventral surface of the penis.
- Penile pain may be present with erection or during sexual intercourse.

MEDICAL THERAPY

- Efficacy of medical therapy for Peyronie's disease has not been definitively established. Clinical trial data on oral and local therapies are scant.
- Peyronie's patients most likely to benefit are those with early-stage disease.[29,40]
- Oral systemic therapies for Peyronie's disease include:
  - Potassium aminobenzoate (POTABA)
  - Tamoxifen
  - Acetyl-L-carnitine
  - Colchicine
  - Vitamin E.
- Intralesional injection therapy into Peyronie's plaque includes:
  - Collagenase
  - Steroids
  - Calcium channel blockers (verapamil)
  - Interferon alpha 2b.

SURGICAL THERAPY

- Surgical treatment reserved for those patients with severe curvature or narrowing that interferes with sexual intercourse.[30,41,42]
- Penile reconstruction should be performed once the disease has stabilized, typically 12–18 months after onset.
- Detailed evaluation of penile vascular status (duplex Doppler ultrasound) and erectile function is recommended before surgical intervention.

5

ERECTILE DYSFUNCTION AND PEYRONIE'S DISEASE

- Surgical reconstruction is divided into three categories:
  - Tunical shortening procedures – Nesbit procedure or plication of tunica[43–45]
  - Tunical lengthening procedures – incising or excising plaque on shortened side and placement of graft material; indicated in patients with severe penile curvature or hourglass deformities[46–48]
  - Prosthetic procedures – reserved for patients with severe erectile dysfunction that doesn't respond to medical therapy; incising or excising plaque during prosthetic placement.[49]
- Complications include penile shortening, penile hematoma, penile narrowing/induration, uretheral injury, glans numbness, and erectile dysfunction.

REFERENCES

1. Lewis RW: Epidemiology of erectile dysfunction. Urol Clin North Am 28:209–16, vii, 2001.
2. Laumann EO, Paik A, Rosen RC: Sexual dysfunction in the United States: prevalence and predictors. JAMA 281:537–44, 1999.
3. Bivalacqua TJ, Usta MF, Champion HC, Kadowitz PJ, Hellstrom WJ: Endothelial dysfunction in erectile dysfunction: role of the endothelium in erectile physiology and disease. J Androl 24 (Suppl):S17–37, 2003.
4. Lue TF: Erectile dysfunction. New Engl J Med 342:1802–13, 2000.
5. Nicolosi A, Moreira ED Jr, Villa M, Glasser DB: A population study of the association between sexual function, sexual satisfaction and depressive symptoms in men. J Affect Disord 82:235–43, 2004.
6. Feldman HA, Goldstein I, Hatzichristou DG, Krane RJ, McKinlay JB: Impotence and its medical and psychosocial correlates: results of the Massachusetts Male Aging Study. J Urol 151:54–61, 1994.
7. Ayta IA, McKinlay JB, Krane RJ: The likely worldwide increase in erectile dysfunction between 1995 and 2025 and some possible policy consequences. BJU Int 84:50–6, 1999.
8. Nelson C, McLemore T: The National Ambulatory Medical Care Survey: 1975–81 and 1985. Vital Health Stat 13:1–50, 1988.
9. Melman A, Gingell JC: The epidemiology and pathophysiology of erectile dysfunction. J Urol 161:5–11, 1999.
10. Giuliano FA, Rampin O, Benoit G, Jardin A: Neural control of penile erection. Urol Clin North Am 22:747–66, 1995.
11. Andersson KE: Neurophysiology/pharmacology of erection. Int J Impot Res 13 (Suppl 3):S8–S17, 2001.
12. Burnett AL: Role of nitric oxide in the physiology of erection. Biol Reprod 52:485–9, 1995.
13. Andersson KE: Erectile physiological and pathophysiological pathways involved in erectile dysfunction. J Urol 170:S6–S14, 2003.
14. Christ GJ, Wang HZ, Venkateswarlu K, Zhao W, Day NS: Ion channels and gap junctions: their role in erectile physiology, dysfunction, and future therapy. Mol Urol 3:61–73, 1999.
15. Boolell M, Allen MJ, Ballard SA et al: Sildenafil: an orally active type 5 cyclic GMP-specific phosphodiesterase inhibitor for the treatment of penile erectile dysfunction. Int J Impot Res 8:47–52, 1996.
16. Hakim LS, Goldstein I: Diabetic sexual dysfunction. Endocrinol Metab Clin North Am 25:379–400, 1996.
17. McKinlay JB: The worldwide prevalence and epidemiology of erectile dysfunction. Int J Impot Res 12 (Suppl 4):S6–S11, 2000.
18. Miralles-Garcia JM, Garcia-Diez LC: Specific aspects of erectile dysfunction in endocrinology. Int J Impot Res 16 (Suppl 2):S10–12, 2004.

19. Goldstein I, Lue TF, Padma-Nathan H et al: Oral sildenafil in the treatment of erectile dysfunction. Sildenafil Study Group. New Engl J Med 338:1397–404, 1998.
20. Hellstrom WJ, Gittelman M, Karlin G et al: Vardenafil for treatment of men with erectile dysfunction: efficacy and safety in a randomized, double-blind, placebo-controlled trial. J Androl 23:763–71, 2002.
21. Brock GB, McMahon CG, Chen KK et al: Efficacy and safety of tadalafil for the treatment of erectile dysfunction: results of integrated analyses. J Urol 168:1332–6, 2002.
22. Carson CC, Lue TF: Phosphodiesterase type 5 inhibitors for erectile dysfunction. BJU Int 96(3):257–80, 2005.
23. Truss MC, Becker AJ, Schultheiss D, Jonas U: Intracavernous pharmacotherapy. World J Urol 15:71–7, 1997.
24. Padma-Nathan H, Hellstrom WJ, Kaiser FE et al: Treatment of men with erectile dysfunction with transurethral alprostadil. Medicated Urethral System for Erection (MUSE) Study Group. New Engl J Med 336:1–7, 1997.
25. Salvatore FT, Sharman GM, Hellstrom WJ: Vacuum constriction devices and the clinical urologist: an informed selection. Urology 38:323–7, 1991.
26. Montorsi F, Deho F, Salonia A et al: Penile implants in the era of oral drug treatment for erectile dysfunction. BJU Int 94:745–51, 2004.
27. Lotan Y, Roehrborn CG, McConnell JD, Hendin BN: Factors influencing the outcomes of penile prosthesis surgery at a teaching institution. Urology 62:918–21, 2003.
28. Montague DK, Angermeier KW, Lakin MM: Penile prosthesis infections. Int J Impot Res 13:326–8, 2001.
29. Hellstrom WJ, Bivalacqua TJ: Peyronie's disease: etiology, medical, and surgical therapy. J Androl 21:347–54, 2000.
30. Gholami SS, Gonzalez-Cadavid NF, Lin CS, Rajfer J, Lue TF: Peyronie's disease: a review. J Urol 169:1234–41, 2003.
31. Davis CJ Jr: The microscopic pathology of Peyronie's disease. J Urol 157:282–4, 1997.
32. Lindsay MB, Schain DM, Grambsch P et al: The incidence of Peyronie's disease in Rochester, Minnesota, 1950 through 1984. J Urol 146:1007–9, 1991.
33. Sommer F, Schwarzer U, Wassmer G et al: Epidemiology of Peyronie's disease. Int J Impot Res 14:379–83, 2002.
34. Dominguez-Malagon HR, Alfeiran-Ruiz A, Chavarria-Xicotencatl P, Duran-Hernandez MS: Clinical and cellular effects of colchicine in fibromatosis. Cancer 69:2478–83, 1992.
35. Jarow JP, Lowe FC: Penile trauma: an etiologic factor in Peyronie's disease and erectile dysfunction. J Urol 158:1388–90, 1997.
36. El-Sakka AI, Hassoba HM, Pillarisetty RJ, Dahiya R, Lue TF: Peyronie's disease is associated with an increase in transforming growth factor-beta protein expression. J Urol 158:1391–4, 1997.
37. Bivalacqua TJ, Diner EK, Novak TE et al: A rat model of Peyronie's disease associated with a decrease in erectile activity and an increase in inducible nitric oxide synthase protein expression. J Urol 163:1992–8, 2000.
38. Nachtsheim DA, Rearden A: Peyronie's disease is associated with an HLA class II antigen, HLA-DQ5, implying an autoimmune etiology. J Urol 156:1330–4, 1996.
39. Usta MF, Bivalacqua TJ, Jabren GW et al: Relationship between the severity of penile curvature and the presence of comorbidities in men with Peyronie's disease. J Urol 171:775–9, 2004.
40. Jack GS, Gonzalez-Cadavid N, Rajfer J: Conservative management options for Peyronie's disease. Curr Urol Rep 6:454–60, 2005.
41. Kendirci M, Hellstrom WJ: Critical analysis of surgery for Peyronie's disease. Curr Opin Urol 14:381–8, 2004.
42. Hellstrom WJ, Usta MF: Surgical approaches for advanced Peyronie's disease patients. Int J Impot Res 15 (Suppl 5):S121–4, 2003.
43. Coughlin PW, Carson CC 3rd, Paulson DF: Surgical correction of Peyronie's disease: the Nesbit procedure. J Urol 131:282–5, 1984.

5

ERECTILE DYSFUNCTION AND PEYRONIE'S DISEASE

44. Pryor JP: Correction of penile curvature and Peyronie's disease: why I prefer the Nesbit technique. Int J Impot Res 10:129–31, 1998.
45. Ralph DJ, al-Akraa M, Pryor JP: The Nesbit operation for Peyronie's disease: 16-year experience. J Urol 154:1362–3, 1995.
46. Lue TF, El-Sakka AI: Venous patch graft for Peyronie's disease. Part I: technique. J Urol 160:2047–9, 1998.
47. El-Sakka AI, Rashwan HM, Lue TF: Venous patch graft for Peyronie's disease. Part II: outcome analysis. J Urol 160:2050–3, 1998.
48. Leungwattanakij S, Bivalacqua TJ, Reddy S, Hellstrom WJ: Long-term follow-up on use of pericardial graft in the surgical management of Peyronie's disease. Int J Impot Res 13:183–6, 2001.
49. Carson CC: Penile prosthesis implantation in the treatment of Peyronie's disease. Int J Impot Res 10:125–8, 1998.

Neurourology, urodynamics, and urogynecology

Matthew E Nielsen and E James Wright

SUMMARY

- Voiding is the culmination of a complex, exquisitely coordinated neuromuscular system under voluntary control but subsuming numerous visceral reflex arcs acting independently of volitional awareness or control.
- Urine storage and emptying are active processes.
- Urinary continence is maintained by anatomic support structures and neuromuscular control mechanisms.
- Urodynamic testing provides manometric, neuromuscular, and perceptual information to inform the practitioner approaching a patient with voiding dysfunction.
- Goals of therapy for neurogenic voiding dysfunction include preservation of renal function, adequate urinary continence, and maximum independence/ease of care.

6

NEUROUROLOGY

VOIDING FUNCTION

- Normal voiding function enlists the faculties of all levels of the nervous system, from higher cortical centers (brain) to primitive autonomic reflex arcs (sacral spinal cord).
- Normal bladder function allows for:
  - Changes in volume while maintaining low pressure to normal capacity of 350–500 ml
  - The ability to sense fullness
  - The ability to voluntarily initiate and effectively complete voiding of the stored volume.
- The outlet mechanism:
  - The internal sphincter is composed of smooth muscle at the bladder neck
  - The external sphincter is composed of skeletal muscle adjacent to the urogenital membrane.
- Normal voiding is coordinated by the pontine micturition center through sacral parasympathetic nerves, resulting in detrusor contraction and sphincteric relaxation. Cerebral cortical centers are involved in the sensation of bladder filling and the volitional control of voiding (medial pons) and storage (lateral pons) through downstream neurologic pathways.[1]
  - Disruption of the transmission of pontine control (e.g. in spinal cord injury or multiple sclerosis) may result in discoordination of this reflex, or detrusor-sphincter dyssynergia (DSD).
- Urine storage is an active process facilitated by sympathetic stimulation of the outlet mechanism and suppression of the parasympathetic stimulation of the detrusor.

NEUROPHARMACOLOGY OF VOIDING

- The neuropharmacology of voiding is governed by autonomic and somatic nerves.
- Adrenergic/sympathetic (beta-2 receptors relax the bladder body, alpha-1 receptors contract the bladder neck and external sphincter).
- Cholinergic/parasympathetic (M2 muscarinic postganglionic receptors mediate smooth muscle contraction in the detrusor).
- Nicotinic cholinergic receptors mediate voluntary striated muscle contraction.

PATHOLOGICAL CONDITIONS AFFECTING LOWER URINARY TRACT FUNCTION

- International Continence Society functional classification of neuromuscular dysfunction:
  - Detrusor: normal vs hyperreflexic vs hyporeflexic
  - Striated sphincter: normal vs hyperactive vs incompetent
  - Sensation: normal vs hyperactive vs hyposensitive.
- Cerebral lesions [e.g. from cerebrovascular accident (CVA), dementia, tumor, head injury]:
  - May affect the transmission of normal sensation and volitional control
  - Spontaneous (disinhibited) coordinated voiding.
- Suprasacral lesions generally result in spastic neuropathic bladder characterized by:
  - Reduced capacity
  - High voiding pressures with associated detrusor hypertrophy
  - Involuntary detrusor contractions (hyperreflexia) and spasticity or dyssynergia of striated muscle at the outlet
  - Loss of inhibition from higher centers.
- Parkinson's disease:
  - Voiding dysfunction in 35–70%; urgency, frequency, nocturia, and urge incontinence in 50–70%
  - Urodynamics typically reveal detrusor hyperreflexia with sphincter synergia
  - May have pseudodyssynergia or poor sphincter control
  - Caution is required when considering prostatectomy for patients with obstructive symptoms, as the neurologic disease may impose sphincter control problems precipitating incontinence.
- Multiple sclerosis:
  - Demyelinating process most commonly involves posterior and lateral columns of the cervical spinal cord
  - 50–90% complain of voiding symptoms at some time (10% initial presenting symptomatic complaint), with three general clinical syndromes:
    - Detrusor hyperreflexia with sphincter synergia (38%)
    - Detrusor hyperreflexia with striated sphincter dyssynergia (29%)
    - Detrusor areflexia (26%)
  - Conservative management is the rule, and should be undertaken in concert with the treating neurologist.

- Spinal dysraphisms: myelomeningocele/spina bifida – congenital failure of the formation of the neural arch:
  - Classically present with leakage due to areflexic bladder with open bladder neck resulting in urge and/or stress urinary incontinence
  - The minority (10–15%) have detrusor-striated sphincter dyssynergia
  - Recommended to obtain urodynamic studies (with particular attention to detrusor leak point pressure) to assure safety of upper tracts.
- Intervertebral disc disease:
  - Majority of herniated discs at L3/L4, L4/L5, L5/S1[2]
  - A common medicolegal referral
  - 1–18% of cases may have an element of voiding dysfunction (most commonly areflexia with normal compliance, resulting in retention, hesitancy, straining to void)
  - Severe cases may result in the loss of voluntary anal or urethral sphincter control
  - May be associated with sensory loss (S1/S2: lateral foot, S2/S4: perineal)
  - Laminectomy may not reverse dysfunction (controversy in literature – 60% vs 22% in two large studies); prelaminectomy urodynamics are ideal, but not always possible.
- Peripheral neuropathy (e.g. diabetes, pernicious anemia, posterior spinal cord lesions):
  - May result in loss of sensory input to the detrusor motor nucleus, abrogating reflex stimulation and resulting in atony
  - Loss of detrusor tone results in 'flaccid' low pressure bladder with minimal contractility, increased capacity, and elevated postvoid residual.

PATTERNS OF NEUROGENIC DYSFUNCTION

Detrusor-sphincter dyssynergia

- Classically seen in spinal cord injury. Risk of upper tract injury secondary to complications of ureteral reflux (antireflux mechanism of intramural ureter can be overcome at >40 cmH$_2$O pressure).[3]
- Striated (external) sphincter dyssynergia typically seen in suprasacral cord lesions.
- Smooth (internal) sphincter dyssynergia may be seen with lesions above T7 or T8.
- Causes functional obstruction with poor emptying and high detrusor pressure.
- Concomitant detrusor hyperactivity results in dysfunction of filling/storage as well as the emptying failure associated with increased outlet resistance.

Spinal shock

- Flaccid paralysis below the level of injury immediately following insult (including smooth muscle).
- Smooth muscle paralysis results in bladder overfilling (overflow incontinence) and constipation/fecal impaction; bladder neck closed/competent.
- Gradual recovery of reflex activity (hyperactive) in weeks–months following injury.

- Striated muscle reflexes precede smooth muscle reflexes (i.e. retention initially predominates).
- Periodic urodynamic evaluation required in recovery phase to follow progression/risk stratify:
  - Low-pressure storage managed with intermittent catheterization
  - High-pressure storage/overactive detrusor managed initially with anticholinergics, may proceed to sphincterotomy, botox injection, augmentation, and/or diversion
  - Generally recommended to avoid irreversible surgical options – within the first 12 months of injury.

Autonomic dysreflexia

- High spinal cord lesions (above T6) may result in the triggering of high sympathetic outflow (sweating, bradycardia, and hypertension – sometimes severe, carrying risk of CVA) from autonomic or somatic stimulation (e.g. overdistension of the bladder, lower extremity spasm, catheter insertion, or other instrumentation).
- Addressing the precipitating factor(s), e.g. insertion of a catheter, treating the blood pressure, may be lifesaving.

TREATMENT

- Preservation or restoration of the low-pressure reservoir function of the bladder is critical.
- Facilitate the preservation of renal function and urinary continence.
- Options include anticholinergic medications, catheterization [ideally clean intermittent catheterization, to avoid the complications of indwelling catheters (e.g. infections, strictures, erosion, stones)] and in more severe cases, invasive procedures, including sphincterotomy, augmentation, or diversion.

URODYNAMIC TESTING

GENERAL INFORMATION

- Urodynamic testing provides a graphical representation of neuromuscular activity of the bladder, sphincter, and pelvic floor musculature.
- Allows dynamic study of urine storage and evacuation.
- In spite of their objective nature, urodynamic findings must always be interpreted in the context of a patient's history and symptoms.
- Urodynamics provides a framework for the functional classification of voiding dysfunction: e.g. failure to empty vs failure to store, as a consequence of bladder and/or outlet dysfunction.
- Whereas empiric treatment may be guided by symptoms, urodynamics may suggest potential high-risk sequelae of certain conditions necessitating specific attention.
- Examples of urodynamic risk factors:
  - Impaired compliance or high pressure (especially >40 cmH$_2$O) detrusor overactivity present throughout filling

- Elevated detrusor leak point pressure (>40 cmH$_2$O), e.g. from DSD (risk of reflux damage to renal units)
- Poor emptying (risk of overdistension, infection of retained urine) with high storage pressures (risk of reflux of infected urine).

STORAGE/FILLING PHASE

Cystometrogram (CMG)

- Evaluation of bladder storage and sensation.
- Pressure–volume relationships (accommodation of filling and voiding).
- Volume information (total capacity and postvoid residual).
- Volitional control of initiating and inhibiting detrusor contraction.
- Stability and coordination of detrusor contraction with voiding.
- First sensation of fullness at 100–200 ml; normal capacity = 400–500 ml.
- Leak point pressures: a measure of intrinsic sphincter function:
  - Abdominal leak point pressure (ALPP): ability of bladder outlet to resist changes in abdominal pressure
  - Proposed definitions: ALPP<60 cmH$_2$O = intrinsic sphincter deficiency; 60–90 = probable component of ISD, >90 = no ISD[4]
  - Detrusor leak point pressure: lowest detrusor pressure at which urine leakage occurs in the absence of either a detrusor contraction or increased abdominal pressure. Typically associated with impaired compliance.
- Bladder compliance can be decreased by neuromuscular pathology or increased collagenous connective tissue (including an increase in the ratio of type III:type I collagen).[5]

EMPTYING PHASE

Voiding pressure–flow studies

- Simultaneous measurement of detrusor pressure and flow rate.
- Urethral sphincter or pelvic floor electromyography (EMG) assesses striated muscle activity extrinsic to the urethral lumen.
- Postvoid residual.
- Uroflowmetry provides information on the flow of urine from the urethra:
  - Normal peak flow rates: 20–25 ml/s (male) and 20–30 ml/s (female)
  - Shape of the curve itself can be informative
  - Mechanical obstruction is typically reflected by prolonged flow time and sustained low flow rate
  - Absent detrusor activity is typically reflected by a sawtooth pattern of nonsustained spurts of reduced flow, reflecting abdominal straining.
- The micturition reflex: coordinated steps to accomplish normal voiding.
- Relaxation of striated urethral sphincter (EMG silences).
- Contraction of detrusor.
- Opening of bladder neck and urethra.
- Onset of urine flow.

URINARY INCONTINENCE

General information

- Population estimates find prevalence of incontinence 10–40%.
- Stress incontinence most common, accounts for approx. 50% of cases.
- Urge incontinence second most common type, approx. 10–15%.

Pathophysiology

- International Continence Society has promulgated definitions that serve as a conceptual framework:[6]
  - Stress urinary incontinence (SUI): involuntary leakage on effort or exertion, or on sneezing or coughing (seen on examination as synchronous leakage with exertion/effort or coughing). SUI may be seen urodynamically as incontinence in the absence of a detrusor contraction (with synchronous abdominal contraction)
  - May be thought of as a urethral dysfunction in two general categories:
    - Urethral hypermobility (reflecting dysfunction of normal periurethral support mechanisms) – essentially a problem of female anatomy. Female urethral continence is maintained by a combination of the striated sphincter and passive anatomic coaptation via transmission of abdominal pressure to the urethra, supported by its attachments to pelvic floor musculature and connective tissue.[7–9] Loss of this posteroinferior 'hammock' support to the urethra (resulting in urethral hypermobility) allows leakage of urine with increases in abdominal pressure
    - Intrinsic sphincter deficiency: poor coaptation (may be at the level of mucosal 'seal' or of the sphincter itself); defined by abdominal leak point pressure in Urodynamic testing section, above
  - Urge urinary incontinence: involuntary leakage accompanied by or immediately preceded by urgency
  - DOI (detrusor overactivity incontinence) may be seen urodynamically as incontinence due to involuntary detrusor contraction during filling cystometry
  - May be thought of as bladder dysfunction
  - Mixed urinary incontinence: incontinence with urgency and also precipitated by exertion, sneezing, and coughing.

Evaluation

- Consider whether the complaint represents an established, stereotypical pattern or whether it may be an acute, transient finding.
- In cases of transient urinary incontinence, one may consider whether there is an obvious treatable cause that may be addressed without extensive urologic evaluation:
  - Examples of this include delirium, infection, atrophic vaginitis/urethritis, medications (e.g. diuretics), endocrine causes (e.g. diabetes), restricted mobility, fecal impaction.[10]

- Historical clues: urologic, Ob/Gyn, neurologic, medical/surgical histories; history of pelvic trauma, radiation, or surgery; length, severity, and characterization of symptoms; associated bowel problems:
  - A voiding and intake and/or incontinence diary may be informative in the characterization of type and severity of specific complaints.
- Physical exam: attention to structure and function.
- Neurologic exam: evaluate overall mental status and mobility; focused exam of lumbar and sensory distribution (lower extremity deep tendon reflexes, bulbocavernosus reflex, anal wink).
- Women: attempt to demonstrate SUI on exam; thorough pelvic exam, with specific attention to evidence of menopausal atrophy, pelvic organ prolapse, Q-tip test to evaluate urethral mobility:
  - NB: evaluation in standing position may be more physiologic in terms of demonstrating pelvic organ prolapse and SUI.
- Cystoscopy not routinely indicated; rather, may be informative when specifically indicated (hematuria, prior surgery, etc.).
- Urodynamics may provide additional functional information to characterize the underlying defect(s).

Treatment

- Behavioral modification: (Kegel exercises, pelvic floor biofeedback, devices (e.g. weighted cones) strengthen urethral support and may facilitate recruitment of an additional voluntary compensatory mechanism (demonstrated in placebo-controlled trials to offer benefit, though may not be expected to overcome profound degrees of dysfunction).
- Medications: antidepressants: imipramine (tricyclic), estrogen replacement controversial; may not address pathophysiology of significant SUI or DOI.
- Bulking agents (e.g. submucosal collagen) may be helpful in select cases of intrinsic sphincter deficiency (ISD); may require repeat injections (without boosters, success rates 1–3 years: 71%–58%–46%).[11]
- Surgery (reviewed by AUA Female Stress Urinary Incontinence Guidelines Panel)[12] (no randomized controlled studies available for panel review).
- Conclusion: retropubic suspensions and transvaginal slings have the best long-term outcomes.
- Retropubic suspensions: mean 84% cure, 90% dry at 48+ months.
- Sling procedures: mean 83% cure, 87% dry at 48+ months.
- Poorer long-term results for transvaginal suspensions and anterior repairs.
- Suspensions reinforce/strengthen existing support structures.
- Slings introduce new structural support system.

VESICOVAGINAL FISTULA

- Classically presents with continuous urinary drainage from the vagina.
- Most commonly associated with birth trauma in developing countries.
- In the developed world, most commonly iatrogenic (75% associated with hysterectomy).
- Risk of fistula after hysterectomy 0.1–0.2%.[13]
- Becomes apparent after days–weeks following surgery.
- Cystoscopy and retrograde pyelography to rule out (or localize) ureteral involvement.

6

NEUROUROLOGY, URODYNAMICS, AND UROGYNECOLOGY

- Surgical approach may be abdominal or vaginal; helpful to impose uninvolved tissue [Martius flap (vascularized labial tissue), peritoneum, or gracilis muscle].
- Repair is complicated by previous radiation or history of carcinoma (r/o recurrent malignancy).

URETHRAL DIVERTICULUM

- 1–5% incidence in the general population; 1/3 of patients have history of recurrent UTI.[14]
- Classically present with 3 D's: dysuria (50%), postvoid dribbling (25%), and dyspareunia (10%).
- Anterior vaginal mass +/− tenderness on pelvic exam.
- Approximately 60% have genuine SUI; may also have leakage from intermittent drainage of diverticulum.
- Diagnosis by physical exam, cystourethroscopy, urethrography (sensitive in up to 95% of cases).
- Endoscopic incision is not recommended; transvaginal excision and reconstruction of urethra within periurethral fascia is standard of care.

REFERENCES

1. Blaivas JG: Non-traumatic neurogenic voiding dysfunction in the adult. AUA Update Series, Vol IV. Houston, TX: American Urological Association Office of Education, Lessons 11 and 12, 1985, pp 1–16.
2. Appell RA: Voiding dysfunction and lumbar disc disorders. Probl Urol 7(1):41–53, 1993.
3. Sullivan M, Yalla SV: Spinal cord injuries and other forms of myeloneuropathies. Probl Urol 6(4):643–58, 1992.
4. McGuire EJ, Fitzpatrick CC, Wan J et al: Clinical assessment of urethral sphincter function. J Urol 150:1452, 1993.
5. Landau EH, Jayanthi VR, Churchill BM et al: Loss of elasticity in dysfunctional bladders: Urodynamic and histochemical correlation. J Urol 152:702, 1994.
6. Abrams P, Cardoza L, Fall M et al: The standardization of terminology in lower urinary tract function: report from the standardization subcommittee of the International Continence Society. Urology 61:37, 2003.
7. Constantinou CE, Govan DE: Spatial distribution and timing of transmitted and reflexly generated urethral pressures in healthy women. J Urol 127:964, 1982.
8. DeLancey JO: Structural aspects of urethrovesical function in the female. Neurourol Urodynam 7:509, 1988.
9. Tanagho EA: The ureterovesical junction: anatomy and physiology. In: Chishold GD, Williams DI, eds. Scientific Foundation of Urology. Chicago: Year Book Medical, 1982, pp 295–404.
10. Resnick NM: Transient incontinence. Medical Grand Rounds 3:81, 1984.
11. Herschorn S, Steele DJ, Radomski SB: Followup of intraurethral collagen for female stress urinary incontinence. J Urol 156(4):1305–9, 1996.
12. Leach GE, Dmochowski RR, Appell RA et al: Female Stress Urinary Incontinence Guidelines Panel summary report on surgical management of female stress incontinence. The American Urological Association. J Urol 158(3):875–80, 1997.
13. Harris WJ: Early complications of abdominal and vaginal hysterectomy. Obstet Gynecol Surv 50:795–805, 1995.
14. Aldridge CW, Beaton JH, Nanzig RP: A review of office urethroscopy and cystometry. Am J Obstet Gynecol 131:432–5, 1978.

Benign prostatic hyperplasia

Matthew B Gretzer

SUMMARY

- Benign prostatic hyperplasia (BPH) is uncontrolled, non-malignant growth of the prostate characterized by hyperplasia of epithelial and stromal cells within the transition zone.
- Clinically, BPH typically presents with lower urinary tract symptoms (LUTS).
- The differential diagnosis of LUTS includes BPH, urinary infection, primary bladder dysfunction, prostatitis/chronic pelvic pain, urethral stricture, urolithiasis, and bladder carcinoma.
- Prostate size does not necessarily correlate with the severity of LUTS.
- The AUA/IPSS Symptom Index should be used as a measure for grading symptom severity, determining need for therapy, and assessing response to therapy.
- Due to the variability of the impact of LUTS on quality of life among men with BPH, the patient's perception of the severity of the condition remains a primary determinant in the selection of management options.
- Common therapies include watchful waiting, alpha-blockers, 5 alpha-reductase inhibitors, transurethral microwave therapy (TUMT), radiofrequency transurethral needle ablation (TUNA), electrosurgical or laser transurethral resection, and open prostatectomy.

GENERAL PRINCIPLES

PROSTATE ANATOMY

- The prostate is composed of glandular (70%) and fibromuscular stromal (30%) elements.
- Stromal elements are composed of smooth muscle and are continuous with the capsule.
  - Alpha-1A adrenergic receptors are predominately in the stroma and contribute to the contraction and increased tone of prostatic smooth muscle.[1,2]
- Glandular elements are divided into 3 distinct zones: transition, central, and peripheral (Figure 7.1).[1]
- Transition zone:
  - 5–10% of the glandular prostate surrounds the urethra proximal to the ejaculatory ducts
  - Commonly the site of BPH
  - 20% of adenocarcinomas originate in this zone
  - Clinically, the prostate is described as having two lateral lobes, separated by a central sulcus, and a median lobe that may project into the bladder. While these lobes do not correspond to histologically defined structures, they may be related to transition zone hypertrophy laterally and centrally.

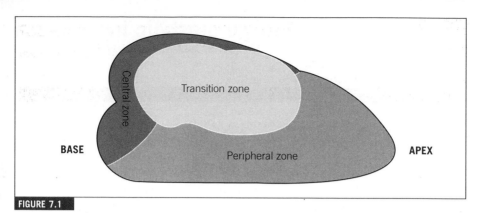

FIGURE 7.1

Glandular zones of the prostate.

- Central zone:
  - Constitutes 25% of the glandular prostate
  - Extends to the base of the bladder
  - 1–5% of adenocarcinomas arise in the central zone.
- Peripheral zone:
  - 70% of glandular prostate
  - 70% of adenocarcinomas arise in this zone.

PRESENTATION AND EPIDEMIOLOGY

- BPH is characterized by non-malignant prostate growth.
- It typically presents clinically with lower urinary tract symptoms (LUTS) (Table 7.1).
- Prevalence:
  - United States (men $\geq$ 60 years): 40%
  - United States (men $\geq$ 80 years): 90%
  - Global (men $\geq$ 60 years): >50%.
- While histological evidence illustrates the development of hyperplastic nodules in men as young as 40 years, the symptomatic effects of this process are more commonly experienced by men between the 5th and 8th decades of life.[3]
- Androgens do not cause BPH, but are necessary for BPH development.
- Obesity is potentially associated with BPH.[3]

TABLE 7.1

TRADITIONAL CLASSIFICATION OF LOWER URINARY TRACT SYMPTOMS (LUTS)

Irritative	Obstructive
Frequecy	Weak stream
Urgency	Intermittency
Nocturia	Hesitancy
Dysuria	Incomplete voiding
	Postvoid dribbling
	Straining to void

ETIOLOGY

- BPH results from hyperplasia of epithelial and stromal cells within the periurethral transition zone.[1]
- The cause remains unclear. Current theories include roles for androgens, estrogens, stromal–epithelial interactions, local growth factors, and testosterone and its active metabolite dihydrotestosterone (DHT) during puberty and aging.[4]
- With age, decreased Leydig cell testosterone production results in a relative increase in estrogen levels. Estrogens have been shown to augment DHT receptor synthesis and potentiate its effects on prostate growth.[1,4,5]
- Alterations of DHT levels may also augment the effect of local growth factors within the prostate, affecting the balance between cell proliferation and apoptosis, and bring about alterations in paracrine activity that affect the homeostasis between epithelial and stromal cells and contribute to BPH development.[1,4]

PATHOPHYSIOLOGY

- Prostate size does not necessarily correlate with the severity of LUTS, and it is likely that complex interactions of prostatic and urethral smooth muscle tone with bladder dysfunction contribute to the generation of symptoms.[1,6]
- Hyperplastic tissue may induce mechanical outflow obstruction to produce obstructive symptoms.
- Stimulation of sympathetic innervation of the stromal elements may also contribute to obstructive symptoms.[1,6]
- Compensatory changes in bladder function due to prolonged obstruction, compounded by age-related changes in bladder and nervous system function, may lead to irritative symptoms and are often recognized as the most bothersome of BPH-related complaints.[1,6]

DIAGNOSIS AND EVALUATION

DIAGNOSIS

- Due to the lack of symptom specificity, a goal of the work-up for a man with LUTS is to determine whether the symptoms are secondary to BPH.[1,6,7]
- Other potential causes of LUTS include neurogenic bladder, diabetes, infection, urethral stricture, urolithiasis, bladder carcinoma/CIS (carcinoma in situ).

INITIAL EVALUATION[7]

- Comprehensive medical history (Figure 7.2):
  - Assessment of comorbid medical problems
  - Surgical history
  - Voiding history.
- Physical examination:
  - Abdominal exam
  - DRE (digital rectal examination)
  - Complete neurological exam.

7

BENIGN PROSTATIC HYPERPLASIA

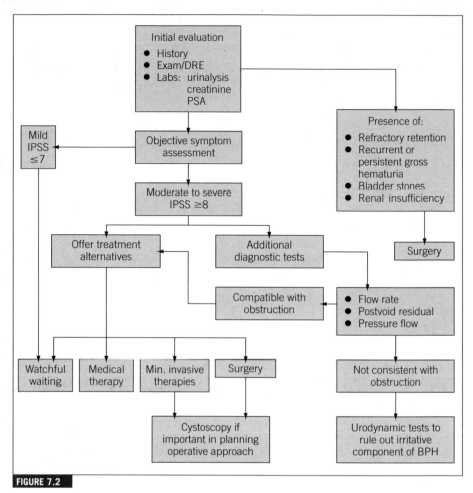

FIGURE 7.2

Algorithm for BPH diagnosis and treatment (based on AUA Practice Guidelines).[7]

- Urinalysis:
  - Glucose, red cells, white cells, presence of urinary infection.
- Cytology:
  - Recommended as option for men with primarily irritative symptoms
  - May also be considered in men with tobacco history or other risk factors for urothelial carcinoma.
- PSA (prostate-specific antigen):
  - Recommended for men with at least 10-year life expectancy and/or those for whom results would potentially change treatment
  - Also useful to establish a baseline if considering management with 5-alpha-reductase inhibitor therapy.
- Creatinine:
  - Not recommended during initial evaluation of routine/standard patients
  - May help establish diagnosis of renal insufficiency in men with longstanding obstruction or signs/symptoms of renal disease, thus affecting determination of initial therapeutic approach.

- AUA/IPSS Symptom Index:
  - See Appendix 1
  - Symptoms classified as mild (0–7), moderate (8–19), and severe (20–35)
  - Should not be used to establish the diagnosis of BPH, but rather as a tool to grade symptom severity and assess response to therapy or detect symptom progression
  - Potentially helpful in distinguishing between obstructive and irritative LUTS during history and physical exam.
- Cystoscopy:
  - Not required in the absence of a specific indication (i.e. hematuria or potential urethral stricture)
  - Often performed prior to interventional therapy to assess the bladder for effects of obstruction (such as cellules, diverticula, and trabeculation) and/or to evaluate for the presence of bladder neck contracture, urethral stricture, bladder tumors, and calculi
  - May also provide anatomic assessment (i.e. prostatic urethra and median lobe) for planning prior to minimally invasive procedures.
- Other tests:
  - Measurement of urinary flow rates, postvoid residual urine volumes, pressure-flow urodynamic studies, and ultrasound are optional
  - May aid with diagnosis in men with complex medical histories, such as neurological diseases, and those considering invasive therapy.

TREATMENT

GENERAL PRINCIPLES

- Due to the variability of the impact of LUTS on quality of life among men with BPH, the patient's perception of the severity (or bother) of the condition is a primary determinant in the selection among management options.[7]
- Four primary categories of treatment options:
  1. Watchful waiting
  2. Medical therapy
  3. Minimally invasive therapies
  4. Surgical therapy.
- Indications for surgery:[7]
  - Refractory retention
  - Any of the following if clearly related to BPH:
    - Recurrent UTIs (urinary tract infections)
    - Persistent gross hematuria
    - Renal insufficiency
    - Bladder stones.

WATCHFUL WAITING

- May consider for uncomplicated patients with mild or moderate symptoms but with low degree of bother.
- Men undergoing delayed therapy require periodic follow-up to monitor for any changes in symptom level, physical exam, and/or laboratory values that may indicate the need for active intervention.[1,6–8]

7

BENIGN PROSTATIC HYPERPLASIA

- Potential complications of BPH progression include urinary retention, renal insufficiency, UTI, and bladder calculi.

MEDICAL THERAPY

Alpha adrenergic antagonists[7,9–11]

- Currently include doxazosin (Cardura), terazosin (Hytrin), tamsulosin (Flomax), and afluzosin (Xatral XL).
- Relax prostatic stromal, capsular, and bladder neck smooth muscle.[9–11]
- Alpha-1A receptors are the primary subtype of alpha receptor present in the prostate. Of the alpha blockers, tamsulosin and afluzosin are selective for the alpha-1A receptor.[9–11]
- Alpha blockers do not affect serum PSA.[7]
- While differences among the adverse-event profiles have been documented among the alpha blockers, no single alpha blocker has shown to be superior, and they have all have demonstrated up to 50% reduction in symptom scores.[7]
- Doxazosin and terazosin require dose titration to minimize postural hypotension, and if therapy is interrupted it is recommended to resume these drugs at the initial dosing regimen.
- Tamsulosin and afluzosin may be added to pre-existing hypertension therapy.
- Potential adverse effects include postural hypotension, drowsiness, dizziness, headache, nasal congestion, and retrograde ejaculation. Up to 10% of men are unable to tolerate this medication.

5-Alpha-reductase inhibitors[7,12–16]

- Currently include finasteride (Proscar) and dutasteride (Avodart).
- 5-alpha-reductase inhibitors prevent the conversion of intraprostatic testosterone to its active metabolite, dihydrotestosterone (DHT).
  - Serum and intraprostatic DHT levels will decrease, but not to castrate levels, since type I receptors in skin and liver will not be affected[12–14]
  - Serum testosterone levels will increase or remain unchanged.
- Two isoenzymes exist for 5-alpha-reductase: type I and type II. Type II is the most common in the prostate.[16]
- 5-alpha-reductase inhibitor therapy reduces serum PSA concentration by approximately 50%, but will generally not affect percent free PSA.
- Long-term use may reduce the risk of acute urinary retention and subsequent need for invasive therapy.[12–15]
  - Reduces prostate size and symptom severity
  - Not recommended for men with LUTS without prostate enlargement.[7]
- Combination therapy with alpha blockers has been shown to delay clinical progression and reduce long-term risk of retention and need for surgery compared with alpha blocker monotherapy.[15]
- May improve hematuria secondary to BPH.
- Side effects include impotence, decreased libido, and changes in ejaculate volume.

Phytotherapies[17-19]

- *Serenoa repens* (saw palmetto):
  - Some data suggest clinical effectiveness in men with BPH
  - Mechanism of action unknown, but is associated histologically with induction of atrophy and epithelial contraction
  - Saw palmetto alone does not generally affect PSA concentration; however, some ingredients in combination therapies may possess anti-androgenic activity that could potentially decrease PSA
  - Common dose for BPH is 320 mg (lipophilic ingredients) daily.
- *Pygeum africanum* (African plum, Tadenan):
  - Used in combination with beta-sitosterol (Harzol) and with saw palmetto by many men with BPH.
- Others:
  - *Radix urticae* (Bazoton)
  - Mepartricin (Ipertrofan).

MINIMALLY INVASIVE THERAPIES

Transurethral microwave therapy (TUMT)[7,20 25]

- TUMT uses microwave energy in the range of 800–1300 MHz to heat and produce coagulative necrosis within the transition and central zones of the prostate.
- Involves placement of a catheter fitted with a microwave antenna situated within the prostatic urethra. Microwave energy penetrates the prostate and radiates heat.
  - The production of coagulative necrosis depends on both the temperature achieved and the duration of therapy
- Routinely performed in an office/clinic setting with minimal sedation.
- Efficacy:
  - In the average patient, generally more effective than medical therapy but less effective than surgery[7]
  - In sham control studies, substantial improvements in IPSS and peak flow rates were observed 12 weeks after therapy, suggesting that maximal improvement is not achieved until that time[24]
  - Long-term efficacy studies have demonstrated that 67% of men treated with TUMT were without need of further therapy at 5 years.[25]
- Potential adverse events include pain, irritative voiding symptoms, urinary retention, and urethral sloughing.
  - Confirm proper placement of rectal temperature sensor and urethral catheter, and monitor patient during therapy
  - Do not oversedate patients or use spinal or general anesthesia (patient perception of pain allows for prevention of excessive overheating of tissue)
  - Newer devices provide penile and bulbar urethra cooling capable of reducing pain, reducing risk of urethral sloughing, and potentially enhancing microwave radiation and heat penetration (thus achieving adequate necrosis of BPH tissue in shorter periods of treatment).

7

BENIGN PROSTATIC HYPERPLASIA

- Contraindications:
  - Prostatic urethral length <3.5 cm
  - Presence of median lobe
  - Prior pelvic radiation (increased rate of rectal fistula).

Transurethral needle ablation (TUNA)[7,26–30]

- TUNA uses low-level radiofrequency (RF) energy delivered to the prostate parenchyma through needles inserted transurethrally.
- A monopolar RF signal of 490 kHz produces tissue heating due to tissue resistance to current as it flows from the active electrode to the indifferent or return electrode. Accurate prostate volume assessment prior to therapy aids accurate needle length selection for optimal treatment.
- Commonly used in men with a prominent median lobe, prostates <40 g, and primarily irritative voiding symptoms.
- Local anesthesia in the form of Xylocaine (lidocaine) jelly and oral analgesia/sedation.
  - This therapy requires accurate needle placement to achieve effective outcomes.
- Efficacy:
  - Similar to TUMT: generally more effective than medical therapy but less effective than surgery[7]
  - AUA Symptom Index improves by 77% and peak flows increase by 6 ml/s at 12 months[28–30]
  - Reoperation required in 13–14% of patients within 2 years.
- Potential adverse events include postoperative urinary retention (13–42%) and irritative voiding symptoms (40%, persisting for up to 2 weeks).

Prostatic urethral stents[7,31,32]

- Expandable, meshed metal or polyurethane devices deployed into the prostatic urethra under fluoroscopic and/or endoscopic guidance.
- Act by partially relieving mechanical obstruction of the urethra by prostatic tissue.
- Role in patients whose medical conditions allow other forms of treatment, or in those without urinary retention, is unclear.
- Should be considered only in high-risk patients, particularly those with urinary retention.[7]
- Potential adverse events include stent encrustation, occlusion, and perineal pain/discomfort with voiding.

SURGERY

Transurethral resection of the prostate (TURP)[7,33–35]

- For decades, TURP has been the gold standard for surgical management of BPH. Remains a reference standard by which the efficacies of newer modalities are often measured.
- It involves resection of adenomatous tissue with an electrocautery wire loop.
- It is usually performed under spinal or general anesthesia, and typically involves an overnight hospital stay.

- Efficacy:
  - Chance of improvement in patient symptoms: 88% (95% CI 70–96%)
  - Magnitude of reduction in AUA Symptom Index: 85%.
- Potential perioperative adverse effects include TUR syndrome (2%), hematuria (>5%), UTI (>5%), and urinary retention (5%).
- TUR syndrome:[33]
  - Cause: hyponatremia secondary to absorption of hypotonic irrigating fluid
  - Presentation: mental status changes, nausea, vomiting, hypotension, oliguria, and visual disturbances
  - Treatment: diuretics (furosemide) and *slow* IV infusion of 3% saline solution
  - Should not occur with use of bipolar cautery, which utilizes saline irrigation.
- Hematuria – if persistent venous bleeding occurs after insertion of catheter at end of procedure:
  - Fill catheter balloon with 50 ml of fluid (i.e. overinflate)
  - Place catheter on traction for up to 7 minutes.[33]
- Potential long-term adverse effects include retrograde ejaculation (75%), erectile dysfunction (1%), urinary incontinence (1%), and bladder neck contraction (1%).

Transurethral electrovaporization of the prostate (TUVP)[7,36,37]

- Involves a technique similar to TURP:
  - Employs a rollerball electrode that is rolled over the prostatic tissue
  - Cutting current is set to a higher power than TURP
  - Combines electrosurgical vaporization with tissue desiccation, which ideally provides for accurate resection of tissue with less blood loss.
- Potential advantages compared to TURP include minimal intraoperative and postoperative bleeding.
- Potential disadvantages include lack of a tissue specimen for cancer diagnosis, slightly longer operative times, and potentially higher rates of irritative voiding symptoms (dysuria) and episodes of postoperative urinary retention.
- Efficacy:
  - Short-term results are similar to TURP
  - Long-term comparative trials are lacking.

Transurethral incision of the prostate (TUIP)[7,38,39]

- Involves division of the prostatic capsule at the bladder neck with one or two cuts using a Collings knife.
- Ideally, redirects the compressive force of the hyperplastic tissue away from the urethra.
- TUIP may be performed in less time than TURP, and is associated with a lower incidence of bleeding and retrograde ejaculation.
- Intended for men with small prostates (<30 g).
- Efficacy:
  - Similar to TURP in select patients
  - However, may be associated with higher rates of reoperation.

Laser ablation[7,40–43]

- Laser therapy employs laser energy to produce coagulation or vaporization of prostate tissue through generation of temperatures ranging from 60°C to 90°C for coagulation and >100°C for vaporization.
- Transurethral laser coagulation:
  - Uses a right-angle laser fiber, introduced transurethrally, that does not come into contact with prostate tissue
  - Technically simple
  - Efficacy is similar to TURP
  - Has potentially higher rates of postoperative urinary retention (21%) than TURP.
- Transurethral laser vaporization:
  - Similar to transurethral electrovaporization
  - Laser fiber comes into contact with prostate tissue
  - Short-term efficacy similar to TURP
  - Has potentially higher rates of postoperative urinary retention (21%) than TURP
  - Potentially useful in patients at high bleeding risk.

Open prostatectomy[7,44]

- Intact removal of the prostatic adenoma using either a suprapubic (i.e. transvesicle) or retropubic (extravesicle, through the capsule of the prostate) surgical approach.
- Appropriate choice for men with large bladder stones and/or diverticulae that need concomitant repair.
- Normally reserved for men with large prostates (>70–100 g).

REFERENCES

1. Roerhrborn CG, McConnell JD: Etiology, pathophysiology, and natural history of benign prostatic hyperplasia. In: Walsh PC, Retik AB, Vaughan ED, Wein AJ, eds. Campbell's Urology, Vol 2, 8th edn. Philadelphia: WB Saunders, 2002, pp 1297–336.
2. Beduschi MC, Beduschi R, Oesterling JE: Alpha-blockade therapy for benign prostatic hyperplasia: from a nonselective to a more selective alpha-1A-adrenergic antagonist. Urology 51:861, 1998.
3. Guess HA, Arrighi HM, Metter EJ et al: The cumulative prevalence of prostatism matches the autopsy prevalence of benign prostatic hyperplasia. Prostate 17:241, 1990.
4. McConnell JD: Prostatic growth: new insights into hormonal regulation. Br J Urol 76: 5–10, 1995.
5. Barrack ER, Berry SJ: DNA synthesis in the canine prostate: effects of androgen induction and estrogen treatment. Prostate 1045–56, 1987.
6. McConnell JD, Barry MJ, Bruskewitz RC et al: Benign prostatic hyperplasia: diagnosis and treatment. Clinical Practice Guideline, Number 8. Rockville, MD, Agency for Health Care Policy and Research, Public Health Service, US Department of Health and Human Services, 1994.
7. AUA Practice Guidelines Committee: AUA Guideline on Management of Benign Prostatic Hyperplasia (2003). Chapter 1: Diagnosis and treatment recommendations. J Urol 170(2):530, 2003.
8. Barry MJ, Fowler FJ Jr, O'Leary MP et al: The American Urological Association Symptom Index for benign prostatic hyperplasia. J Urol 148:1549, 1992.
9. Lepor H: Alpha-adrenergic blockers for the treatment of benign prostatic hyperplasia. In: Lepor H, ed. Prostatic Diseases. Philadelphia: WB Saunders, 2000, pp 297–307.

10. Narayan P, Tewari A: Overview of alpha-blocker therapy for benign prostatic hyperplasia. Urology 51(4a):38, 1998(suppl).
11. Beduschi MC, Beduschi R, Oesterling JE: Alpha-blockade therapy for benign prostatic hyperplasia: from a nonselective to a more selective alpha-1A-adrenergic antagonist. Urology 51:861, 1998.
12. Finasteride Study Group: Finasteride(MK-906) in the treatment of benign prostatic hyperplasia. Prostate 22:291–9, 1993.
13. Nickel JC, Fradet Y, Boake RC et al: Efficacy and safety of finasteride therapy for benign prostatic hyperplasia: results of a 2 year randomized controlled trial (The PROSPECT STUDY). Can Med Assoc J 155:1251, 1996.
14. Kaplan SA, Holtgrewe L, Bruskewitz R et al: Comparison of the efficacy and safety of finasteride in older versus younger men with benign prostatic hyperplasia: The Proscar Longterm Efficacy and Safety Study Group (PLESS). Urology 57:1073–7, 2001.
15. McConnell JD, Roehrborn CG, Bautista OM: The long-term effect of doxazosin, finasteride, and combination therapy on the clinical progression of benign prostatic hyperplasia. New Engl J Med 349:2387–98, 2003.
16. Russell DW, Wilson JD: Steroid 5alpha-reductase: two genes/two enzymes. Ann Rev Biochem 63:25, 1994.
17. Marks LS, Partin AW, Epstein JI et al: Effects of saw palmetto herbal blend in men with symptomatic benign prostatic hyperplasia. J Urol 163(5):1451–6, 2000.
18. Wilt TJ, Ishani A, Stark G et al: Saw Palmetto extracts for the treatment of benign prostatic hyperplasia: a systematic review. JAMA 280:1604, 1998.
19. Boyle P, Robertson C, Lowe F et al: Meta analysis of clinical trials of Permixon in the treatment of symptomatic benign prostatic hyperplasia. Urology 55:533–9, 2000.
20. Blute ML: Transurethral microwave thermotherapy: minimally invasive therapy for benign prostatic hyperplasia. Urol 50:163–6, 1997.
21. Devonec M, Berger N, Fendler JP, Joubert P et al: Thermoregulation during transurethral microwave thermotherapy: experimental and clinical fundamentals. Eur Urol 23 Suppl 1:63–7, 1993.
22. Djaven B, Larson T, Blute M, Marberger M: Transurethral microwave thermotherapy: What role should it play versus medical management in the treatment of benign prostatic hyperplasia. Urology 52(6):935–47, 1998.
23. Larson TR, Blute ML, Tri JL et al: Contrasting heating patterns and efficacy of the Prostatron and Targis microwave antennae for thermal treatment of benign prostatic hyperplasia. Urology 51:908–15, 1998.
24. de la Rosette JJMCH, d' Anacona FCH, Debruyne FMJ: Current status of thermotherapy treatment of the prostate. J Urol; 157:430–8, 1997.
25. D'Ancona FC, Francisca EA, Witjes WP et al: High-energy thermotherapy versus transurethral resection in the treatment of benign prostatic hyperplasia: results of prospective randomized study with 1-year of follow-up. J Urol 158:120–5, 1997.
26. Issa MM, Oesterling JE: Transurethral needle ablation (TUNA): an overview of radiofrequency thermal therapy for the treatment of benign prostatic hyperplasia. Curr Opin Urol 6:20–7, 1996.
27. Chapple CR, Issa MM, Woo H: Transurethral needle ablation (TUNA): a critical review of radiofrequency thermal therapy in the management of benign prostatic hyperplasia. Eur Urol 35:110–28, 1999.
28. Naslund M, Perez-Marrero R, Roehrborn CG et al: Intermediate term outcomes of TUNA for BPH: 36-month results of the TUNA vs TURP U.S. randomized study. J Urology 161(4 suppl): 389. Abstract 1511, 1999.
29. Roerborn CG, Sisal M, Bruskewitz RC et al: Transurethral needle ablation for benign prostatic hyperplasia: 12-month results of a prospective multi-center U.S. study. Urology 51:415–21, 1998.
30. Ramon J, Lynch TH, Eardley I et al: Transurethral needle ablation of the prostate for the treatment of benign prostatic hyperplasia: a collaborative multi-centre study. Br J Urol 80:128–35, 1997.
31. Oesterling JE, Kaplan SA, Epstein HB et al: The North American experience with the UroLume endoprosthesis as a treatment for benign prostatic hyperplasia: long-term results. Urology 44:353–62, 1994.

7

BENIGN PROSTATIC HYPERPLASIA

32. Badlani GH, Press SM, Defalco A et al: Urolume endourethral prosthesis for the treatment of urethral stricture disease: long-term results of the North American Multicenter UroLume Trial. Urology 45:846–56, 1995.
33. Fitzpatrick JM, Mebust WK: Minimally invasive and endoscopic management of benign prostatic hyperplasia. In: Walsh PC, Retik AB, Vaughan ED, Wein AJ, eds. Campbell's Urology, Vol 2, 8th edn. Philadelphia: WB Saunders, 2002, p 1379.
34. Mebust WK, Holtgrewe HL, Cocket ATK, Peters PC, and Writing Committee. Transurethral prostatectomy: immediate and postoperative complications. A cooperative study of 13 participating institutions evaluating 3885 patients. J Urol 141:243–7, 1989.
35. Wasson JH, Reda DJ, Bruskewitz RC et al: A comparison of transurethral surgery with watchful waiting for moderate symptoms of benign prostatic hyperplasia. New Engl J Med 138:195–8, 1987.
36. Patel A, Fuchs GJ, Gutierrez-Aceves J et al: Prostate heating patterns comparing electrosurgical transurethral resection and vaporization: a prospective randomized study. J Urol 157:169–72, 1997.
37. Kaplan SA, Laor E, Fatal M, Te AE: Transurethral resection of the prostate versus transurethral electrovaporization of the prostate: a blinded, prospective comparative study with 1-year follow-up. J Urol 159:454–8, 1997.
38. Orandi A: Transurethral incision of the prostate. J Urol 110:229, 1973.
39. Orandi A: Transurethral incision of the Prostate (TUIP): 646 cases in 15 years – a chronological appraisal. Br J Urol 57:703, 1985.
40. Zlotta AR, Schulman CC: Interstitial laser coagulation for the treatment of benign prostatic hyperplasia using local anesthesia only. BJU Int 88:341–2, 1999.
41. Keoghane SR, Lawrence KC, Gray AM et al: A double blind randomized controlled trial and economic evaluation of transurethral resection vs. contact laser vaporization for benign prostatic enlargement: a 3-year follow-up. Br J Urol 85:74–8, 2000.
42. Costello AJ, Shaffer BS, Crowe MR: Second generation delivery options for laser prostatic ablation. Urology 43:262–6, 1994.
43. Costello AJ, Kabalin JN: Side-firing Neodynium:YAG laser prostatectomy. Eur Urol 35:138–46, 1999.
44. Han M, Alfert HJ, Partin AW: Retropubic and suprapubic open prostatectomy. In: Walsh PC, Retik AB, Vaughn ED et al, eds: Campbell's Urology, Vol 2, 8th edn. Philadelphia: WB Saunders, 2002, p 1423.

APPENDIX 1: AUA/IPSS SYMPTOM INDEX

Question	Never (0)	Less than 1 in 5 times (1)	Less than half the time (2)	Half the time (3)	More than half the time (4)	Almost all the time (5)
Over the last month, how often have you had a sensation of not emptying your bladder competely after you finished urinating?	0	1	2	3	4	5
Over the last month, how often have you had to urinate again less than 2 hours after you finished urinating?	0	1	2	3	4	5
Over the last month, how often have you found you stopped and started again several times when you urinated?	0	1	2	3	4	5
Over the last month, how often have you found it difficult to postpone urination?	0	1	2	3	4	5
Over the last month, how often had you had a weak urinary stream?	0	1	2	3	4	5
Over the last month, how often had you had to push or strain to begin urination?	0	1	2	3	4	5
Over the last month, how many times did you get up to urinate from the time you went to bed at night until the time you got up in the morning?	None	1 time	2 times	3 times	4 times	5 times

If you were to spend the rest of your life with your urinary condition just the way it is now, how would you feel about that? Scale of 0–6 (from delighted to terrible).

BENIGN PROSTATIC HYPERPLASIA　7

APPENDIX 2: COMMON MEDICAL THERAPIES FOR BPH[7,45]

Class	Primary adverse events	Medication	Dose
Alpha adrenergic antagonists	• Orthostatic hypertension • Dizziness • Asthenia (tiredness) • Ejaculatory dysfunction • Nasal congestion	Doxazosin (Cardura)	• Begin at 1mg daily • Titrate upwards once per week as tolerated (2 mg, 4 mg, 8 mg) to maximum dose of 8 mg daily
		Terazosin (Hytrin)	• Begin at 1 mg daily • Titrate upwards once per week as tolerated (2 mg, 5 mg, 10 mg) to maximum dose of 10 mg daily
		Tamsulosin (Flomax)	• Begin at 0.4 mg daily • May titrate as tolerated to maximum dose of 0.8 mg daily
		Alfuzosin (Uroxatral)	• 10 mg daily • Titration not required
5-Alpha-reductase inhibitors	• Decreased libido • Ejaculatory dysfunction • Erectile dysfunction • Gynecomastia	Finasteride (Proscar)	• 5 mg daily
		Dutasteride (Avodart)	• 0.5 mg daily

Interstitial cystitis and chronic pelvic pain

Matthew E Nielsen

SUMMARY

- Interstitial cystitis (IC)/chronic pelvic pain syndrome is a chronic, often unrecognized, lower urinary tract disease.
- Primary symptoms include one or more of the following: urinary frequency, urinary urgency, and pelvic pain. Other symptoms include nocturia, dysuria, dyspareunia, and testicular, scrotal, and perineal pain.[1-4]
- IC is much more common than previously thought. Based on recent data, as many as 1 in 5 women in the United States may be affected.[5,6]
- A substantial number of men diagnosed with chronic prostatitis actually have IC.[7,8]
- IC is potentially caused by bladder epithelial dysfunction, which leads to diffusion of urinary solutes (potassium) into the bladder interstitium, tissue injury, and inappropriate afferent nerve stimulation.[9-12]
- Evaluation should include history with validated symptom questionnaire, physical examination, urinalysis, and urine culture. Additional tests include the potassium sensitivity test,[10] cystoscopy, and urodynamics.
- Several efficacious treatments exist, including pentosan polysulfate, hydroxyzine, amitriptyline, and intravesical heparin.
- Urinary diversion should be considered only in patients with severe disease refractory to less-invasive therapies.

EPIDEMIOLOGY

- IC is more common among women than men.[1-3]
- The prevalence for both sexes has been rising steadily over the last 20 years.
- Most investigators agree that IC is much more common than previously believed.
  - Data suggest that at least 1 million and possibly as many as 25 million individuals in the United States are affected[5-8,13]
  - In recent US screening studies involving almost 5000 US patients, **17.5–25% of females had probable IC**.[5,6]
- At least 6–8% of men initially diagnosed with prostatitis actually have IC.[7,8]

PATHOPHYSIOLOGY

- The sine qua non of IC is inappropriate stimulation of sensory nerves in the bladder and urethra.
- There are at least two types of sensory nerves involved: small unmyelinated C-fibers (mediating pain) and A delta fibers (mediating urgency).
  - These fibers may activate independently or in combination to produce IC symptoms.
- Hypothesized mechanisms of inappropriate nerve stimulation in IC include chronic infection, autoimmune disorders, vasculogenic disorders, and primary neurological dysfunction.[14,15]

- **Increasing evidence suggests that IC may be caused by a 'leaky' bladder epithelium**.
  - Increased epithelial permeability at the bladder surface potentially allows caustic urinary solutes – primarily potassium – to diffuse into the bladder interstitium, where they may injure tissue, stimulate sensory nerves, and generate symptoms[9–12]
  - A new paradigm – called lower urinary dysfunctional epithelium (LUDE) – proposes that IC, chronic pelvic pain, urethritis, and chronic prostatitis all result from leaky epithelium and should therefore be considered as different manifestations of the same pathophysiological process[10]
  - The epithelial leak model forms the rationale for treatment with pentosan polysulfate and intravesical heparin (see Treatment section)[16]
  - The central role of urinary potassium in the epithelial leak model forms the basis for the potassium sensitivity test (see Additional Evaluation section).[9,10]
- Mast cells:
  - Mast cell mediators stimulate sensory nerves[17]
  - Mast cell activity is increased in IC patients, with increased mast cell mediators present in the urine[18]
  - IC symptom flares may increase during allergy season.[3,19]
- Other mediators:
  - Urine in IC has been reported to contain increased levels of inflammatory mediators, growth factors, and antiproliferative factor (APF)[20,21]
  - These compounds may potentially produce symptoms and/or tissue injury.[10]

PRESENTATION

SYMPTOMS

- Urinary frequency, urinary urgency, and pelvic pain are the principal symptoms.
  - **Bladder pain associated with IC may refer to the lower abdomen, lower back, inguinal region, penis, scrotum, labia, vagina, perineum, or proximal thighs**.[1–4]
- Nocturia.[1–4]
- Dyspareunia:
  - May occur in males as well as females[3,4,22]
  - Other symptoms (i.e. urinary frequency and urgency) may flare after sexual activity.[3,4,19,22]
- Dysuria.

DIAGNOSTIC PEARLS

- The NIDDK diagnostic criteria were developed for research protocols **and are not useful in routine clinical urology since they will fail to identify the majority of IC patients**.[23–25]
- **It is not necessary for patients to have both frequency/urgency and pelvic pain to make a diagnosis**.[26]
  - Many IC patients with frequency/urgency have no pelvic pain, and many with pelvic pain have no frequency/urgency.[4]

- In females, consider a diagnosis of IC for:
  - A patient who has been previously diagnosed with, and failed therapy for, recurrent UTI (2 or more within 1 year), overactive bladder, urethral syndrome, urethritis, vulvodynia, vulvovestibulitis, endometriosis, yeast vaginitis, or gynecologic chronic pelvic pain
  - Lower urinary tract symptoms associated with sexual activity.
- For males, consider a diagnosis of IC for:
  - A patient who has been previously diagnosed with, and failed antibiotic therapy for, chronic bacterial prostatitis (NIH type 2) and/or chronic epididymitis
  - Any patient previously diagnosed with chronic non-bacterial prostatitis (NIH type 3a or 3b)
  - Chronic episodes of painful ejaculation
  - Chronic scrotal and/or testicular pain in the absence of any other identifiable etiology.

BASIC EVALUATION

Basic evaluation of a patient suspected of having IC should include the following:

HISTORY

- Symptoms should be quantified with the Pelvic Pain and Urgency/Frequency (PUF)[5] or O'Leary Sant[27] validated questionnaires.
  - Some data suggest that the PUF questionnaire (Figure 8.1) is the most sensitive for detecting patients with IC.[28]
- Voiding log:
  - Very useful
  - A 1- or 2-day duration is normally sufficient
  - >7 voids in a day is abnormal[2,3]
  - Patients should record volume of each void, as smaller volumes are associated with IC.[2,3]

PHYSICAL EXAMINATION

- Typical findings – females:
  - Anterior vaginal wall tenderness
  - Pelvic muscle tenderness.
- Typical findings – males:
  - Prostate and/or bladder base tenderness
  - Scrotal, testicular, epididymal, and/or spermatic cord tenderness without physical abnormalities.

URINALYSIS

- Typically will contain no bacteria (except perhaps skin flora from contamination) and no WBCs.
- 10–25% of younger patients (<40 years) may have benign microhematuria (<5 RBC/HPF).

INTERSTITIAL CYSTITIS AND CHRONIC PELVIC PAIN

8

PELVIC PAIN and URGENCY/FREQUENCY
PATIENT SYMPTOM SCALE

Please circle the answer that best describes how you feel for each question.

		0	1	2	3	4	SYMPTOM SCORE	BOTHER SCORE
1	How many times do you go to the bathroom during the day?	3–6	7–10	11–14	15–19	20+		
2	a. How many times do you go to the bathroom at night?	0	1	2	3	4+		
	b. If you get up at night to go to the bathroom, does it bother you?	Never Bothers	Occasionally	Usually	Always			
3	a. Do you now or have you ever had pain or symptoms during or after sexual intercourse?		Never	Occasionally	Usually	Always		
	b. Has pain or urgency ever made you avoid sexual intercourse?		Never	Occasionally	Usually	Always		
4	Do you have pain associated with your bladder or in your pelvis (vagina, labia, lower abdomen, urethra, perineum, testes, or scrotum)?		Never	Occasionally	Usually	Always		
5	a. If you have pain, is it usually			Mild	Moderate	Severe		
	b. Does your pain bother you?		Never	Occasionally	Usually	Always		
6	Do you still have urgency after going to the bathroom?		Never	Occasionally	Usually	Always		
7	a. If you have urgency, is it usually			Mild	Moderate	Severe		
	b. Does your urgency bother you?		Never	Occasionally	Usually	Always		
8	Are you sexually active? Yes____ No____							

SYMPTOM SCORE = (1, 2a, 3a, 4, 5a, 6, 7a)	
BOTHER SCORE = (2b, 3b, 5b, 7b)	
TOTAL SCORE (Symptom Score + Bother Score) =	

©2000 C. Lowell Parsons, M.D

Total score ranges from 1 to 35.
A total score of 10–14 = 74% likelihood of positive PST; 15–19 = 76%; 20 or above = 91% likelihood of positive PST.

Revised 11/17/2003

FIGURE 8.1

Pelvic Pain and Urgency/Frequency (PUF) patient symptom scale.

URINE CULTURE

- For females, sterile catheterized urine sample is required.
- Typically will be negative, although may be positive for low ($\leq 10^2$) levels of flora.

ADDITIONAL EVALUATION

Additional evaluation of the patient suspected of having IC may include:

POTASSIUM SENSITIVITY TEST (PST)

- The first new diagnostic test for IC in 75 years.[9]
- A positive test strongly suggests the presence of IC.[10]

- In clinical studies the PST is positive:
  - In 80% of patients diagnosed with IC[10]
  - In 80% of women with gynecologic pelvic pain[10]
  - In 76% of men with chronic non-bacterial prostatitis[8]
  - In <1.5% of normal controls.[10]
- See Figure 8.2 for protocol.

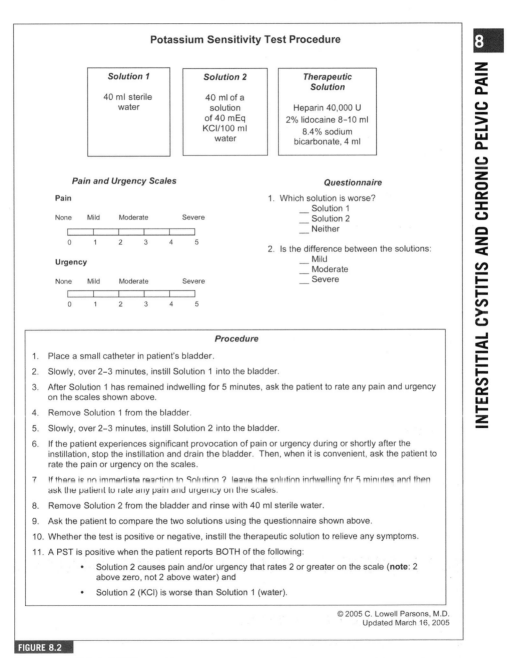

Potassium Sensitivity Test Procedure

Solution 1	*Solution 2*	*Therapeutic Solution*
40 ml sterile water	40 ml of a solution of 40 mEq KCl/100 ml water	Heparin 40,000 U 2% lidocaine 8–10 ml 8.4% sodium bicarbonate, 4 ml

Pain and Urgency Scales

Pain

None Mild Moderate Severe

0   1   2   3   4   5

Urgency

None Mild Moderate Severe

0   1   2   3   4   5

Questionnaire

1. Which solution is worse?
   ___ Solution 1
   ___ Solution 2
   ___ Neither

2. Is the difference between the solutions:
   ___ Mild
   ___ Moderate
   ___ Severe

Procedure

1. Place a small catheter in patient's bladder.
2. Slowly, over 2–3 minutes, instill Solution 1 into the bladder.
3. After Solution 1 has remained indwelling for 5 minutes, ask the patient to rate any pain and urgency on the scales shown above.
4. Remove Solution 1 from the bladder.
5. Slowly, over 2–3 minutes, instill Solution 2 into the bladder.
6. If the patient experiences significant provocation of pain or urgency during or shortly after the instillation, stop the instillation and drain the bladder. Then, when it is convenient, ask the patient to rate the pain or urgency on the scales.
7. If there is no immediate reaction to Solution 2, leave the solution indwelling for 5 minutes and then ask the patient to rate any pain and urgency on the scales.
8. Remove Solution 2 from the bladder and rinse with 40 ml sterile water.
9. Ask the patient to compare the two solutions using the questionnaire shown above.
10. Whether the test is positive or negative, instill the therapeutic solution to relieve any symptoms.
11. A PST is positive when the patient reports BOTH of the following:
    - Solution 2 causes pain and/or urgency that rates 2 or greater on the scale (**note**: 2 above zero, not 2 above water) and
    - Solution 2 (KCl) is worse than Solution 1 (water).

© 2005 C. Lowell Parsons, M.D.
Updated March 16, 2005

FIGURE 8.2

Potassium sensitivity test (PST) procedure.

INTERSTITIAL CYSTITIS AND CHRONIC PELVIC PAIN

8

CYSTOSCOPY

GENERAL CONCEPTS

- If hematuria is present, consider diagnostic cystoscopy to rule out other urinary tract abnormalities.
- Cystoscopy under general anesthesia:
  - Traditionally required for a diagnosis of IC[23]
  - However, recent clinical data have not supported this concept, and **the vast majority of patients with IC symptoms will have normal or non-specific cystoscopic findings**[29,30]
  - **Therefore, cystoscopy under general anesthesia is not required in the evaluation of suspected IC patients.**[26]

CYSTOCOPIC FINDINGS ASSOCIATED WITH IC

- Hunner's ulcer:[31]
  - Erythematous epithelial lesion, similar in endoscopic appearance to bladder carcinoma in situ, characteristic of severe IC
  - Biopsy may show non-specific inflammatory changes
  - Usually present only in patients with severe disease (approximately <1% overall).[2]
- Glomerulations:
  - Punctate vascular bladder lesions that appear with filling of the bladder[1]
  - A non-specific finding that is present in approximately 39–45% of IC patients, but may also be present in up to 39% of asymptomatic controls.[29,32,33]

URODYNAMICS[15,34]

- Useful for distinguishing IC from other lower urinary tract voiding disorders.
- Characteristic cystometrogram (CMG) findings:
  - Sensory urgency symptoms occurring at <150 ml[15]
  - Functional capacity <350 ml.[15]

TREATMENT

MEDICAL THERAPY

Pentosan polysulfate (Elmiron)

- Principle is to restore epithelial function and prevent leak of urinary solutes (i.e. potassium) into the bladder interstitium.[16]
- Efficacy has been consistently demonstrated in numerous clinical trials and meta-analysis of clinical trials.[35–40]
- 65–70% of all patients will improve significantly within 8 months of beginning therapy.[39,40]
- Dose:
  - 100 mg orally three times per day[41,42]
  - Alternatively, may consider 200 mg orally twice per day **(off-label use)**.[42]
- Contraindications and warnings:[41]
  - Contraindications: pentosan polysulfate allergy
  - Warnings: none.

Intravesical heparin

- Principle is to restore epithelial function and prevent leak of urinary solutes.[16,43]
  - Should be reserved for more severe patients or those failing oral therapy[42]
  - 20 000 to 40 000 units, self-administered by patient, one or more times per day[42]
  - Use total volume of 10 ml.[42]

Amitriptyline

- May reduce urgency and pain sensations.[44,45]
- Dose: 25–100 mg orally once at bedtime.[42]

Hydroxyzine

- Effective at reducing mast cell-associated flares in symptoms, which are seen in about 60% of patients.[46–48]
- Dose: 10–25 mg orally once at bedtime.[42]

Other agents

- Pyridium:
  - May be used for mild symptomatic relief
  - Dose: 100–200 mg orally up to three times per day.
- Intravesical dimethyl sulfoxide (DMSO):[49]
  - Mechanism of action is unclear[45]
  - Up to 50% of patients will respond[42]
  - Protocol: 50 ml once per week for 6–8 weeks[42]
  - May cause significant pain flares during instillation.
- Intravesical therapeutic solution:
  - New therapy that **acutely relieves bladder symptoms**[50]
  - 94% of patients will obtain immediate relief for 2–40 hours[50]
  - Should be performed in conjunction with other therapies[50]
  - Protocol: mix 40 000 units of heparin with 8 ml of 2% lidocaine and 3 ml of 8.4% sodium bicarbonate. Instill in bladder and leave 20–30 minutes[50]
  - May be performed three times per week for several weeks[50]
  - In severe cases, may be self-administered by patients at home 1–3 times per day.[50]

SURGICAL THERAPY

- Cystoscopic hydrodistension under anesthesia:[51]
  - Dilate bladder by filling with water at 80 cmH$_2$0 for 1–3 minutes
  - Relieves symptoms in about 50–60% of patients
  - Relief typically lasts 6–10 months.
- Sacral neuromodulation:
  - Involves implantation of a device that stimulates the sacral nerve
  - The principle is to alleviate symptoms by inhibition of afferent nerve signals
  - In the short term, alleviates symptoms in some patients with refractory IC[52,53]
  - However, long-term results have been disappointing.[54]

8

INTERSTITIAL CYSTITIS AND CHRONIC PELVIC PAIN

- Augmentation cystoplasty:
  - Not effective and should not be performed.[15]
- Cystectomy and urinary diversion:
  - Should be performed only in severe patients who have failed all conservative therapy.[14,15]

TREATMENT PEARLS

- Medical therapy (notably pentosan polysulfate) may take time to work, especially in severe patients.
  - Substantial symptomatic improvements may take a year or more to appear.[50]
- Therefore, when reviewing a treatment plan in a patient who is not responding to medical therapy during the first 12 months of treatment, add more treatments if necessary, but do not stop the initial therapy.[50]
- Avoid narcotics if possible.
- Dietary modifications:
  - Data are scant regarding potential efficacy at reducing symptoms[14]
  - However, some investigators believe that reducing coffee and potassium-rich foods (citrus, tomatoes, chocolate) is helpful, but not for long-term benefit.[14]

REFERENCES

1. Hand JR: Interstitial cystitis, a report of 223 cases. J Urol 61:291–310, 1949.
2. Parsons CL: Interstitial cystitis: clinical manifestations and diagnostic criteria in over 200 cases. Neurourol Urodyn 9:241–50, 1990.
3. Koziol JA, Clark DC, Gittes RF, Tan EM: The natural history of interstitial cystitis: a survey of 374 patients. J Urol 149:465–9, 1993.
4. Parsons CL, Zupkas P, Parsons JK: Intravesical potassium sensitivity in patients with interstitial cystitis and urethral syndrome. Urology 57:428–33, 2001.
5. Parsons CL, Dell J, Stanford EJ et al: Increased prevalence of interstitial cystitis: previously unrecognized urologic and gynecologic cases identified using a new symptom questionnaire and intravesical potassium sensitivity. Urology 60:573–8, 2002.
6. Parsons CL, Tatsis V: Prevalence of interstitial cystitis in young women. Urology 64:866–70, 2004.
7. Parsons CL, Albo ME: Intravesical potassium sensitivity in prostatitis patients. J Urol 168:1054–7, 2002.
8. Parsons CL, Rosenberg MT, Sassani P et al: Quantifying symptoms in men with interstitial cystitis/prostatitis, and its correlation with potassium-sensitivity testing. BJU Int 95:86–90, 2005.
9. Parsons CL, Greenberger M, Gabal L, Bidair M, Barme G: The role of urinary potassium in the pathogenesis and diagnosis of interstitial cystitis. J Urol 159:1862–7, 1998.
10. Parsons CL: Prostatitis, interstitial cystitis, chronic pelvic pain, and urethral syndrome share a common pathophysiology: lower urinary dysfunctional epithelium and potassium recycling. Urology 62:976–82, 2003.
11. Parsons CL, Lilly JD, Stein P: Epithelial dysfunction in nonbacterial cystitis (interstitial cystitis). J Urol 145:732–5, 1991.
12. Lilly JD, Parsons CL: Bladder surface glycosaminoglycans as a human epithelial permeability barrier. Surg Gynecol Obstet 171:493–6, 1990.
13. Jones CA, Nyberg L: Epidemiology of interstitial cystitis. Urology 49 (Suppl 5A):2–9, 1997.
14. Moldwin RM, Sant GR: Interstitial cystitis: a pathophysiology and treatment update. Clin Obstet Gynecol 45:259–72, 2002.

15. Parsons CL: Interstitial cystitis: new concepts in pathogenesis, diagnosis, and management. In: Drutz HP, Herschorn S, Diamant NE, eds. Female Pelvic Medicine and Reconstructive Pelvic Surgery. London: Springer-Verlag, 2003, pp 199–211.
16. Parsons CL: Epithelial coating techniques in the treatment of interstitial cystitis. Urology 49(Suppl 5A):100–4, 1997.
17. Theoharides TC, Kempuraj D, Sant GR: Mast cell involvement in interstitial cystitis: a review of human and experimental evidence. Urology 57(Suppl 1):47–55, 2001.
18. Letourneau R, Pang X, Sant GR et al: Intragranular activation of bladder mast cells and their association with nerve processes in interstitial cystitis. Br J Urol 77:41–54, 1996.
19. Koziol JA: Epidemiology of interstitial cystitis. Urol Clin North Am 21:7–71, 1994.
20. Erickson DR: Urine markers of interstitial cystitis. Urology 57(Suppl 6A):15–21, 2001.
21. Keay SK, Szekely Z, Conrads TP et al: An antiproliferative factor from interstitial cystitis patients is a frizzled 8 protein-related sialoglycopeptide. Proc Natl Acad Sci USA 101:11803–8, 2004.
22. Forrest JB, Vo Q: Observations on the presentation, diagnosis, and treatment of interstitial cystitis in men. Urology 57(Suppl 6A):26–9, 2001.
23. Gillenwater JY, Wein AJ: Summary of the National Institute of Arthritis, Diabetes, Digestive and Kidney Diseases Workshop on Interstitial Cystitis, National Institutes of Health, Bethesda, Maryland, August 28–29, 1987. J Urol 140:203–6, 1988.
24. Wein AJ, Hanno PM, Gillenwater JY: Interstitial cystitis: an introduction to the problem. In: Hanno PM, Staskin DR, Krane RJ, Wein AJ, eds. Interstitial Cystitis. London: Springer-Verlag, 1990, pp 3–15.
25. Hanno PM, Landis JR, Matthews-Cook Y et al: The diagnosis of interstitial cystitis revisited: lessons learned from the National Institutes of Health Interstitial Cystitis Database study. J Urol 161:553–7, 1999.
26. Nickel JC: Interstitial cystitis: the paradigm shifts. International consultations on interstitial cystitis. Rev Urol 6:200–2, 2004.
27. O'Leary MP, Sant GR, Fowler FJ Jr et al: The interstitial cystitis symptom index and problem index. Urology 49(Suppl 5A):58–63, 1997.
28. Moldwin RM, Kushner L: The diagnostic value of interstitial cystitis questionnaires. Presented at Research Insights into Interstitial Cystitis: A Basic and Clinical Science Symposium, Alexandria, Virginia, October 30 to November 1, 2003.
29. Waxman JA, Sulak PJ, Kuehl TJ: Cystoscopic findings consistent with interstitial cystitis in normal women undergoing tubal ligation. J Urol 160:1663–7, 1998.
30. Ottem DP, Teichman JM: What is the value of cystoscopy with hydrodistension for interstitial cystitis? Urology 66:494–9, 2005.
31. Hunner GL: A rare type of bladder ulcer in women: report of cases. Boston Med Surg J 172:660–4, 1915.
32. Messing E, Pauk D, Schaeffer A et al: Associations among cystoscopic findings and symptoms and physical examination findings in women enrolled in the Interstitial Cystitis Data Base (ICDB) Study. Urology 49(Suppl 5A):81–5, 1997.
33. Tomaszewski JE, Landis JR, Russack V et al: Biopsy features are associated with primary symptoms in interstitial cystitis: results from the Interstitial Cystitis Database Study. Urology 57(Suppl 1):67–81, 2001.
34. Nigro DA, Wein AJ, Foy M et al: Associations among cystoscopic and urodynamic findings for women enrolled in the Interstitial Cystitis Data Base (ICDB) Study. Urology 49(Suppl 5A):86–92, 1997.
35. Parsons CL, Benson G, Childs SJ et al: A quantitatively controlled method to prospectively study interstitial cystitis and which demonstrates the efficacy of pentosan polysulfate. J Urol 150:845–8, 1993.
36. Mulholland SG, Hanno P, Parsons CL et al: Pentosan polysulfate sodium for therapy of interstitial cystitis. A double-blind placebo-controlled clinical study. Urology 35:552–8, 1990.
37. Parsons CL, Mulholland SG: Successful therapy of interstitial cystitis with pentosan polysulfate. J Urol 138:513–16, 1987.

38. Holm-Bentzen M, Jacobsen F, Nerstrom B et al: A prospective double-blind clinically controlled multicenter trial of sodium pentosan polysulfate in the treatment of interstitial cystitis and related painful bladder disease. J Urol 138:503–7, 1987.
39. Hanno PM. Analysis of long-term Elmiron therapy for interstitial cystitis. Urology 49(S5A):93–9, 1997.
40. Nickel JC, Barkin J, Forrest J et al: Elmiron Study Group. Randomized, double-blind, dose-ranging study of pentosan polysulfate sodium for interstitial cystitis. Urology 65(4):654–8, 2005.
41. Pentosan polysulfate sodium: Mosby's Drug Consult. St. Louis: Mosby, 2005.
42. Parsons CL: Current strategies for managing interstitial cystitis. Expert Opin Pharmacother 5:287–93, 2004.
43. Parsons CL, Housley T, Schmidt JD et al: Treatment of interstitial cystitis with intravesical heparin. Br J Urol 73:504–7, 1994.
44. Hanno PM, Buehler J, Wein AJ: Use of amitriptyline in the treatment of interstitial cystitis. J Urol 141:846–8, 1989.
45. van Ophoven A, Pokupic S, Heinecke A, Hertle L: A prospective, randomized, placebo controlled, double-blind study of amitriptyline for the treatment of interstitial cystitis. J Urol 172:533–6, 2004.
46. Theoharides TC: Hydroxyzine in the treatment of interstitial cystitis. Urol Clin N Am 21:113–19, 1994.
47. Theoharides TC, Sant GR: Hydroxyzine therapy for interstitial cystitis. Urology 49:108–10, 1997.
48. Minogiannis P, El-Mansoury M, Betances JA, Sant GR, Theoharides TC: Hydroxyzine inhibits neurogenic bladder mast cell activation. Int J Immunopharmacol 10:553–63, 1998.
49. Stewart BH, Persky L, Kiser WS: The use of dimethylsulfoxide (DMSO) in the treatment of interstitial cystitis. J Urol 98:671–2, 1967.
50. Parsons CL: Successful downregulation of bladder sensory nerves with combination of heparin and alkalinized lidocaine in patients with interstitial cystitis. Urology 65(1):45–8, 2005.
51. Hanno PM, Wein AJ: Conservative therapy of interstitial cystitis. Semin Urol 9:143–7, 1991.
52. Whitmore KE, Payne CK, Diokno AC, Lukban JC: Sacral neuromodulation in patients with interstitial cystitis: a multicenter clinical trial. Int Urogynecol J Pelvic Floor Dysfunct 14:305–8; discussion 308–9, 2003.
53. Peters KM, Konstandt D: Sacral neuromodulation decreases narcotic requirements in refractory interstitial cystitis. BJU Int 93:777–9, 2004.
54. Elhilali MM, Khaled SM, Kashiwabara T, Elzayat E, Corcos J: Sacral neuromodulation: long-term experience of one center. Urology 65:1114–17, 2005.

Renal transplantation and renovascular hypertension

Danil V Makarov

SUMMARY

- Kidney transplant decreases morbidity and mortality among patients with kidney failure, but exchanges the problems of end-stage renal disease (ESRD) for those of chronic immunosuppression.
- Types of immunosuppression include antibodies (daclizumab, basiliximab, thymoglobulin, and OKT3), calcineurin blockers (cyclosporine and tacrolimus), steroids, mTOR inhibitors (sirolimus and everolimus), and antimetabolites (mycophenolate mofetil).
- Renovascular hypertension is hypertension resulting from a renal arterial lesion that is relieved by correction of the offending lesion or removal of the kidney. The hypertension is related to increased angiotensin expression.
- The prevalence of renovascular hypertension among the general hypertensive population is 0.5–5%.
- At least 70% of renovascular lesions are atherosclerotic.
- Other types of lesions include intimal fibroplasia, medial fibroplasia, perimedial fibroplasia, and fibromuscular hyperplasia.
- Treatment for renovascular hypertension includes medical management, angioplasty, angioplasty with stent, and surgical revascularization.

RENAL TRANSPLANTATION

GENERAL INFORMATION

- Preferred form of renal replacement therapy.[1]
- Cost-effective vs dialysis if graft survival >2 years.[2]
- Exchanges the problems of ESRD for those of immunosuppressed transplant recipients, but with decreased morbidity and mortality.[3]
- Isograft: a graft of tissue that is obtained from a donor genetically identical to the recipient.
- Xenograft: a type of tissue graft in which the donor and recipient are of different species.
- Allograft: a graft of tissue obtained from a donor of the same species as – but with a different genetic make-up from – the recipient, as a tissue transplant between two humans.[4]

BASIC IMMUNOLOGY

Cellular immunity

- T cells:
  - Detect processed antigen via the T-cell receptor
  - An antigen-presenting cell must give second signal when activated
  - Produces cytokines
  - Kills infected cells via interactions with cell surface molecules.[5–8]

- B cells:
  - Detect tertiary structures of antigens
  - IgD and IgM antibodies act as receptors
  - Need cytokine signals from T cells for activation
  - Produce antibodies when activated.[6,7,9,10]

Humoral immunity

- Antibodies:
  - Produced by activated B cell
  - Mediate complement fixation.[6,7]

Innate immunity

- Non-specific, constitutional responses.
- Physical barriers, macrophages, monocytes, PMNs, complement, NK cells.
- No improvement with repeated exposure.[11]

T vs B cells

- MHC:
  - Combination of various HLA haplotypes creates genetic variability
  - Improves chances of population survival against new pathogens.
- MHC Class I:
  - HLA A, B, C
  - Expressed by most nucleated cells
  - Binds to CD8 on T lymphocytes
  - Presents intracellular peptides.
- MHC Class II:
  - HLA DR, DP, DQ
  - Expressed by specialized antigen-presenting cells (APCs): dendritic cells, macrophages, and endothelial cells.[6,7]

TYPES OF IMUNOSUPPRESSION

Antibodies

- Block antigen from being recognized by recipient T cells.
- Given at the time of surgery:
  - Daclizumab and basiliximab
  - Block IL-2 receptor
  - Minimal side-effect profile.[12,13]
- Given at surgery or at time of rejection:
  - Thymoglobulin and OKT3
  - Stimulate cytokine release
  - May cause ARDS, SIRS, leukopenia
  - Require antiviral and anti-PCP prophylaxis.[7,14]

Calcineurin blockers

- Block the activation of calcineurin after antigen binds TCR.
- Cyclosporine and tacrolimus (FK-506).
- Prevent rejection.
- Must monitor levels to attain target trough.
- Nephrotoxic.

- Induce hypertension.
- More cosmetic changes (hypertrichosis and gingival hyperplasia) with cyclosporine.[15]
- More neurotoxicity and diabetes with tacrolimus.
- In meta-analysis, tacrolimus better at preventing rejection and reducing graft loss.[16]

Steroids

- IL-1 blocked at normal doses.
- IL-2 blocked at high dose.
- Administered by high-dose 'pulse,' then tapered to minimize side effects.

Mammalian target of rapamycin (mTOR) inhibitors

- Sirolimus, everolimus.
- Blocks T-cell activation by inhibiting progression from G1 to S phase.[17]
- Allow withdrawal of cyclosporine and preservation of renal function.[18]

Antimetabolites

- Mycophenolate mofetil [now more commonly used than Imuran (azathioprine)].
- Prevents and treats rejection.
- Causes leukopenia and GI upset.
- Effective when combined with calcineurin blocker and steroids.[7,19]

TREATMENT OF ACUTE REJECTION

- Banff I (cellular):
  - Steroid pulse.
- Banff II–III (resistant or vascular):
  - OKT3, thymoglobulin
  - Phasmapheresis if antibodies are present
  - IVIG, anti-B cell antibodies.[1,7]

RECIPIENT EVALUATION

The following recipient factors should be considered:
- Presence of active infection.
- Renal malignancy:
  - Incidental: no waiting period after definitive treatment
  - Symptomatic: wait 2 years after treatment.
- Bladder, prostate, or testis malignancy:
  - Wait 2 years after treatment.
- Primary disease recurrence:
  - High risk, high consequence: focal segmental glomerulosclerosis and hemolytic uremic syndrome
  - High risk, low consequence: diabetes and IgA nephropathy
  - Very low risk
  - Autosomal dominant polycystic kidney and vesicoureteral reflux.[20]
- Bladder function:
  - Clean intermittent catheterization may be performed safely and effectively post-transplant

RENAL TRANSPLANTATION AND RENOVASCULAR HYPERTENSION

9

- Anastomoses to augmented bladders or diversions generally have good outcomes
- Transurethral resection of the prostate in a patient with ESRD and oliguria ('dry TURP') is associated with increased risk of strictures.
- Technical aspects:
  - Identify safe vessel for anastomosis; beware of steal
  - Reconstruction of atherosclerotic vessels may be necessary.[21]
- Social support and/or financial resources.[1,7,22]

DONOR EVALUATION

Cadaveric

- Cadaveric criteria allow double kidneys at extremes of age and non-heart beating donors.
- Zero mismatch list factors: waiting time, antibody levels, and other factors (i.e. recipient age).[23]

Living

- >50% of kidney transplants are from living donors.
- Poorly matched living donor fares better than well-matched cadaveric.[24]
- Mortality = 0.03%.
- Major morbidity = 0.2%.[24]
- Minor morbidity = 8%.[25]
- For the donors, is not associated with an increased risk of renal failure or hypertension, but is associated with asymptomatic proteinuria.[26]
- <1% later regretted the donation.[27]

SURGERY

- Renal vasculature variations:
  - Preserve lower pole artery to supply the ureter if possible
  - Use Carrel patch in cadaveric donors <6 years old
  - Small lower pole vessel: may anastomose end-to-end to inferior epigastric artery.[28]
- Lower urinary tract:
  - Extravesical ureteroneocystostomy is normally performed.[29]
- Native nephrectomy – indications for excision:
  - Suspicion of malignancy
  - Large size (i.e. autosomal dominant polycystic kidney)
  - Grade 4–5 vesicoureteral reflux
  - Massive proteinuria
  - Intractable hypertension
  - Recurrent stones or urinary tract infection (UTI).[30]
- Laparoscopic donor:
  - Advantages: small incision, shorter stay, less pain, faster return to work
  - Disadvantages: increased Operating Room time, shorter vessels, right side technically challenging.[25]

RENOVASCULAR HYPERTENSION

CLINICAL DEFINITION

- Hypertension (HTN) resulting from a renal arterial lesion that is relieved by correction of the offending lesion or removal of the kidney.[31]

PATHOPHYSIOLOGY

- Angiotensin II:
  - Autoregulates glomerular filtration rate (GFR)
  - Increases efferent arteriole resistance
  - Maintains GFR in face of hypoperfusion.
- In the affected kidney:
  - There is increased renin release with Na retention due to decreased perfusion caused by the renal artery lesion.
- For unilateral disease, in the unaffected contralateral kidney:
  - Renin is suppressed
  - Na is secreted.[31,32]

Acute phase

- Euvolemia.
- Angiotensin II-dependent vasoconstriction creates hypertension.
- Hypertension may be controlled by:
  - Arterial repair
  - Angiotensin-converting enzyme (ACE) inhibitor therapy
  - Angiotensin II antagonists.

Chronic phase

- Prolonged hypertension damages the non-ischemic kidney.
- Na^+ and fluid retention increase as natriuresis declines.
- Hypertension becomes volume-dependent.
- Hypertension can be treated by Na^+ depletion *and* surgery.
  - Surgery alone may become ineffective.[31,33]

EPIDEMIOLOGY AND CLASSIFICATION

Prevalence: 0.5–5% of general hypertensive population.[34]

ATHEROSCLEROSIS

- 70–90% of all renovascular lesions.[35]
- Renal manifestation of systemic vascular disease.
- Involves proximal 2 cm of renal artery.
- Distal involvement rare.
- 40% of those with high-grade stenosis may occlude completely.[36]
- Often contributes to loss of renal function and ESRD.[31,35]
- These patients have 12% 5-year survival on hemodialysis (poorest of all ESRD patients).[37]

FIBROMUSCULAR DYSPLASIA

- Accounts for approximately one-third of renovascular lesions.
- Four major manifestations.

Intimal fibroplasia

- Occurs primarily in children and young adults.
- Pathology demonstrates circumferential collagen accumulation inside the internal elastic lamina.
- Angiography demonstrates smooth, focal stenosis in proximal to mid vessel.
- Non-operative management results in progressive obstruction and ischemic atrophy.

Medial fibroplasia

- Comprises 80–90% of fibromuscular dysplasias.[35]
- Commonly affects 25–50-year-old women.
- Often bilateral involvement.
- Arteriography demonstrates string of beads appearance of distal renal artery or its branches.
- Low risk of disease progression with medical management.

Perimedial fibroplasia

- Generally affects 15–30-year-old women.
- Renal artery is only site of occurrence.
- Pathology demonstrates tightly stenotic collagen 'collar' replacing media.
- Non-operative management results in progressive obstruction, leading to ischemic renal atrophy.

Fibromuscular hyperplasia

- Rarest form of fibromuscular dysplasia.
- Affects children and young adults.
- Represents a true hyperplasia of arterial wall smooth muscle.
- Arteriography demonstrates smooth stenosis.
- Progresses to obstruction.[31,33,35,38]

PRESENTATION, EVALUATION, AND DIAGNOSIS

CLINICAL FEATURES

- New-onset HTN presenting prior to age 30 or after age 55.
- Sudden onset HTN.
- Family history of HTN.
- HTN resistant to medical therapy.
- Malignant hypertension.
- HTN in association with pulmonary edema, hypercholesterolemia, generalized atherosclerotic disease, chronic renal failure, or history of smoking.[39]

CLINICAL SIGNS

- Severe HTN.
- Epigastic bruit.

- Severe hypertensive retinopathy.
- Generalized atherosclerotic disease.
- Proteinuria.
- Hypokalemia.[33]
- Azotemia worsening with medical management of HTN.[31]
- Risk factors for renal artery stenosis (evaluated in patient undergoing cardiac catheterization).
- Advanced age.
- Female sex.
- Coronary artery disease.
- Peripheral vascular disease.
- History of congestive heart failure (CHF).
- Elevated creatinine.[40]

WORK-UP

Imaging

- Captopril renogram:
  - Ischemic kidney dependent on function of angiotensin II to maintain GFR
  - ACE inhibitor will stop production of angiotensin II and will decrease GFR in stenotic kidney
  - Manifests as asymmetric uptake on radionuclide renogram
  - Sensitivity 85–90% and specificity 93–98%.[31,33]
- Duplex renal ultrasound.
  - Documents flow velocities, non-invasively and without administration of iodinated contrast dye
  - Peak systolic flows >180 cm/s are abnormal
  - Categories of stenosis are normal, mild (<60% stenosis) and severe (>60%)
  - Sensitivity 75–98% and specificity 90–100%.[31,41]
- CT angiography:
  - Images main renal artery and some early branches well
  - Better availability than magnetic resonance angiography (MRA)
  - Requires large volume of iodinated contrast
  - Sensitivity and specificity >95%.[33,42]
- Magnetic resonance angiography:
  - Gadolinium–DTPA used to enhance blood signal is non-invasive and uses no iodinated contrast
  - Demonstrates main renal artery well
  - Image quality worse than angiography
  - Sensitivity and specificity >90%.[39,43]
- Renal arteriography:
  - Gold standard
  - Requires arterial puncture, arterial catheters, radiation and iodinated contrast infusion
  - May result in renal impairment
  - May be performed more safely using CO_2 gas and digital subtraction imaging
  - May proceed immediately to percutaneous angioplasty.[31]

9

RENAL TRANSPLANTATION AND RENOVASCULAR HYPERTENSION

Functional testing

- Captopril test:
  - Measurement of peripheral renin before and after captopril administration
  - Peripheral renin will increase more substantially in patients with RVH as compared to those with essential HTN
  - Sensitivity 75% and specificity 89%
  - Low sensitivity makes this test less useful as a general screen.[31]
- Renal vein renin:
  - Hypersecretion of renin from affected kidney suppresses renin secretion from the contralateral kidney
  - >50% elevation in renin level defines ischemic kidney and confirms presence of renovascular hypertension.[31]
- Diagnostic algorithm:
  - High suspicion → angiography as first test
  - Low suspicion → captopril renography
  - If positive, proceed to angiography
  - If indeterminate, may proceed to imaging modality (U/S, CT, or MR).[31,39]

TREATMENT AND PROGNOSIS

MEDICAL MANAGEMENT

- Appropriate for patients with:
  - Medial fibroplasia or atherosclerotic stenosis, not intimal or perimedial fibroplasias
  - Unilateral stenosis
  - Creatinine >2.5 mg/dl
  - Renal artery <7 cm long
  - Proteinuria >1 g/day.
- Optimal regimen includes:
  - Aggressive blood pressure control
  - Lipid-lowering agents
  - Antiplatelet therapy
  - Smoking cessation.[33,35,39]

INTERVENTIONAL RADIOLOGY

Angioplasty

- First-line therapy for fibromuscular dysplasia:
  - May improve HTN in up to 80%
  - Restenosis (~30%) easily retreated.[38]
- Less success for atherosclerosis:
  - Lower cure rate, higher restenosis (especially with ostial lesions)
  - Outcome of balloon angioplasty alone not different from medical management.[44]
- Complications 10–20%:
  - Renal dysfunction, puncture site hematoma, pseudoaneurysm, intimal dissection, atheroembolic shower, arterial rupture.[35,39]

Angioplasty with stent

- Indicated for:
  - Poor results with angioplasty alone
  - Restenosis after angioplasty
  - Management of angioplasty complications such as dissection or intimal flap
  - Ostial lesion.[31]
- Complications:
  - Lower incidence of dissection and intimal tear
  - Restenosis 6–38%
  - Lower cure rates with atherosclerotic lesions
  - Mortality <3%.[45]

Clinical parameters associated with poor outcomes

- Renal size <8 cm.
- Creatinine >3–4 mg/dl.
- Comorbid cause of renal dysfunction (i.e. diabetes, amyloidosis).
- Long-standing essential HTN.
- Bilateral renal artery stenosis.
- Long-standing renal dysfunction.
- Extensive burden of atherosclerosis.[39]

SURGICAL REVASCULARIZATION

- Typically reserved for patients with:
  - Concurrent aortic aneurysm dissection
  - Renal artery aneurysm
  - Failed angioplasty/stenting.
- Highly effective therapy for fibromuscular dysplasia:
  - 50–60% cure rate
  - Failure rate <10%.
- Less effective for atherosclerotic disease.[39]

Procedures

- If aorta is healthy:
  - Aortorenal bypass with free graft of autologous hypogastic artery or saphenous vein
  - Aortorenal bypass with PTFE (polytetrafluoroethylene) graft if autologous tissue is unavailable
  - Endarterectomy.[35]
- If severe aortic atherosclerosis is present:
  - Splenorenal bypass for left renal artery (RA)
  - Hepatorenal bypass for right RA.[31]
- Partial or total nephrectomy reserved for patients with:
  - Severe renal atrophy
  - Uncorrectable renovascular lesions
  - Renal infarct
  - Severe arteriolar nephrosclerosis.[46]

RENAL TRANSPLANTATION AND RENOVASCULAR HYPERTENSION

9

REFERENCES

1. Barry JM: Renal transplantation. In: Walsh PC, Retik AB, Vaughan ED, Wein AJ, eds. Campbell's Urology, 8th edn. Philadelphia: WB Saunders, 2002, pp 345–76.
2. Winkelmayer WC, Weinstein MC, Mittleman MA et al: Health economic evaluations: the special case of end-stage renal disease treatment. Med Decis Making 22:417, 2002.
3. Schnuelle P, Lorenz D, Trede M et al: Impact of renal cadaveric transplantation on survival in end-stage renal failure: evidence for reduced mortality risk compared with hemodialysis during long-term follow-up. J Am Soc Nephrol 9:2135, 1998.
4. The Columbia Encyclopedia, 6th edn, 2005.
5. Nishimura MI, Roszkowski JJ, Moore TV et al: Antigen recognition and T-cell biology. Cancer Treat Res 123:37, 2005.
6. Flechner SM, Finke JH, Fairchild RL: Basic principles of immunology in urology. In: Walsh PC, Retik AB, Vaughan ED, Wein AJ, eds. Campbell's Urology, 8th edn. Philadelphia: WB Saunders, 2002, pp 307–44.
7. Shoskes D: Renal transplantation. Presented at the American Urologic Association Annual Review Course, Dallas, TX, June 12, 2005.
8. Davis MM, Bjorkman PJ: T-cell antigen receptor genes and T-cell recognition. Nature 334:395, 1988.
9. Ollila J, Vihinen M: B cells. Int J Biochem Cell Biol 37:518, 2005.
10. Parker DC: T cell-dependent B cell activation. Annu Rev Immunol 11:331, 1993.
11. Hoffmann JA, Kafatos FC, Janeway CA et al: Phylogenetic perspectives in innate immunity. Science 284:1313, 1999.
12. Morris JA, Hanson JE, Steffen BJ et al: Daclizumab is associated with decreased rejection and improved patient survival in renal transplant recipients. Clin Transplant 19:340, 2005.
13. Boggi U, Vistoli F, Signori S et al: Efficacy and safety of basiliximab in kidney transplantation. Expert Opin Drug Saf 4:473, 2005.
14. Goggins WC, Pascual MA, Powelson JA et al: A prospective, randomized, clinical trial of intraoperative versus postoperative Thymoglobulin in adult cadaveric renal transplant recipients. Transplantation 76:798, 2003.
15. Margreiter R, Pohanka E, Sparacino V et al: Open prospective multicenter study of conversion to tacrolimus therapy in renal transplant patients experiencing ciclosporin-related side-effects. Transpl Int 18:816, 2005.
16. Webster AC, Woodroffe RC, Taylor RS et al: Tacrolimus versus ciclosporin as primary immunosuppression for kidney transplant recipients: meta-analysis and meta-regression of randomised trial data. BMJ 331:810, 2005.
17. Taylor AL, Watson CJ, Bradley JA: Immunosuppressive agents in solid organ transplantation: mechanisms of action and therapeutic efficacy. Crit Rev Oncol Hematol 56:23, 2005.
18. Oberbauer R, Kreis H, Johnson RW et al: Long-term improvement in renal function with sirolimus after early cyclosporine withdrawal in renal transplant recipients: 2-year results of the Rapamune Maintenance Regimen Study. Transplantation 76:364, 2003.
19. van Gelder T, Shaw LM: The rationale for and limitations of therapeutic drug monitoring for mycophenolate mofetil in transplantation. Transplantation 80:S244, 2005.
20. Hariharan S, Adams MB, Brennan DC et al: Recurrent and de novo glomerular disease after renal transplantation: a report from renal allograft disease registry. Transplant Proc 31:223, 1999.
21. Pfeiffer T, Sandmann W, Luther B et al: Vascular surgery for recipient preparation, improvement of graft quality and acceptability, and therapy of ischemic graft damage in kidney transplantation. Transplant Proc 34:2219, 2002.
22. Kasiske BL, Ramos EL, Gaston RS et al: The evaluation of renal transplant candidates: clinical practice guidelines. Patient Care and Education Committee of the American Society of Transplant Physicians. J Am Soc Nephrol 6:1, 1995.
23. Light JA: A 25 year history of kidney transplantation at the Washington Hospital Center. Clin Transpl 159–68, 1998.

24. Koller H, Mayer G: Evaluation of the living kidney donor. Nephrol Dial Transplant 19(Suppl 4):iv41, 2004.
25. Su LM, Ratner LE, Montgomery RA et al: Laparoscopic live donor nephrectomy: trends in donor and recipient morbidity following 381 consecutive cases. Ann Surg 240:358, 2004.
26. Goldfarb DA, Matin SF, Braun WE et al: Renal outcome 25 years after donor nephrectomy. J Urol 166:2043, 2001.
27. Fehrman-Ekholm I, Brink B, Ericsson C et al: Kidney donors don't regret: follow-up of 370 donors in Stockholm since 1964. Transplantation 69:2067, 2000.
28. Berardinelli L: Technical problems in living donor transplantation. Transplant Proc 37:2449, 2005.
29. Pleass HC, Clark KR, Rigg KM et al: Urologic complications after renal transplantation: a prospective randomized trial comparing different techniques of ureteric anastomosis and the use of prophylactic ureteric stents. Transplant Proc 27:1091, 1995.
30. Darby CR, Cranston D, Raine AE et al: Bilateral nephrectomy before transplantation: indications, surgical approach, morbidity and mortality. Br J Surg 78:305, 1991.
31. Novick AC: Renovascular hypertension. In: Walsh PC, Retik AB, Vaughan ED, Wein AJ, eds. Campbell's Urology, 8th edn. Philadelphia: WB Saunders, 2002 pp 229–71.
32. Welch WJ: The pathophysiology of renin release in renovascular hypertension. Semin Nephrol 20:394, 2000.
33. Olin JW: Renal artery disease: diagnosis and management. Mt Sinai J Med 71:73, 2004.
34. Greco BA, Breyer JA: Atherosclerotic ischemic renal disease. Am J Kidney Dis 29:167, 1997.
35. Safian RD, Textor SC: Renal-artery stenosis. New Engl J Med 344:431, 2001.
36. Zierler RE, Bergelin RO, Isaacson JA et al: Natural history of atherosclerotic renal artery stenosis: a prospective study with duplex ultrasonography. J Vasc Surg 19:250, 1994.
37. Baboolal K, Evans C, Moore RH: Incidence of end-stage renal disease in medically treated patients with severe bilateral atherosclerotic renovascular disease. Am J Kidney Dis 31.971, 1998.
38. Slovut DP, Olin JW: Fibromuscular dysplasia. New Engl J Med 350:1862, 2004.
39. Bloch MJ, Basile J: Clinical insights into the diagnosis and management of renovascular disease. An evidence-based review. Minerva Med 95:357, 2004.
40. Harding MB, Smith LR, Himmelstein SI et al: Renal artery stenosis: prevalence and associated risk factors in patients undergoing routine cardiac catheterization. J Am Soc Nephrol 2:1608, 1992.
41. Mollo M, Pelet V, Mouawad J et al: Evaluation of colour duplex ultrasound scanning in diagnosis of renal artery stenosis, compared to angiography: a prospective study on 53 patients. Eur J Vasc Endovasc Surg 14:305, 1997.
42. Wittenberg G, Kenn W, Tschammler A et al: Spiral CT angiography of renal arteries: comparison with angiography. Eur Radiol 9:546, 1999.
43. Leung DA, Hoffmann U, Pfammatter T et al: Magnetic resonance angiography versus duplex sonography for diagnosing renovascular disease. Hypertension 33:726, 1999.
44. van Jaarsveld BC, Krijnen P, Pieterman H et al: The effect of balloon angioplasty on hypertension in atherosclerotic renal-artery stenosis. Dutch Renal Artery Stenosis Intervention Cooperative Study Group. New Engl J Med 342:1007, 2000.
45. van de Ven PJ, Kaatee R, Beutler JJ et al: Arterial stenting and balloon angioplasty in ostial atherosclerotic renovascular disease: a randomised trial. Lancet 353:282, 1999.
46. Oskin TC, Hansen KJ, Deitch JS et al: Chronic renal artery occlusion: nephrectomy versus revascularization. J Vasc Surg 29:140, 1999.

9

RENAL TRANSPLANTATION AND RENOVASCULAR HYPERTENSION

Cystic diseases of the kidney

Ioannis M Varkarakis

SUMMARY

- Simple renal cyst is a common, benign condition usually detected incidentally.
- The Bosniak classification system is used to distinguish simple cysts from complex renal cysts and cystic renal cell carcinoma.
- Acquired renal cystic disease occurs in patients with renal failure and is characterized by bilateral cortical and/or medullary cysts. It is associated with an increased risk of renal cell carcinoma.
- Autosomal dominant polycystic kidney disease is an inherited disease of the collecting duct characterized by multiple large renal cysts, progressive renal insufficiency, and extrarenal manifestations including hepatic cysts and cerebral artery aneurysm. Treatment is supportive care.
- Autosomal recessive polycystic kidney disease is an inherited disease associated with cystic dilatation of the collecting ducts and characterized by large, hyperechogenic kidneys, hepatic fibrosis, renal insufficiency, respiratory distress, and hypertension. Treatment is supportive care.

10

SIMPLE RENAL CYST

GENERAL INFORMATION

- Present in 50% of people aged >50 years.
- Frequency increases with age.
- Characterized by a fluid-filled, epithelial-lined cavity in the renal parenchyma or on the surface of the kidney.
  - Bordered by a single layer of flattened cuboidal epithelial cells.
- May or may not communicate with the collecting system.
- May be multiple and bilateral.
- May be located near the renal pelvis (peripelvic or parapelvic).

PRESENTATION

- Usually asymptomatic (i.e. incidental finding on abdominal imaging performed for other reasons).
- However, simple renal cysts may also present with pain, hematuria, hypertension, and/or palpable flank mass.
- Infected simple renal cysts may present with fever, pain, and/or systemic signs of infection.

DIAGNOSIS

Ultrasonography

- Classic findings:
  - Absence of internal echoes
  - Well-defined thin smooth wall

- Spherical or ovoid shape
- Increased through-transmission with acoustic enhancement behind the cyst.
- If all of these characteristics are not present or cannot be reliably demonstrated, the cyst may be 'complex' and require further evaluation with abdominal computed tomography (CT) or magnetic resonance imaging (MRI).

Computed tomography

- Useful for evaluation of complex cysts.
- Diagnostic accuracy for a simple cyst close to 100%.
- CT criteria for a simple cyst are similar to those used in ultrasonography:
  - Well-defined thin smooth wall and margins
  - Spherical or ovoid shape
  - Homogeneous content [Hounsfield units (HU) ranging from -10 to $+20$] without enhancement after IV contrast.
- If the cyst fluid is hyperdense ($+20$ to $+90$ HU):
  - For a cyst <3 cm in size, if there is no enhancement it is probably a simple cyst
  - For a cyst >3 cm, even if there is no enhancement, close follow-up or biopsy should be considered.
- Note that at least 1–3% of simple cysts may be calcified.

Magnetic resonance imaging

- Offers little information beyond that available from ultrasound and CT.
  - Potentially more specific in identifying the nature of the cystic fluid.

Bosniak classification system

- Based on abdominal imaging.
- Type I: simple benign cyst as defined by ultrasound and CT criteria (see above); it measures as water density and does not enhance.
- Type II: benign cyst; may contain a few thin septa and/or fine calcifications; <3 cm high attenuation lesions that do not enhance.
- Type IIF: may contain additional septa and/or non-enhancing, thickened calcifications; may minimally enhance; ≥3 cm intrarenal non-enhancing lesions.
- Type III: indeterminate cystic masses; have thickened, irregular enhancing walls and/or septa.
- Type IV: malignant cystic lesions containing enhancing soft tissue elements.

TREATMENT

Bosniak type I or II

- Observation:
  - Recommended approach to asymptomatic patients.
- Percutaneous cyst aspiration, with or without infusion of sclerosing agents:
  - Consider for patients with pain/other symptoms
  - Long-term results are often suboptimal; cysts will frequently recur.
- Laparoscopic cyst decortication:
  - Effective treatment for patients with pain/other symptoms.

Bosniak type III

- Suspicious for malignancy.
- Consider vigilant follow-up vs cyst aspiration with renal biopsy vs surgical excision.

Bosniak type IV

- Assume cystic renal cell carcinoma.
- Treat as renal malignancy (see Chapter 13).

ACQUIRED RENAL CYSTIC DISEASE

10

GENERAL INFORMATION

- Occurs in patients with end-stage renal disease (ESRD).
- Often seen in patients on dialysis, but may occur in patients who are not on dialysis.
  - Appears to be a feature of ESRD rather than a response to dialysis.
- The incidence rises with:
  - Increased duration of ESRD
  - Increased time on dialysis.
- Characterized by bilateral small cysts (0.5–1 cm) located in the cortex and/or medulla.
- Cysts are usually filled with clear straw-colored or hemorrhagic fluid and contain calcium oxalate crystals.
- Prevalence is increased among Blacks and Japanese.
- Occurs in men more frequently than women (male:female ratio is 3:1).
- Cysts may regress after kidney transplantation.

ASSOCIATION WITH RENAL CELL CARCINOMA

- Acquired renal cystic disease is associated with an increased risk of renal cell carcinoma.
  - Estimated 50-fold increase in risk compared with the general population
  - Approximately 4–10% of patients with acquired renal cystic disease will develop renal cell carcinoma.
- The risk of renal cell carcinoma does not change after renal transplantation.

PRESENTATION

- Flank pain:
  - May be secondary to bleeding in or around the kidney, which occurs in up to 50% of patients.
- Hematuria.
- Infected cysts may present with fever, pain, and/or systemic signs of infection.

DIAGNOSIS

Ultrasound, computed tomography, or magnetic resonance imaging

- Characteristic findings:
  - Small hyperechoic kidneys
  - Numerous cysts of various sizes.

CYSTIC DISEASES OF THE KIDNEY

TREATMENT

- Asymptomatic:
  - Expectant management
  - Consider intermittent screening with abdominal imaging because of relatively high risk of renal cell carcinoma.
- Recalcitrant bleeding:
  - Selective embolization vs nephrectomy.
- Infected cyst:
  - Percutaneous or surgical drainage vs nephrectomy.

AUTOSOMAL DOMINANT POLYCYSTIC KIDNEY DISEASE (ADPKD)

GENERAL INFORMATION

- Usually presents after age 30 years.
- Inherited (autosomal dominant) disease of the collecting duct, characterized by multiple large renal cysts and a number of associated anomalies (namely cysts in other organs).
- Incidence is 1 per 500 to 1 per 1000 births.
- There is *no* increased risk of renal cell carcinoma with ADPKD compared with the general population.
- It is an important cause of renal insufficiency.
  - Present in approximately 15% of patients on hemodialysis in the United States
  - Most patients with ADPKD will eventually progress to renal failure.

ETIOLOGY

- There are several theories:
  - Tubular epithelial hyperplasia causing obstruction and weakening of the basement membrane
  - Abnormal, apical placement of Na-K-ATPase in cyst epithelia causing fluid to enter the cyst rather than leave it
  - Defect in the tubular basement membrane
  - Defect in one of the proteins of the supportive extracellular connective tissue matrix.

PATHOLOGY

- Macrosopic:
  - Diffuse cysts, ranging in size from several millimeters to several centimeters, located throughout the cortex and medulla.
- Microscopic:
  - Focal tubular dilatation
  - Epithelial hyperplasia or adenoma formation in the cyst wall
  - Apoptosis in the epithelial lining of the cysts
  - Arteriosclerosis and interstitial fibrosis in advanced renal stage disease.

GENETICS

- Three genes have been identified:
  - PKD1 (90% of cases)

- PKD2 (5–10% of cases)
- PKD3 (a small percentage of patients who have been found to have neither a PKD1 nor a PKD2 gene defect)
- Families with PKD1 and PKD2 have the same major manifestations; those with PKD2 usually have later onset of symptoms and slower progression to renal insufficiency.
- Penetrance is 100%.

PRESENTATION

- Screening with ultrasonography in asymptomatic individuals with a positive family history allows for detection in up to 85% of cases.
- Typically, symptoms occur between ages 30 and 50 years.
  - May rarely present at younger ages.
- Hematuria (microscopic and macroscopic):
  - Occurs in up to 50% of patients
  - Is the presenting symptom in 19–35% of patients.
- Hypertension:
  - Renin-mediated.
- Urinary stones:
  - May occur in 20–30% of patients.
- Renal infections:
  - Occur more commonly in women than men
  - May occur in cysts or as renal parenchymal infections.
- Extrarenal manifestations:
  - Hepatic cysts
  - Congenital hepatic fibrosis with portal hypertension
  - Cerebral artery (Berry) aneurysm (10–40%)
  - Colonic diverticula
  - Mitral valve prolapse.

DIAGNOSIS

- Typically made through combination of positive family history and imaging showing characteristic renal cysts and extrarenal manifestations.
- When there is no positive family history, a presumptive diagnosis can be made from abdominal imaging if bilateral renal cysts are present with 2 or more of the following:
  - Bilateral renal enlargement
  - >3 hepatic cysts
  - Cerebral artery aneurysm
  - Solitary cyst of the arachnoid, pineal gland, pancreas, or spleen.

TREATMENT

- There is no cure for ADPKD.
- Treatment is primarily supportive and should be directed toward management of symptoms and renal failure.
- For treatment of pyelonephritis and/or infected renal cyst, note that lipid-soluble antibiotics (chloramphenicol, fluoroquinolone, trimethoprim–sulfamethoxazole) are more effective for cyst penetration.

10

CYSTIC DISEASES OF THE KIDNEY

- For treatment of cyst-related pain, consider laparoscopic cyst decortication:
  - 80% will be pain-free at 1 year
  - 62% will be pain-free at 2 years.
- For treatment of cyst-related pain, percutaneous aspiration with or without installation of a sclerosing agent may be performed, but is less effective, and recurrence is frequent.

AUTOSOMAL RECESSIVE POLYCYSTIC KIDNEY DISEASE (ARPKD)

GENERAL INFORMATION

- Inherited (autosomal recessive) disease characterized by cystic dilatation of the collecting ducts.
  - Possibly caused by a gene located on chromosome 6.
- Typically diagnosed in neonates; may also be diagnosed in adolescents and young adults.
- Rare:
  - Occurs in 1:5000 to 1:40 000 live births.
- 50% of affected newborns will die within the first few hours of life.
  - Of those that survive the neonatal period, 50% are alive at 10 years of age.

PATHOLOGY

Kidney

- Kidneys retain fetal lobulations.
- Small cysts typically occur throughout the kidney with no normal renal parenchyma.
  - In older children, cysts may be larger and similar to those seen in ADPKD.
- The renal vessels, renal pelvis, and ureter typically appear normal.

Liver

- Severity of hepatic involvement typically increases with age.
- No cysts, but varying degrees of congenital hepatic fibrosis characterized by biliary ectasia and periportal fibrosis.

PRESENTATION

- Respiratory distress (neonates):
  - Due to pulmonary hypoplasia.
- Potter's facies with limb deformities (neonates):
  - Due to oligohydramnios.
- Renal insufficiency:
  - At birth, blood urea nitrogen (BUN) and creatinine may be normal, but will start rising after 48 hours.
- Hypertension.
- Congenital hepatic fibrosis:
  - Older patients may have portal hypertension, esophageal varices, and hepatosplenomegaly.

IMAGING CHARACTERISTICS

Ultrasound

- In utero:
  - Oligohydramnios
  - Empty bladder
  - Large hyperechogenic kidneys.
- In the newborn:
  - Large hyperechogenic kidneys
  - Larger renal cysts are rare in the newborn but may be present in older children.
- With progression of renal failure the kidneys become smaller (in contrast to ADPKD, in which the kidneys remain large).

Intravenous urography

- Calyces, renal pelvis and ureter are usually not visible.
- Delayed films may show characteristic radial or medullary streaking (sunburst pattern) caused by dilated collecting tubules filled with contrast medium.
- Transient nephromegaly mimicking ADPKD in newborns is possible and should be considered. Family history and liver biopsy may help clarify the diagnosis.

TREATMENT

- There is no cure for ARPKD.
- Treatment consists of supportive measures; genetic evaluation and family counseling arc necessary.

10

CYSTIC DISEASES OF THE KIDNEY

FURTHER READING

Bono AV, Lovisolo JA: Renal cell carcinoma – diagnosis and treatment: state of the art. Eur Urol 31 (Suppl 1):47, 1997.

Bosniak MA: The use of the Bosniak classification system for renal cysts and cystic tumors. J Urol 157:1852, 1997.

Dalton D, Neiman J, Grayhack JT: The natural history of simple renal cysts: a preliminary study. J Urol 135:905, 1986.

Glassberg KI: Renal dysgenesis and cystic disease of the kidney. In: Walsh PC, Vaughan ED Jr, Wein AJ, Retik AB, eds. Campbell's Urology, 8th edn. Philadelphia: WB Saunders, 2002, p 1925.

Heidenreich A, Ravery V: European Society of Oncological Urology. Preoperative imaging in renal cell cancer. World J Urol 22:307, 2004.

Hughson MD, Buckwald D, Fox M: Renal neoplasia and acquired cystic kidney disease in patients receiving long-term dialysis. Arch Pathol Lab Med 110:592, 1986.

Kuroda N, Toi M, Hiroi M et al: Review of renal oncocytoma with focus on clinical and pathobiological aspects. Histol Histopathol 18:935, 2003.

Lepor H, Walsh PW: Idiopathic retroperitoneal fibrosis. J Urol 122:1, 1979.

Levine E, Hartman DS, Mellstrup JW et al: Current concepts and controversies in imaging of renal cystic disease. Urol Clin North Am 24:523, 1997.

Nelson CP, Sanda MG: Contemporary diagnosis and management of renal angiomyolipoma. J Urol 168:1315, 2002.

Novick AC, Campbell SC: Renal tumors. In: Walsh PC, Vaughan ED Jr, Wein AJ, Retik AB, eds. Campbell's Urology, 8th edn. Philadelphia: WB Saunders, 2002, p 2672.

Roy S, Dillon MJ, Tropeter RS et al: Autosomal recessive polycystic kidney: long-term outcome of neonatal survivors. Pediatr Nephrol 11:302, 1997.

Schatz SM, Lieber MM: Update on oncocytoma. Curr Urol Rep 4:30, 2003.

Streem SB, Franke JJ, Smith JA. Path physiology of urinary tract obstruction. In: Walsh PC, Vaughan ED Jr, Wein AJ, Retik AB, eds. Campbell's Urology, 8th edn. Philadelphia: WB Saunders, 2002, p 506.

Truong LD, Choi YJ, Shen SS et al: Renal cystic neoplasms and renal neoplasms associated with cystic renal diseases: pathogenetic and molecular links. Adv Anat Pathol 10:135, 2003.

Varkarakis IM, Jarrett TW: Retroperitoneal fibrosis. AUA Update Series 24:18, 2005.

Wilson PD: Polycystic kidney disease. New Engl J Med 350:151, 2004.

Wilson PD: Polycystic kidney disease: new understanding in the pathogenesis. Int J Biochem Cell Biol 36:1868, 2004.

Zerres K, Rudnik-Schoneborn S, Steinkamn C et al: Autosomal recessive polycystic kidney disease. J Mol Med 76:303, 1998.

Angiomyolipoma, oncocytoma, and retroperitoneal fibrosis

Ioannis M Varkarakis

SUMMARY

- Angiomyolipoma is a benign lesion of the kidney characterized by proliferation of blood vessels, adipose tissue, and smooth muscle. It is associated with tuberous sclerosis. Most contain fat. If asymptomatic and <4 cm, treatment is observation. If symptomatic and/or ≥4 cm, treatment is selective embolization or surgery.
- Oncocytoma is a benign lesion of the kidney that represents 3–7% of all renal tumors. On computed tomography (CT) or magnetic resonance imaging (MRI), it has a characteristic central stellate scar. Since it cannot be definitively diagnosed with abdominal imaging, and since it often coexists with renal cell carcinoma, treatment is surgery.
- Retroperitoneal fibrosis is a rare fibrotic disease of the retroperitoneum that encircles and encases retroperitoneal structures. It may be idiopathic or occur secondary to inflammation, malignancy, radiation, abdominal aortic aneurysm, or medications. Initial treatment includes relief of urinary obstruction and biopsy. Subsequent treatment options include corticosteroids, tamoxifen, and ureterolysis.

ANGIOMYOLIPOMA

GENERAL INFORMATION

- Angiomyolipoma (AML) is a benign, neoplastic lesion of the kidney characterized by proliferation of blood vessels, adipose tissue, and smooth muscle.
- Represents <0.3% of renal tumors.
- Associated with tuberous sclerosis, an inherited, autosomal dominant disorder characterized by mental retardation, epilepsy, adenoma sebaceum, and multiorgan hamartomas.
  - 20% of all AMLs occur in patients with tuberous sclerosis
  - >50% of patients with tuberous sclerosis have AMLs
  - AMLs in patients with tuberous sclerosis are often bilateral, multicentric, and symptomatic
  - Female to male ratio is 2:1.
- Sporadic AML (i.e. individuals without tuberous sclerosis):
  - More commonly occur in middle-aged women
  - Occur more frequently on right (80%) compared with left (20%)
  - Usually single and of larger size.

PATHOLOGY

Macroscopic appearance

- Yellowish gray.
- No capsule.
- No necrosis.
- May have areas of gross hemorrhage.

Microscopic appearance

- Increased quantity of blood vessels, adipose tissue, and smooth muscle elements.
- Positive immunoreactivity for HMB-45:
  - Characteristic for AML
  - Positive reaction rules out sarcoma.

PRESENTATION

- Incidental finding on abdominal imaging in an asymptomatic individual.
- Spontaneous bleed:
  - Occurs in approximately 10% of tumors
  - May be associated with a significant retroperitoneal hematoma with associated flank pain, hematuria, palpable mass, and hypovolemic shock
  - Risk of spontaneous bleeding depends upon size: <4 cm = 13% risk; ≥4 cm = 51% risk
  - Pregnancy is associated with increased risk for bleeding.
- Other symptoms:
  - <4 cm 23% with symptoms, >4 cm 82% with symptoms
  - Pain
  - Anemia
  - Hypertension.

DIAGNOSIS

Ultrasonography

- A well-circumscribed, highly echogenic lesion, often associated with acoustic shadowing.
- Fat may be present.

Computed tomography

- *The presence of even a small amount of fat (HU <10) in the tumor makes the diagnosis of AML.*
  - However, 14% of AMLs do not contain fat.
- AML never has calcifications.

Angiography

- Hypervascular tumors with aneurysmal dilatation.
- Not necessary for diagnosis.

TREATMENT

Observation

- Appropriate for asymptomatic tumors <4 cm with classic radiological features of AML.
- Follow-up imaging every 6–12 months to evaluate growth rate.

Ablative therapy

- Appropriate for tumors that are symptomatic, ≥4 cm, or do not have classic radiological features consistent with AML.
- Options:
  - Selective embolization
  - Partial nephrectomy
  - Radical nephrectomy.

ONCOCYTOMA

GENERAL INFORMATION

- A benign tumor derived from distal tubules.
  - There are very rare reports of malignant/metastatic oncocytomas.
- Constitutes 3–7% of renal tumors.
- Male to female ratio is 2:1.
- Generally presents during the 4th to 6th decades.
- Tends to be asymptomatic.
- Affects left and right kidneys equally.
- Bilateral, multicentric, and metachronous tumors reported in 6–13% of cases.
- Multifocal oncocytomas are sometimes called 'oncocytomatosis.'
- Often coexists with renal cell carcinoma.
- Genetics:
  - May be associated with loss of chromosome 1p and Y, loss of heterozygosity at 14q, or rearrangements at 11q13.

PATHOLOGY

Macroscopic

- Light brown or tan in appearance.
- Well circumscribed with a well-defined capsule.
- Large tumors may have a pathognomonic, central stellate scar.
- Typically not associated with necrosis or hemorrhage.

Microscopic

- Composed of uniform round or polygonal eosinophilic cells, arranged in an organoid, tubulocystic, solid, or mixed growth pattern.
- Many intracellular mitochondria are responsible for characteristic staining properties.
- Some oncocytomas present atypical features such as nuclear atypia, prominent nucleoli, hemorrhage, extension in perinephric fat, and aneuploidy.

ANGIOMYOLIPOMA, ONCOCYTOMA, AND RETROPERITONEAL FIBROSIS

11

EVALUATION

Radiological appearance

- CT:
  - Central stellate scar.
- Angiography:
  - Spoke-wheel pattern of feeding arteries
  - Lucent rim sign.
- MRI:
  - Well-defined capsule
  - Central stellate scar
  - Distinctive intensities on T1 and T2 images.

Renal biopsy

- Limited value because oncocytoma may occur in association with renal cell carcinoma in 7–32% of cases.
- Also may be difficult to distinguish oncocytoma from renal cell carcinoma.

TREATMENT

- Because it cannot be definitively distinguished from renal cell carcinoma with current imaging modalities, and because it may be associated with renal cell carcinoma, treatment recommendations are the same as those for renal cell carcinoma (see Chapter 14).

FOLLOW-UP

- Since oncocytoma is generally a benign tumor, follow-up need not be as intensive as for renal cell carcinoma.
- Consider closer follow-up for large or multifocal tumors, or if renal sparing surgery is performed.

RETROPERITONEAL FIBROSIS (RF)

GENERAL INFORMATION

- A rare fibrotic disease of the retroperitoneum that encircles and encases retroperitoneal structures.
- Usually starts at the level of the 4th–5th lumbar vertebrae. May envelope the aorta and inferior vena cava (IVC).
- May extend from the aortic bifurcation superiorly to the renal arteries and laterally beyond the outer edge of the psoas muscle to envelope the ureters.
  - In 15% of cases, the fibrosis extends outside the retroperitoneum
  - Fibrosis typically surrounds the aorta first and then extends around the ureters, which are often the first organs to be functionally compromised.
- The idiopathic form is also known as 'Ormond's disease' or 'fibrous retroperitonitis.'
- Presents most commonly in the 5th to 6th decades.
- It is 2–3 times more common in men than women.

ETIOLOGY

- Idiopathic (70%).
- Secondary (30%):
  - Any retroperitoneal inflammatory process (i.e. urinoma, hematoma, abscess)
  - Malignancy (lymphoma is the most common)
  - Postoperative
  - Post radiotherapy
  - Aortic aneurysm
  - Chemicals, including asbestos and talcum powder
  - Medications, including β-blockers, LSD, methysergide, methyldopa, hydralazine, and pergolide.

PATHOLOGY

- Macroscopic:
  - Dense, hard mass with a woody consistency.
- Microscopic:
  - Areas of collagen with distinct areas of non-specific chronic inflammation.

PRESENTATION

- Depends upon the retroperitoneal organs that are functionally affected.
- May present as non-specific systemic complaints: malaise, anorexia, weight loss, moderate pyrexia, nausea/vomiting.
- Symptoms consistent with ureteral obstruction, such as flank pain.
- Lower extremity edema secondary to IVC compression.
- Hypertension, intestinal ischemia, and claudication secondary to compression of the renal, iliac, and mesenteric arteries, respectively.

DIAGNOSIS

Physical exam

- Unrevealing most of the time.

Ultrasonography

- Hydronephrosis.
- Hypoechoic periaortic mass.

Computed tomography of abdomen with urogram

- Unilateral or bilateral hydronephrosis.
- Proximal ureteral dilatation (middle and distal ureter spared).
- Medial ureteral deviation (at the level of L4–5).
- Extrinsic compression of urinary system with lack of intrinsic obstruction.
- Fibrotic retroperitoneal plaque.

Magnetic resonance imaging of the abdomen and pelvis

- Similar findings to CT.
- Useful in patients with renal insufficiency.

Retrograde or antegrade pyelography

- Rarely used.

Labs

- Non-specific.
- Erythrocyte sedimentation rate (ESR) is usually elevated.

TREATMENT

General

- Preservation of renal function with:
  - Percutaneous nephrostomy tubes or
  - Ureteral catheters (characteristically advanced without resistance).
- Discontinuation of offending medications or chemicals.
- CT-guided percutaneous biopsy to evaluate for malignancy.
- Spontaneous resolution has been reported but is rare.

Medical management

- May consider as primary therapy in all patients after exclusion of malignancy.
  - While there are no large clinical trials, numerous case reports support efficacy of corticosteroids.
- Also appropriate for patients who are high-risk surgical candidates.
- May also consider as adjuvant therapy for surgery.
- **Corticosteroids**:
  - 20–60 mg of prednisolone on alternate days for 6–8 weeks, then taper down over several weeks.
- **Immunosuppressants**:
  - Should be avoided in elderly and uremic patients
  - May be used alone or in combination with glucocorticoids
  - Include azathioprine, cyclophosphamide, penicillamine, and mycophenolate mofetil.
- **Tamoxifen:**
  - Reported in combination with corticosteroids or alone after corticosteroids fail
  - Data on effectiveness are scant.

Ureterolysis

- May be performed via open or laparoscopic approaches.
- Laparoscopic procedures more challenging but associated with less morbidity.
- Technical aspects:
  - Dissection should begin at the distal, non-dilated ureter
  - Even if the disease involves one ureter, treatment of both ureters should be considered
  - Once the ureters are freed, they may be intraperitonealized or wrapped in omentum or laterally placed with retroperitoneal fat interposed between the ureters and the fibrosis

- Ureteral stents are removed after the obstruction has resolved (usually within 6–8 weeks).
- Long-term follow up is necessary as late recurrence can occur.
- Potential complications:
  - Ureteral injury
  - Urine leak
  - Late intestinal obstruction.

Other procedures

- Repair of any associated aortic aneurysms.
- Excision of the involved ureteral segment with reanastomosis.
  - Boari flap if lower 1/3 is involved.
- Renal autotransplantation.
- Uretral replacement with ileum or appendix.
- Nephrectomy.

11

FURTHER READING

Bono AV, Lovisolo JA: Renal cell carcinoma – diagnosis and treatment: state of the art. Eur Urol 31 (Suppl 1):47, 1997.

Bosniak MA: The use of the Bosniak classification system for renal cysts and cystic tumors. J Urol 157:1852, 1997.

Dalton D, Neiman J, Grayhack JT: The natural history of simple renal cysts: a preliminary study. J Urol 135:905, 1986.

Glassberg KI: Renal dysgenesis and cystic disease of the kidney. In: Walsh PC, Vaughan ED Jr, Wein AJ, Retik AB, eds. Campbell's Urology, 8th edn. Philadelphia: WB Saunders, 2002, p 1925.

Heidenreich A, Ravery V: European Society of Oncological Urology. Preoperative imaging in renal cell cancer. World J Urol 22:307, 2004.

Hughson MD, Buckwald D, Fox M: Renal neoplasia and acquired cystic kidney disease in patients receiving long-term dialysis. Arch Pathol Lab Med 110:592, 1986.

Kuroda N, Toi M, Hiroi M et al: Review of renal oncocytoma with focus on clinical and pathobiological aspects. Histol Histopathol 18:935, 2003.

Lepor H, Walsh PW: Idiopathic retroperitoneal fibrosis. J Urol 122:1, 1979.

Levine E, Hartman DS, Mellstrup JW et al: Current concepts and controversies in imaging of renal cystic disease. Urol Clin North Am 24:523, 1997.

Nelson CP, Sanda MG: Contemporary diagnosis and management of renal angiomyolipoma. J Urol 168:1315, 2002.

Novick AC, Campbell SC: Renal tumors. In: Walsh PC, Vaughan ED Jr, Wein AJ, Retik AB, eds. Campbell's Urology, 8th edn. Philadelphia: WB Saunders, 2002, p 2672.

Roy S, Dillon MJ, Tropeter RS et al: Autosomal recessive polycystic kidney: long-term outcome of neonatal survivors. Pediatr Nephrol 11:302, 1997.

Schatz SM, Lieber MM: Update on oncocytoma. Curr Urol Rep 4:30, 2003.

Streem SB, Franke JJ, Smith JA. Path physiology of urinary tract obstruction. In: Walsh PC, Vaughan ED Jr, Wein AJ, Retik AB, eds. Campbell's Urology, 8th edn. Philadelphia: WB Saunders, 2002, p 506.

Truong LD, Choi YJ, Shen SS et al: Renal cystic neoplasms and renal neoplasms associated with cystic renal diseases: pathogenetic and molecular links. Adv Anat Pathol 10:135, 2003.

Varkarakis IM, Jarrett TW: Retroperitoneal fibrosis. AUA Update Series 24:18, 2005.

Wilson PD: Polycystic kidney disease. New Engl J Med 350:151, 2004.

Wilson PD: Polycystic kidney disease: new understanding in the pathogenesis. Int J Biochem Cell Biol 36:1868, 2004.

Zerres K, Rudnik-Schoneborn S, Steinkamn C et al: Autosomal recessive polycystic kidney disease. J Mol Med 76:303, 1998.

ANGIOMYOLIPOMA, ONCOCYTOMA, AND RETROPERITONEAL FIBROSIS

Prostate cancer: localized

Misop Han and J Kellogg Parsons

SUMMARY

- Prostate cancer is the most common non-skin cancer and the second leading cause of cancer mortality in US men.
- Screening involves digital rectal examination (DRE) and serum prostate-specific antigen (PSA) testing.
- Diagnosis of prostate cancer is made from transrectal ultrasound-guided prostate needle biopsy.
- Staging (TNM) and grading (Gleason score) information is directly associated with prognosis.
- Treatment for clinically localized prostate cancer should be individualized, based on the aggressiveness of the tumor, patient life expectancy, and patient preference.
- Definitive, curative therapy should be considered in men with localized prostate cancer and greater than 10 years of life expectancy.
- Treatments for localized prostate cancer include expectant management, radical prostatectomy, radiation, and cryosurgery.

GENERAL INFORMATION

EPIDEMIOLOGY

- The most common visceral cancer in US men (~232 000 cases in 2005).[1]
- The second leading cause of cancer death in US men (~30 000 deaths in 2005).[1]
- The prevalence of prostate cancer increases with age:[1]
  - Autopsy study (from 1 in 4 men in the 4th and 5th decades to 3 in 4 in the 9th decade)[2-4]
  - 1 in 6 of men are diagnosed with prostate cancer during their lifetime.[1]
- Marked disparity between prevalence and incidence rates.
- Marked variability exists in the natural history of prostate cancer.
- Widespread screening using DRE and serum PSA began in the 1980s.[5,6]
  - Substantial stage migration has occurred as a result
  - The incidence of local-regional disease has substantially increased, while the incidence of metastatic disease has substantially decreased.[1,7]
- A significant decrease in prostate cancer-specific mortality is at least partly due to aggressive screening and effective treatment in the past two decades.

PROSTATE-SPECIFIC ANTIGEN

- PSA is a serine protease, produced by prostatic epithelium and periurethral glands, that liquefies seminal coagulum.[8]
- Serum PSA level may be elevated in prostatitis, benign prostatic hyperplasia, or prostate cancer.[9]
- The risk of prostate cancer increases as serum PSA level increases.[10-13]

- PSA expression is strongly influenced by androgens.
  - Decreased androgens are associated with decreased PSA.
- PSA levels will decrease with use of 5α-reductase inhibitors (i.e. finasteride and dutasteride) by ~50%.
- There are three major types of PSA assays: total PSA, free PSA, and complexed PSA.
- Total PSA is the most common assay and is usually referred to simply as PSA.
  - Total PSA equals the sum of free PSA (~10–30%) and complexed PSA (~70–90%) present in serum.
- Free PSA:
  - An isoform of PSA that is not bound to serum proteins
  - Percent free PSA = (free PSA/total PSA) × 100
  - Percent free PSA is more specific for prostate cancer detection than total PSA
  - Lower percent free PSA is associated with an increased probability of prostate cancer (Table 12.1).
- Complexed PSA:
  - An isoform of PSA that is bound to serum proteins, primarily the protease inhibitor α_1-antichymotrypsin[14–16]
  - Is more specific for prostate cancer detection than total PSA and as specific as percent free PSA
  - Higher complexed PSA is associated with an increased probability of prostate cancer.
- PSA velocity:
  - The change in PSA concentration per unit time
  - In screening populations, PSA velocity >0.75 ng/ml/year is associated with an increased risk of prostate cancer
  - In men diagnosed with prostate cancer, PSA velocity >2.0 ng/ml/year is associated with an increased risk for prostate cancer-specific mortality following surgery (10-fold) or external beam radiation (12-fold).[18,19]

TABLE 12.1

PROBABILITY OF PROSTATE CANCER ON PROSTATE NEEDLE BIOPSY* BY PERCENT FREE PSA (fPSA) FOR TOTAL PSA OF 4–10 NG/ML

Percent fPSA (%)	Probability of prostate cancer (%)
0–10	56
10–15	28
15–20	20
20–25	16
>25	8

*Based on sextant (6-core) biopsy.[17]

DIAGNOSIS

PROSTATE-SPECIFIC ANTIGEN AND PROSTATE CANCER SCREENING

- A highly controversial issue.
- Recommendations for screening vary widely.
  - Annual screening generally recommended beginning at age 40–45 years for African-Americans or those with a positive family history and beginning at age 50 years for all others
  - No consensus as to when to stop screening.
- Traditional cut-off for performing biopsy is ≥4.0 ng/ml.
- Recent data also suggest considering biopsy in men:
  - With PSA of 2.6–4.0 ng/ml
  - With PSA velocity >0.75 ng/ml/year over a period of at least 18 months.

PROSTATE BIOPSY

- Primary test for diagnosing prostate cancer.
- It is performed based on:
  - Abnormal PSA parameters (see above)
  - And/or abnormal DRE.
- Transrectal ultrasound (TRUS)-guided is the most common method.
  - Performed with local anesthesia and periprocedural oral antibiotics.
- Typically 8–12 cores are taken, emphasizing sampling of the lateral peripheral zone.
- Potential complications include urinary infection, hematuria, rectal bleeding, urinary retention, and vasovagal reaction.

PROSTATE BIOPSY PATHOLOGY

Gleason score

- Also called the Gleason sum.
- The most common method for grading prostate cancer.
- The system assigns a score from 1 to 5 for each area of cancer based upon the histopathological pattern of the tumor.
- The Gleason score is the sum of two numbers: (1) the most prevalent Gleason pattern and (2) the second most prevalent pattern present in the biopsy.
  - For example, for a biopsy containing a large tumor area of pattern 4 and a smaller area of pattern 3, the Gleason score is 4 + 3 = 7
  - If the tumor in the specimen contains only one type of pattern, the pattern number is doubled. Thus, the Gleason score of a tumor containing only a Gleason 4 pattern is 4 + 4 = 8.
- Classification:
  - 2–4: Well differentiated
  - 5–6: Moderately differentiated
  - 7: Moderately to poorly differentiated
  - 8–10: Poorly differentiated.

High-grade prostatic intraepithelial neoplasia (HG-PIN)

- A putative precursor lesion of prostate cancer.
- Has been associated with a higher risk of prostate cancer detection in subsequent biopsies.
- Immediate or delayed repeat biopsy is not mandatory, but may be considered.[20]

Atypical small acinar proliferation (ASAP)

- An atypical focus is not a distinct premalignant lesion, but is a suspicious finding associated with an increased risk of cancer on subsequent biopsy.[21]
- Immediate (within 3 months) re-biopsy with increased sampling of the area around atypical focus is indicated.[20]

EVALUATION AND STAGING

CLINICAL STAGING (TNM SYSTEM)

- Based on clinical presentation and DRE.
- Staging work-up for T1 and T2:[20]
  - No further staging required for the majority of these cancers
  - Bone scan if PSA >20 ng/ml or Gleason score ≥8
  - Pelvic CT or MRI if staging nomogram (see below) indicates >20% probability of lymph node involvement or other intraabdominal/pelvic malignancy is suspected.
- Staging work-up for T3 and T4:[20]
  - Bone scan
  - Pelvic CT or MRI.

STAGING NOMOGRAMS

- Include the Partin Tables.
- Useful for guiding treatment.[22,23]
- They utilize parameters obtained at the time of diagnosis (serum PSA level, clinical stage, and biopsy Gleason score) to predict pathological stage.
  - Information regarding pathological stage allows informed decision-making regarding appropriate treatment options.

TREATMENT

Treatment should be individualized based on the aggressiveness of the tumor, patient life expectancy, and patient preference.

EXPECTANT MANAGEMENT

- Strategy is to monitor patients with low-risk disease and intervene with intent to cure if there is evidence of cancer progression.
- There are no formal criteria for patient selection.
  - However, low-grade (Gleason sum <7) and low-volume (<3 biopsy cores positive for cancer and <50% cancer in any one core) cancers are desirable.[24,25]
- Clinical feasibility has been demonstrated in carefully selected patients.[24,25]

- Principles include:
  - PSA and DRE every 6 months
  - Repeat biopsy within 6–18 months of initial diagnosis
  - Repeat biopsy if evidence of progression on exam or serum markers.

RADICAL PROSTATECTOMY

- The first treatment available for prostate cancer.[26,27]
- Reduces local progression, distant metastasis development, and cancer-specific and overall mortality rates compared with watchful waiting.[28]
- Major long-term complications include urinary incontinence, erectile dysfunction, and bladder neck contracture (anastomotic stricture).
  - Bladder neck contracture increases the risk of urinary incontinence.
- Surgical approaches to radical prostatectomy include retropubic, perineal, and laparoscopic (with or without robot assistance).
- Outcomes: 15-year estimates (from the Johns Hopkins retropubic prostatectomy series):[29]
  - PSA-free survival: 66%
  - Metastasis-free survival: 82%
  - Cancer-specific survival: 91%.
- Control outcomes are similar for perineal prostatectomy. Laparoscopic outcomes are not yet mature, but results are likely comparable.

EXTERNAL BEAM RADIATION THERAPY

- Technique:
  - The use of gamma radiation (usually photons) directed at the prostate and surrounding tissue through multiple fields
  - Three-dimensional conformal radiotherapy (3D-CRT) was developed to minimize radiation injury to the bladder and the rectum and to focus the radiation dose to the prostate
  - Intensity-modulated radiation therapy (IMRT) can provide localization of the radiation dose to geometrically complex fields
  - Dose escalation and 3D-CRT improve the treatment results
  - Currently used dosage is 76–80 Gy.
- Direct survival comparisons between surgery and radiation are difficult because definitions for treatment success and failure are different for each treatment.
- Neoadjuvant hormonal therapy and/or combined brachytherapy may be used in high-risk patients.
- Potential complications:
  - Radiation proctitis and/or cystitis
  - Hemorrhagic cystitis
  - Erectile dysfunction, usually delayed (≥ 1 year after therapy)
  - Urinary retention.
- PSA level gradually decreases for up to 2–3 years after radiotherapy.
- PSA 'bounce:'
  - A transient PSA elevation occurring during the first 2 years following radiotherapy

PROSTATE CANCER: LOCALIZED

12

20. NCCN Clinical Practice Guidelines in Oncology. www.NCCN.org. 2005.
21. Chan TY, Epstein JI: Follow-up of atypical prostate needle biopsies suspicious for cancer. Urology 53:351, 1999.
22. Partin AW, Kattan MW, Subong EN et al: Combination of prostate-specific antigen, clinical stage, and Gleason score to predict pathological stage of localized prostate cancer. A multi-institutional update [see comments]. JAMA 277:1445, 1997. [Published erratum appears in JAMA 278(2):118, 1997.]
23. Partin AW, Mangold LA, Lamm DM et al: Contemporary update of prostate cancer staging nomograms (Partin Tables) for the new millennium. Urology 58:843, 2001.
24. Khan MA, Carter HB, Epstein JI et al: Can prostate specific antigen derivatives and pathological parameters predict significant change in expectant management criteria for prostate cancer? J Urol 170:2274, 2003.
25. Carter HB, Walsh PC, Landis P et al: Expectant management of nonpalpable prostate cancer with curative intent: preliminary results. J Urol 167:1231, 2002.
26. Kuchler H: Uber prostatavergrossgrugen. Deutsch Klin 18:458, 1866.
27. Young HH: The early diagnosis and radical cure of carcinoma of the prostate. Johns Hopkins Hosp Bull 16:315, 1905.
28. Bill-Axelson A, Holmberg L, Ruutu M et al: Radical prostatectomy versus watchful waiting in early prostate cancer. New Engl J Med 352:1977, 2005.
29. Han M, Partin AW, Pound CR et al: Long-term biochemical disease-free and cancer-specific survival following anatomic radical retropubic prostatectomy. The 15-year Johns Hopkins experience. Urol Clin North Am 28:555, 2001.
30. Onik G: Image-guided prostate cryosurgery: state of the art. Cancer Control 8:522, 2001.
31. Cytron S, Paz A, Kravchick S et al: Active rectal wall protection using direct transperineal cryo-needles for histologically proven prostate adenocarcinomas. Eur Urol 44:315, 2003.
32. Chang Z, Finkelstein JJ, Ma H et al: Development of a high-performance multiprobe cryosurgical device. Biomed Instrum Technol 28:383, 1994.
33. Long JP, Bahn D, Lee F et al: Five-year retrospective, multi-institutional pooled analysis of cancer-related outcomes after cryosurgical ablation of the prostate. Urology 57:518, 2001.
34. Shariat SF, Raptidis G, Masatoschi M et al: Pilot study of radiofrequency interstitial tumor ablation (RITA) for the treatment of radio-recurrent prostate cancer. Prostate 65:260, 2005.
35. Beerlage HP, Thuroff S, Madersbacher S et al: Current status of minimally invasive treatment options for localized prostate carcinoma. Eur Urol 37:2, 2000.
36. Chapelon JY, Ribault M, Vernier F et al: Treatment of localised prostate cancer with transrectal high intensity focused ultrasound. Eur J Ultrasound 9:31, 1999.

Prostate cancer: metastatic

Ganesh S Palapattu

SUMMARY

- Prostate cancer cells metastasize primarily via the lymphatic system.
- The most common sites are pelvic lymph nodes, bone, lung, and liver.
- In the prostate-specific antigen (PSA) era, metastatic prostate cancer most commonly occurs following progression after primary treatment for localized disease.
- Biochemical recurrence is defined as the presence of a rising PSA level following primary therapy with surgery or radiation. Biochemical recurrence may occur years before the onset of clinical metastatic disease.
- The mainstay of treatment for men with metastatic prostate cancer is androgen deprivation.
- The quickest method to achieve castrate levels of circulating testosterone is orchiectomy.
- Androgen-independent (hormone refractory) prostate cancer is defined as clinical and/or PSA progression that occurs despite androgen deprivation therapy.
- The median time to death following the documentation of androgen-independent disease is 12–16 months.

13

DEFINITION AND PRESENTATION

DEFINITION

- Metastatic prostate cancer is defined as prostate cancer found outside of the prostate and/or prostatic region.
- Prostate cancer most commonly metastasizes via the lymphatic system.
- The most common sites of metastasis, from most to least, are pelvic lymph nodes, bone, lung, and liver.
- It is sometimes referred to as stage D disease based on the Whitmore–Jewett staging system.
- Some men initially present with metastatic disease. However, in the PSA screening era, metastatic disease more frequently occurs following progression after primary treatment for localized disease.

PRESENTATION

- Rising PSA.
  - Poorly differentiated metastases may not produce PSA.[1,2]
- Bone pain and/or fractures.
  - Bone metastases affect over 80% of patients with advanced prostate cancer
  - Bone lesions are typically osteoblastic. Bone scintigraphy with Tc-99m MDP (methylene diphosphonate) radiotracer is highly sensitive, but not very specific, for diagnosis.

- Pelvic and/or lower extremity neurological symptoms secondary to spinal cord compression.
- Urinary tract obstruction.

BIOCHEMICAL RECURRENCE

GENERAL PRINCIPLES

- Definitive treatment of localized prostate cancer should result in either undetectable (after surgery) or very low (after radiation) serum PSA concentrations.
- When serum PSA begins to rise after treatment with surgery or radiation, this is termed biochemical recurrence (also termed PSA-only recurrence, biochemical failure, or PSA failure).
- In some modern series with early data, PSA-free survival appears to be similar between select men with localized disease treated with surgery or radiation.[3]
- After surgery, biochemical recurrence is usually defined as serum PSA ≥0.2 ng/ml on two successive measures or a single measure ≥0.4 ng/ml.
  - Approximately one-quarter to one-half of all men will experience biochemical recurrence within the first 10 years after surgery[4,5]
  - Almost three-quarters of those men who do develop it will do so within the first 2 years[6]
  - After surgery, the median time to onset of clinical metastases is 8 years and the median time to death following metastases is 5 years.[5]
- After radiation therapy, biochemical recurrence is usually defined by criteria established by the American Society for Therapeutic Radiology and Oncology (ASTRO): three consecutive rises in PSA, measured every 3–6 months, with the mid-point date between PSA nadir (the lowest PSA value achieved after the completion of therapy) and first PSA elevation designated as the date of failure.[7]
  - This method attempts to take into account the frequent up and down fluctuations of PSA levels ('bounce') that are often seen following radiation therapy.
- There are two main potential causes of biochemical recurrence: local recurrence and metastatic disease (Figure 13.1).
- Local recurrence is defined as prostate cancer that recurs in the prostatic fossa following definitive primary therapy.
- Local recurrence and metastatic disease may occur simultaneously; however, a distinction is often made in order to direct potential treatment.

POST-TREATMENT LOCAL RECURRENCE

Post-radical prostatectomy

- If PSA begins to rise after surgery, the diagnosis of local recurrence is favored in the presence of surgical pathological stage <T3, no lymph node or seminal vesicle invasion, surgical pathological Gleason score ≤7, negative surgical margins, PSA doubling time >10 months, and/or time of PSA recurrence >2 years from date of prostatectomy.[5]
- Select men with surgical pathological Gleason score = 8, positive surgical margins, and a PSA doubling time >10 months may also have local recurrence.[8]

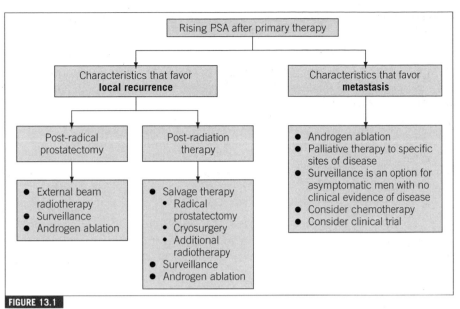

FIGURE 13.1

General schema for approaching the man with a rising prostate-specific antigen (PSA) level after primary therapy (i.e. radical prostatectomy or radiotherapy). Note that local recurrence and metastatic disease can coexist.

- A prostatic fossa biopsy is usually not done, since a negative result does not exclude local recurrence.
- CT scan and bone scan are typically not helpful in determining the location of disease when PSA <20–40 ng/ml.[9,10]
- Treatment options:
  - External beam radiotherapy, termed 'salvage radiotherapy.' Salvage radiotherapy has the highest probability of success in men with PSA <1.5–2.0 ng/ml[8,11]
  - Surveillance
  - Androgen deprivation: the optimal time to initiate in asymptomatic men with a rising PSA is unknown.

POST-RADIATION THERAPY

- With the exception of surgical pathological parameters, the same clinical features that favor local recurrence post-radical prostatectomy may be applied to post-radiation therapy.[3,12]
- Prostate biopsy is not required to make a diagnosis of local recurrence post-radiation therapy but is recommended for men who are candidates for local salvage therapy (see below).[12]
- If prostate biopsy is to be done, it should be performed >18 months from the completion of radiation therapy, since prostate cancer may take up to 18–24 months to dissipate post-radiation therapy.
- Treatment options:
  - Salvage therapy with radical prostatectomy, cryoablation, or additional radiotherapy
  - Surveillance
  - Androgen deprivation.

POST-TREATMENT METASTASES

- Diagnosis:
  - If PSA begins to rise after surgery, the diagnosis of distant metastasis is favored with pathological stage ≥T3, Gleason score ≥8, positive lymph node seminal vesicle invasion, PSA doubling time ≤10 months, and/or time of PSA recurrence <2 years from date of prostatectomy[5,8,13]
  - Imaging may be helpful in asymptomatic men with PSA >20–40 ng/ml.[9] Imaging is indicated for symptomatic men
  - ProstaScint scan (radiolabeled murine monoclonal antibody to prostate-specific membrane antigen – PSMA) may be useful for identifying areas of metastasis in equivocal cases.[14,15]
- Response to therapy is measured by PSA reduction and/or improvement of symptoms.
- Treatment options:
  - Androgen deprivation
  - Chemotherapy
  - Bone-directed therapy.

TREATMENT: ANDROGEN DEPRIVATION

GENERAL PRINCIPLES

- During its initial stages, metastatic prostate cancer is usually 'androgen sensitive.' This means that androgen deprivation therapy causes clinical regression of the cancer.
  - However, most metastatic prostate cancers will eventually become 'androgen independent.' This means that after an initial period of regression, the cancer will progress, regardless of androgen deprivation (Figure 13.2)
  - The median time to disease progression following the initiation of androgen ablation therapy – i.e. the time for the cancer to become androgen independent – is <2 years.
- The median time to death following the documentation of androgen-independent metastatic prostate cancer is 12–16 months.[16]
- Androgen ablation therapy may increase fracture risk, particularly in patients with advanced disease.

LHRH AGONISTS

- Currently include leuprolide, goserelin, and triptorelin.
- Mechanism:
  - Bind in an agonistic fashion to LHRH (luteinizing hormone-releasing hormone) receptors in the pituitary and, after an initial surge of LH (luteinizing hormone) release and testosterone production, suppress further LH release by desensitizing the pituitary.
- Typically achieve castrate (<50 ng/ml) serum testosterone levels within 30 days.
- May be used with an antiandrogen agent, which is termed 'combined androgen blockage.'

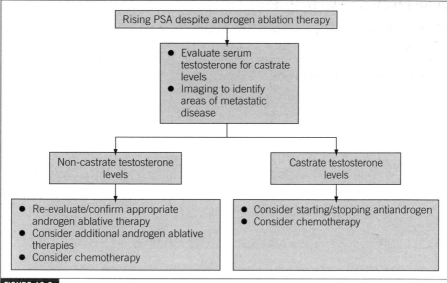

FIGURE 13.2

General outline for the approach to the man with a rising prostate-specific antigen (PSA) level despite androgen ablative therapy. Men with androgen-independent prostate cancer should be considered for clinical trials. Due to the antiandrogen withdrawal phenomenon, the removal of antiandrogen therapy may be associated with a short-lived PSA response in this population.

- Potential adverse effects:
  - May cause a 'flare' or rise in serum testosterone levels 3–4 days after initiation that may exacerbate prostate cancer-related symptoms.[17] Symptoms dissipate in approximately 5–8 days, or may be prevented by concomitant administration of an antiandrogen
  - Breast tenderness, gynecomastia, peripheral edema, hot flashes, diminished libido, erectile dysfunction, and testicular atrophy.

ORCHIECTOMY

- Bilateral orchiectomy will result in castrate levels of testosterone in 3–4 hours. It is the quickest method to achieve castrate levels of circulating testosterone.
- Clinical efficacy is equivalent to an LHRH antagonist.
- Does not affect the production of adrenal androgens [e.g. dehydroepiandrosterone (DHEA)].

LHRH ANTAGONISTS

- Currently include abarelix.
- Mechanism:
  - Block LHRH receptors in the hypothalamus and suppress LH release by the pituitary.
- Unlike LHRH agonists, will not cause a testosterone surge during initiation of therapy.
- Currently not widely used.

ESTROGENS

- Diethylstilbestrol (DES) is most prominent.
- Mechanism:
  - Bind at level of hypothalamus and suppress LHRH secretion.
- Clinical efficacy similar to LHRH antagonists, but not as widely used because of concern for potential cardiovascular adverse events, especially cardiovascular mortality.

ANTIANDROGENS

- Mechanism:
  - Block binding of androgens (testosterone and dihydrotestosterone) to the androgen receptor.
- Two primary types: steroidal and non-steroidal.
- Steroidal:
  - Currently include cyproterone acetate and megestrol
  - Not widely used
  - Also block LH secretion, and therefore are more associated with sexual side effects (see below).
- Non-steroidal:
  - Currently include flutamide and bicalutamide
  - Cause increase in serum testosterone levels, via interfering with endocrine negative feedback, which may also result in increased estrogen levels through amplified conversion of testosterone to estrogen
  - When used as a sole agent, libido and erectile function usually remain unaffected.
- Antiandrogen withdrawal syndrome:
  - Characterized by a decrease in PSA after the cessation of antiandrogen agent[18]
  - Typically lasts for 3–6 months.
- Potential adverse effects:
  - Diarrhea, nausea, vomiting, hepatotoxicity (check LFTs regularly), and gynecomastia
  - For steroidal agents: loss of libido and erectile dysfunction.

ANDROGEN BIOSYNTHESIS INHIBITORS

- Currently include ketoconazole and aminoglutethimide.
- Mechanism:
  - Inhibit enzymatic pathways leading to steroid synthesis.
- Castrate testosterone levels may be observed approximately 8 hours after initiation of therapy.
- May be associated with an escape phenomenon (i.e. rising serum testosterone level) 4–6 weeks after the initiation of therapy.
- May inhibit the cytochrome P450 system.
- Potential adverse effects:
  - Hepatic toxicity, nausea, vomiting, and weakness
  - Decreased corticosteroid levels: corticosteroid supplementation therapy may be required.

TREATMENT: CHEMOTHERAPY

GENERAL PRINCIPLES

- Used to treat androgen-independent prostate cancer.
- Optimal time for administration (i.e. early or late in disease progression) is not known.

MAJOR AGENTS AND MECHANISMS

- Mitoxantrone:
  - Intercalates within DNA and inhibits topoisomerase II.
- Estramustine:
  - A conjugate of estradiol and nitrogen mustard
  - Disrupts microtubule function.
- Taxanes (docetaxel and paclitaxel):
  - Disrupt microtubule function.

EFFICACY

- Mitoxantrone and prednisone compared with prednisone alone decreases pain.
  - No difference in survival.[19]
- Mitoxantrone and hydrocortisone compared with hydrocortisone alone delays time to disease progression.
  - No difference in survival.[20]
- Docetaxel and estramustine compared with mitoxantrone and prednisone improves median survival (18 months vs 16 months), increases time to disease progression, and improves PSA response.[21]
- A docetaxel regimen given every 3 weeks compared with one given every week has significantly better survival (18.9 months vs 17.3 months), pain response, and PSA response.[22]

TREATMENT: BONE METASTASES

- Bisphosphonates:[23]
  - Decrease skeletal complication rates and bone pain
  - Zoledronic acid is the most potent and is approved for treatment of androgen-independent prostate cancer
  - Inhibit cancer cell binding to the bony matrix, osteoclast formation, and bone resorption, and matrix metalloproteinases; may also promote osteoblastic action
  - Potential adverse events: fatigue, anemia, myalgia, fever, and lower extremity edema.
- Radiopharmaceuticals:[23]
  - Decrease pain and delay onset of additional sites of pain
  - Strontium-89 is the most widely used
  - Selectively accumulate in tumor sites, thereby reducing damage to adjacent tissue compared with standard radiotherapy
  - Response rate is >70%
  - May be associated with bone marrow suppression/hematological toxicity.

13

PROSTATE CANCER: METASTATIC

- Endothelin-1 antagonists:[23,24]
  - Endothelin-1 (ET-1), a vasoconstrictor and cell growth modulator, stimulates osteoblasts and growth of bony lesions in patients with metastatic prostate cancer
  - Atrasentan is a selective ETA receptor antagonist which decreases median time to disease progression, incidence of bone pain, and median time to bone pain
  - Currently in phase 3 trials
  - Potential adverse effects: headache, rhinitis, and peripheral edema.
- Local radiotherapy for discrete lesions:
  - Decreases pain
  - May be effective for decreasing neurological symptoms associated with cord compression.
- Affected weight-bearing bones may require orthopedic intervention for stabilization.

REFERENCES

1. Sella A, Konichezky M, Flex D, Sulkes A, Baniel J: Low PSA metastatic androgen-independent prostate cancer. Eur Urol 38:250–4, 2000.
2. Fossa SD, Waehre H, Paus E: The prognostic significance of prostate specific antigen in metastatic hormone-resistant prostate cancer. Br J Cancer 66:181–4, 1992.
3. D'Amico AV, Whittington R, Malkowicz SB et al: Biochemical outcome after radical prostatectomy, external beam radiation therapy, or interstitial radiation therapy for clinically localized prostate cancer. JAMA 280:969–74, 1998.
4. Amling CL, Blute ML, Bergstralh EJ et al: Long-term hazard of progression after radical prostatectomy for clinically localized prostate cancer: continued risk of biochemical failure after 5 years. J Urol 164:101–5, 2000.
5. Pound CR, Partin AW, Eisenberger MA et al: Natural history of progression after PSA elevation following radical prostatectomy. JAMA 281:1591–7, 1999.
6. Dillioglugil O, Leibman BD, Kattan MW et al: Hazard rates for progression after radical prostatectomy for clinically localized prostate cancer. Urology 50:93–9, 1997.
7. Consensus statement: guidelines for PSA following radiation therapy. American Society for Therapeutic Radiology and Oncology Consensus Panel. Int J Radiat Oncol Biol Phys 37:1035–41, 1997.
8. Stephenson AJ, Shariat SF, Zelefsky MJ et al: Salvage radiotherapy for recurrent prostate cancer after radical prostatectomy. JAMA 291:1325–32, 2004.
9. Cher ML, Bianco FJ Jr, Lam JS et al: Limited role of radionuclide bone scintigraphy in patients with prostate specific antigen elevations after radical prostatectomy. J Urol 160:1387–91, 1998.
10. Kane CJ, Amling CL, Johnstone PA et al: Limited value of bone scintigraphy and computed tomography in assessing biochemical failure after radical prostatectomy. Urology 61:607–11, 2003.
11. Tiguert R, Forman JD, Hussain M, Wood DP: Radiation therapy for a rising PSA level after radical prostatectomy. Semin Urol Oncol 17:141–7, 1999.
12. Cox JD, Gallagher MJ, Hammond EH, Kaplan RS, Schellhammer PF: Consensus statements on radiation therapy of prostate cancer: guidelines for prostate re-biopsy after radiation and for radiation therapy with rising prostate-specific antigen levels after radical prostatectomy. American Society for Therapeutic Radiology and Oncology Consensus Panel. J Clin Oncol 17:1155, 1999.
13. Patel A, Dorey F, Franklin J, deKernion JB: Recurrence patterns after radical retropubic prostatectomy: clinical usefulness of prostate specific antigen doubling times and log slope prostate specific antigen. J Urol 158:1441–5, 1997.

14. Ponsky LE, Cherullo EE, Starkey R et al: Evaluation of preoperative ProstaScint scans in the prediction of nodal disease. Prostate Cancer Prostatic Dis 5:132–5, 2002.

15. Brassell SA, Rosner IL, McLeod DG: Update on magnetic resonance imaging, ProstaScint, and novel imaging in prostate cancer. Curr Opin Urol 15:163–6, 2005.

16. Martel CL, Gumerlock PH, Meyers FJ, Lara PN: Current strategies in the management of hormone refractory prostate cancer. Cancer Treat Rev 29:171–87, 2003.

17. Bruchovsky N, Goldenberg SL, Akakura K, Rennie PS: Luteinizing hormone-releasing hormone agonists in prostate cancer. Elimination of flare reaction by pretreatment with cyproterone acetate and low-dose diethylstilbestrol. Cancer 72:1685–91, 1993.

18. Richie JP: Anti-androgens and other hormonal therapies for prostate cancer. Urology 54:15–18, 1999.

19. Tannock IF, Osoba D, Stockler MR et al: Chemotherapy with mitoxantrone plus prednisone or prednisone alone for symptomatic hormone-resistant prostate cancer: a Canadian randomized trial with palliative end points. J Clin Oncol 14:1756–64, 1996.

20. Kantoff PW, Halabi S, Conaway M et al: Hydrocortisone with or without mitoxantrone in men with hormone-refractory prostate cancer: results of the cancer and leukemia group B 9182 study. J Clin Oncol 17:2506–13, 1999.

21. Petrylak DP, Tangen CM, Hussain MH et al: Docetaxel and estramustine compared with mitoxantrone and prednisone for advanced refractory prostate cancer. New Engl J Med 351:1513–20, 2004.

22. Tannock IF, de Wit R, Berry WR et al: Docetaxel plus prednisone or mitoxantrone plus prednisone for advanced prostate cancer. New Engl J Med 351:1502–12, 2004.

23. Nelson JB, Smith MR: Management of bone metastases in patients with prostate cancer. In: Carroll PR, Nelson WG, eds. Report to the Nation on Prostate Cancer. Santa Monica, CA: Prostate Cancer Foundation, 2004, pp 37–43.

24. Carducci MA, Slawin KM, Solit DB: Emerging therapies for prostate cancer. In: Carroll PR, Nelson WG, eds. Report to the Nation on Prostate Cancer. Santa Monica, CA: Prostate Cancer Foundation, 2004, pp 55–63.

13

PROSTATE CANCER: METASTATIC

Renal parenchymal tumors

Edward M Schaeffer

SUMMARY

- The most common type of renal tumor is renal cell carcinoma (RCC).
- RCC accounts for 80–85% of all renal cancers. Incidence and mortality have been increasing. Survival is based on tumor stage.
- Initial evaluation should include complete blood count (CBC), serum electrolytes, liver function tests (LFTs), chest X-ray, and abdominal computed tomography (CT) or magnetic resonance imaging (MRI).
- Treatments for localized RCC include radical nephrectomy, partial nephrectomy, cryosurgery, and radiofrequency ablation.
- Treatments for metastatic RCC include immunotherapy with interferon-alpha or interleukin-2, with or without cytoreductive nephrectomy.
- Other types of kidney tumors include metastatic lesions, sarcomas, juxtaglomerular tumors, and lymphomas.

14

RENAL CELL CARCINOMA

EPIDEMIOLOGY

- Account for 80–85% of all renal cancers.
- ~35 000 new cases per year.[1]
- ~12 000 deaths per year.[1]
- Incidence is increasing[2]
  - From 6.1 per 100 000 persons in 1975 to 9.3 per 100 000 persons in 1995.
- Male to female ratio is 3:2.
- 10–20% higher incidence in African-Americans compared with Caucasians.[2]
- Sporadic tumors are unilateral and unifocal. Bilateral synchronous or asynchronous tumors occur in 2–4% of sporadic RCCs.
- 4% of RCCs are familial.[3]
- Small (<3 cm) lesions now comprise at least 25% of newly diagnosed RCCs.
  - The increased detection is related, in part, to increased use of non-invasive imaging (CT scan and ultrasound). Interestingly, despite earlier detection, the incidences of distant and regional disease and mortality rates are increasing. Reasons for this are unclear.[2,4]
- Risk factors:[5–7]
  - Smoking
  - Obesity
  - Acquired renal cystic disease (30-fold increased risk for dialysis patients with acquired cystic disease).

PRESENTATION

- Advanced tumors have been described as 'internist's tumors' because of the diverse array of presentations.
- Organ-confined tumors are less often symptomatic.

- Classic triad of hematuria, flank pain, and abdominal mass now occurs in <10% of patients.[8]
- >50% of tumors are detected radiographically in contemporary series.
- Presenting symptoms associated with the primary tumor:
  - *Hematuria*
  - Mass – typically appreciated with lower pole masses in thin patients
  - Varicocele: typically on left side, will not decompress when patient is supine
  - Edema, and lower extremity varices associated with vena cava obstruction.
- Presenting symptoms associated with metastases include:
  - Bone pain
  - Neurological symptoms
  - Ascites.
- Paraneoplastic syndromes may occur in up to 20% of RCCs and include:[9]
  - Erythrocytosis (1–5%): due to erythropoietin production by tumor or local hypoxic effect of tumor causing production in surrounding tissue
  - Hypercalcemia (up to 13%): due to parathyroid hormone-related protein production by tumor and metastatic bone lesions
  - Hepatic dysfunction, also called Stauffer's syndrome (3–20%): associated with increased alkaline phosphatase (the most common abnormality), increased transaminases, increased prothrombin time, and hypoalbuminemia;[10] these should normalize after tumor resection, and persistent dysfunction is suggestive of metastatic disease
  - Amyloidosis
  - Anemia (30–80%)
  - Cachexia.

INITIAL EVALUATION

- Physical exam.
- Laboratory studies:
  - CBC
  - Serum electrolytes
  - LFTs.
- Imaging for staging.

IMAGING

- Chest X-ray or chest CT.
- Ultrasound:
  - Excellent screening tool for renal cystic disease
  - Criteria for simple cyst: smooth walls, anechogenic, and increased through transmission[11,12]
  - Not useful in staging for RCC.
- Abdominal CT with IV contrast – Triphasic:
  - Enhancement >10 Hounsfield units (HU) consistent with malignancy in most cases
  - An enhancement threshold of at least 15–20 HU may be more appropriate for small (4.5 cm) lesions[13]
  - Adenopathy ≥2 cm indicates likely metastatic disease
  - Adenopathy <2 cm may be inflammatory.[14]

- MRI with gadolinium:
  - Consider for renal insufficiency/failure or allergy to IV contrast dye.

FINE NEEDLE ASPIRATION OR BIOPSY

- Recommended indications:[15]
  - Concern for renal abscess – flank pain, recurrent urinary tract infection (UTI), fevers
  - History of primary non-renal malignancy.

STAGING

- TNM staging for renal cell carcinoma[16]
  - T: Primary tumor
    - Tx: Primary tumor cannot be assessed
    - T0: No evidence of primary tumor
    - T1: Tumor <7.0 cm in greatest diameter, confined to kidney
    - T2: Tumor >7.0 cm in greatest diameter, confined to kidney
    - T3
      - a: Tumor invades adrenal gland or perinephric structures
      - b: Tumor extends into renal vein or inferior vena cava (IVC) below diaphragm
      - c: Tumor extends into IVC above diaphragm
    - T4: Tumor invades beyond Gerota's fascia

  - N: Regional lymph nodes
    - Nx: Regional nodes cannot be assessed
    - N0: No regional node metastasis
    - N1: Metastasis in a single regional lymph node
    - N2: Metastasis in more than one regional node

  - M: Distant metastasis
    - Mx: Distant metastasis cannot be assessed
    - M0: No distant metastasis
    - M1: Distant metastasis

- IVC involvement:
  - Incidence 4–10%
  - Should perform MRI to evaluate extent
  - Generally portends a worse prognosis
  - If thrombus extends into the right atrium, resection may require circulatory arrest.
- Five-year survival by stage (Table 14.1).

TABLE 14.1

FIVE-YEAR SURVIVAL BY STAGE

Stage	Description	5-Year survival[17]
I	Local T1 tumor	95%
II	Local T2 tumor	85%
III	Node (N1) positive and/or T3 tumor	45–69%*
IV	T4 tumor and/or N2 positive and/or distant metastasis	5–20%

*Stage IIIa has similar 5-year survival to stage II disease.

GRADING

- Fuhrman grading system[18] is most often used.
  - Based on nuclear features (diameter and form) and presence of nucleoli
  - Scored 1–4: 1 = well differentiated, 4 = poorly differentiated
  - Grade correlates with prognosis: grades 3 and 4 have worse prognosis than 1 or 2.

HISTOLOGICAL CLASSIFICATION[3]

- Clear cell:
  - Comprise 70–80% of RCCs
  - Gross appearance: yellow
  - Very vascular
  - ~70% have Von Hippel–Lindau (VHL) mutation
  - Cell origin: proximal tubule
  - Associated with 3p loss.
- Papillary:
  - Comprise 10–15% of RCCs
  - Hypovascular
  - Stellate scar on CT is classic finding
  - Cell origin: proximal tubule
  - Associated with 7, 17 gain, Y loss
  - Associated with c-MET mutations.
- Chromophobe:
  - Comprise 4–5% of RCCs
  - Cell origin: collecting duct.
- Collecting duct:
  - Rare, aggressive subtype
  - Typically present at advanced stage with poor prognosis
  - Cell origin: collecting duct.
- Medullary:
  - Rare, aggressive subtype
  - Associated with sickle cell trait
  - Typically present at advanced stage
  - Poor prognosis.

TREATMENT FOR LOCALIZED RENAL CELL CARCINOMA

Radical nephrectomy

- Gold standard.
- Basic principles: removal of kidney with investing (Gerota's) fascia, regional lymphadenectomy, and ipsilateral adrenalectomy.
- Lymphadenectomy includes dissection of tissue surrounding ipsilateral great vessel from level of renal hilum to inferior mesenteric artery. It improves staging, but benefits to survival are debated;[19,20] potentially may improve response to immunotherapy.[20]
- May consider not performing ipsilateral adrenalectomy for lower pole lesions or lesions <4 cm.[21]

- General surgical approaches include open retroperitoneal, open transperitoneal, laparoscopic retroperitoneal, and laparoscopic transperitoneal.
- For flank incisions, care should be taken to spare the intracostal nerves during access.
- A thoracoabdomial approach may provide better exposure for large, upper pole lesions.
- Open midline incision can be extended to include a sternotomy for access to the intrathoracic IVC and/or atrium for cases with large IVC thrombi.
- Tumor infarction may be performed preoperatively in patients with large tumors and difficult anatomy (or used for palliation in patients with unresectable disease).

Partial nephrectomy

- Basic principle: excision of tumor with margin of normal renal parenchyma.
- Indications: solitary kidney, bilateral tumors, renal insufficiency.
- May also be considered for mass <4 cm with normal contralateral kidney.[15]
- Risks include local and locoregional recurrence (0–5% in most series).[15]
- Laparoscopic partial nephrectomy: combines benefits of laparascopy with renal parenchymal preservation; early oncological data are promising.[22]

Energy ablative techniques: general principles

- Emerging technologies.
- Basic principle of tumor control: tumor necrosis via extremes of temperature.
- May be performed with open, laparoscopic, or percutaneous approaches.
- Currently used as treatment for small (<4 cm) peripheral tumors, mostly in individuals with advanced age and/or extensive comorbidity.

Energy ablative techniques: cryosurgery

- Ultrasound- and/or visually guided insertion of cooled probe into mass.
- Goal: several (2 or 3) freeze–thaw cycles that cool tissue to at least −40°C and achieve tissue necrosis.
- Ice ball size may be monitored ultrasonically.
- Post-procedure surveillance with serial imaging (CT or MRI).
- Tumors will enhance on CT/MRI scan postoperatively if not entirely destroyed; any increase in size of lesion is suspicious for local recurrence.[23,24]

Energy ablative techniques: radiofrequency ablation (RFA)

- CT or ultrasound-guided insertion of RF probe into mass.
- Energy transmission heats tissue (goal temperature 105–110°C) with resultant tissue necrosis.
- Post-procedure surveillance with serial imaging (CT or MRI) scan.[25]
- A halo of fat may surround area of RF ablation on CT/MRI postoperatively; any increase in size of lesion is suspicious for local recurrence.

14

RENAL PARENCHYMAL TUMORS

RECOMMENDED FOLLOW-UP PROTOCOLS AFTER SURGICAL TREATMENT OF LOCALIZED RENAL CELL CARCINOMA[15]

- Based on pathological stage.
- These are recommendations only; preferred follow-up protocols may vary by individual center.
- Radical nephrectomy:
  - T1: exam, blood tests (CBC, creatinine, LFTs) every year
  - T2: exam, blood tests, chest X-ray every year; abdominal CT every 2 years
  - T3: exam, blood tests, chest X-ray every 6 months for 3 years and abdominal CT at 1 year; if no recurrence, then continue with same protocol as T2.
- Partial nephrectomy:
  - T1: exam, blood tests (CBC, creatinine, LFTs) every year
  - T2: exam, blood tests, chest X-ray every year; abdominal CT every 2 years
  - T3: exam, blood tests, chest X-ray, and abdominal CT every 6 months for 3 years; if no recurrence, then continue with same protocol as T2.

TREATMENT FOR METASTATIC RENAL CELL CARCINOMA

- ~30% of newly diagnosed cases of RCC are metastatic.[15]
- Associated with extremely poor survival (50% 1 year, 0–30% 5 years).
- Common sites include lung, bone, liver, brain, and ipsilateral or contralateral kidney.
- Resection of solitary synchronous or metachronous metastatic lesions can improve prognosis.[26]
- RCC is generally chemotherapy-resistant.
- Radiation therapy is used for palliation of metastatic lesions – typically bone lesions.
- Systemic immunotherapy with alpha-interferon or interleukin-2 (IL-2):
  - Overall response rates are ~20%, with 4% complete responses[27]
  - Favorable responses occur in asymptomatic patients who have had a nephrectomy, have good performance status, non-bulky disease, and metastases in lungs or soft tissue.[27]
- Randomized trials suggest that nephrectomy (open or laparoscopic) prior to immunotherapy (or 'cytoreductive nephrectomy') improves survival compared with immunotherapy alone.[28–31]

HEREDITARY SYNDROMES ASSOCIATED WITH RENAL CELL CARCINOMA

Von Hippel–Lindau sydrome

- Characterized by hemoangioblastomas of the central nervous system, renal tumors and cysts, pancreatic tumors and cysts, pheochromocytomas and inner ear tumors.
- *VHL* gene located on chromosome 3p26.[3]
- Autosomal dominant disorder.
- *VHL* is a tumor suppressor gene; the gene product targets proteins for degradation, including HIF (hypoxia-inducible factor), a transcription factor that regulates angiogenesis.
- RCC occurs in 50% of individuals with the VHL mutation.
- RCC typically presents during the third to fifth decades with multifocal lesions.

Hereditary papillary renal cell carcinoma (HPRCC)

- Characterized by papillary renal tumors.[32]
- The *HPRCC* gene is located on chromosome 7q31 and encodes c-MET, a growth factor receptor.[3]
- Due to the slow-growing nature of papillary tumors, typically present during the sixth to seventh decades.

Hereditary leiomyomatosis renal cell carcinoma (HLRCC)

- Characterized by cutaneous leiomyomatosis, uterine fibroids, and papillary RCC.[33,34]
- The *HLRCC* gene is located on chromosome 1q42 and encodes fumarate hydratase, an enzyme in the Kreb's cycle.[34]
- Hereditary papillary RCC is reported in ~20% of affected families.
- Papillary tumors in this syndrome are aggressive and metastasize early.

Birt–Hogg–Dubé syndrome

- Characterized by cutaneous hair follicle tumors, pulmonary cysts, and renal tumors (clear cell, papillary, chromophobe, and oncocytoma).
- Chromophobe is the most common type of renal tumor.[3]
- Fibrofolliculomas of the skin are characteristic. Skin tags may also be present. 15–30% of patients with cutaneous lesions will develop renal tumors.[35]
- 25% of individuals present with a history of spontaneous pneumothorax.[3]

OTHER RENAL MALIGNANCIES

METASTATIC LESIONS

- Lung is the most common primary.

SARCOMA

- Constitute 1–2% of all renal malignancies.
- Leiomyosarcoma is the most common subtype.[36]
- May be difficult to distinguish from an RCC with sarcomatoid features.
- Other findings suggestive of sarcoma include a large mass without adenopathy and the presence of fat or bone in the lesion.
- Treatment is radical nephrectomy with wide excision. Resection of adjacent involved organs indicated as margin status and grade are the most important prognostic variables.[36]

JUXTAGLOMERULAR CELL TUMOR

- Rare renal parenchymal tumor of the renin-producing juxtaglomerular cell.
- Elevated renin is associated with hypertension, hyperaldosteronism, and hypokalemia.
- Typically presents during the second to third decades of life.
- Treatment is surgical excision. Unless another etiology is also present, hypertension should remit or resolve after resection.
- There have been no reported recurrences after resection or metastases.

14

RENAL PARENCHYMAL TUMORS

LYMPHOMAS[37,38]

- Primary renal lymphomas are extremely rare.
- Kidney may be involved by either direct extension or hematogenous spread. Suspect lymphoma if the mass appears infiltrating or multifocal, there is diffuse adenopathy, or evidence of systemic disease.
- Biopsy warranted if lymphoma suspected.

REFERENCES

1. Cancer Facts and Figures 2004. American Cancer Society, 2004.
2. Chow WH, Devesa SS, Warren JL, Fraumeni JF Jr: Rising incidence of renal cell cancer in the United States. JAMA 281:1628 31, 1999.
3. Pavlovich CP, Schmidt LS, Phillips JL: The genetic basis of renal cell carcinoma. Urol Clin North Am 30:437–54, vii, 2003.
4. Parsons JK, Schoenberg MS, Carter HB: Incidental renal tumors: casting doubt on the efficacy of early intervention. Urology 57:1013–15, 2001.
5. Brennan JF, Stilmant MM, Babayan RK, Siroky MB: Acquired renal cystic disease: implications for the urologist. Br J Urol 67:342–8, 1991.
6. Chow WH, Gridley G, Fraumeni JF Jr, Jarvholm B: Obesity, hypertension, and the risk of kidney cancer in men. New Engl J Med 343:1305–11, 2000.
7. Yu MC, Mack TM, Hanisch R, Cicioni C, Henderson BE: Cigarette smoking, obesity, diuretic use, and coffee consumption as risk factors for renal cell carcinoma. J Natl Cancer Inst 77:351–6, 1986.
8. Jayson M, Sanders H: Increased incidence of serendipitously discovered renal cell carcinoma. Urology 51:203–5, 1998.
9. Sufrin G, Chasan S, Golio A, Murphy GP: Paraneoplastic and serologic syndromes of renal adenocarcinoma. Semin Urol 7:158–71, 1989.
10. Rosenblum SL: Paraneoplastic syndromes associated with renal cell carcinoma. J S C Med Assoc 83:375–8, 1987.
11. Bosniak MA: The small (less than or equal to 3.0 cm) renal parenchymal tumor: detection, diagnosis, and controversies. Radiology 179:307–17, 1991.
12. Curry NS: Small renal masses (lesions smaller than 3 cm): imaging evaluation and management. AJR Am J Roentgenol 164:355–62, 1995.
13. Maki DD, Birnbaum BA, Chakraborty DP et al: Renal cyst pseudoenhancement: beam-hardening effects on CT numbers. Radiology 213:468–72, 1999.
14. Studer UE, Scherz S, Scheidegger J et al: Enlargement of regional lymph nodes in renal cell carcinoma is often not due to metastases. J Urol 144:243–5, 1990.
15. Walsh PC (ed.): Campbell's Urology. Philadelphia: WB Saunders, 2004, p 3954.
16. Guinan P, Sobin LH, Algaba F et al: TNM staging of renal cell carcinoma: Workgroup No. 3. Union International Contre le Cancer (UICC) and the American Joint Committee on Cancer (AJCC). Cancer 80:992–3, 1997.
17. Thrasher JB, Paulson DF: Prognostic factors in renal cancer. Urol Clin North Am 20:247–62, 1993.
18. Fuhrman SA, Lasky LC, Limas C: Prognostic significance of morphologic parameters in renal cell carcinoma. Am J Surg Pathol 6:655–63, 1982.
19. Minervini A, Lilas L, Morelli G et al: Regional lymph node dissection in the treatment of renal cell carcinoma: is it useful in patients with no suspected adenopathy before or during surgery? BJU Int 88:169–72, 2001.
20. Pantuck AJ, Zisman A, Dorey F et al: Renal cell carcinoma with retroperitoneal lymph nodes: role of lymph node dissection. J Urol 169:2076–83, 2003.
21. Siemer S, Lehmann J, Kamradt J et al: Adrenal metastases in 1635 patients with renal cell carcinoma: outcome and indication for adrenalectomy. J Urol 171:2155–9; discussion 2159, 2004.
22. Allaf ME, Bhayani SB, Rogers C et al: Laparoscopic partial nephrectomy: evaluation of long-term oncological outcome. J Urol 172:871–3, 2004.
23. Gill IS, Novick AC, Meraney AM et al: Laparoscopic renal cryoablation in 32 patients. Urology 56:748–53, 2000.

24. Sewell PE, Howard JC, Shingleton WB, Harrison RB: Interventional magnetic resonance image-guided percutaneous cryoablation of renal tumors. South Med J 96:708–10, 2003.
25. Gervais DA, McGovern FJ, Arellano RS, McDougal WS, Mueller PR: Renal cell carcinoma: clinical experience and technical success with radio-frequency ablation of 42 tumors. Radiology 226:417–24, 2003.
26. O'Dea MJ, Zincke H, Utz DC, Bernatz PE: The treatment of renal cell carcinoma with solitary metastasis. J Urol 120:540–2, 1978.
27. Bukowski RM: Immunotherapy in renal cell carcinoma. Oncology (Huntingt) 13:801–10; discussion 810, 813, 1999.
28. Finelli A, Kaouk JH, Fergany AF et al: Laparoscopic cytoreductive nephrectomy for metastatic renal cell carcinoma. BJU Int 94:291–4, 2004.
29. Flanigan RC, Salmon SE, Blumenstein BA et al: Nephrectomy followed by interferon alfa-2b compared with interferon alfa-2b alone for metastatic renal-cell cancer. New Engl J Med 345:1655–9, 2001.
30. Mickisch GH, Garin A, van Poppel H, de Prijck L, Sylvester R: Radical nephrectomy plus interferon-alfa-based immunotherapy compared with interferon alfa alone in metastatic renal-cell carcinoma: a randomised trial. Lancet 358:966–70, 2001.
31. Rabets JC, Kaouk J, Fergany A et al: Laparoscopic versus open cytoreductive nephrectomy for metastatic renal cell carcinoma. Urology 64:930–4, 2004.
32. Zbar B, Glenn G, Lubensky I et al: Hereditary papillary renal cell carcinoma: clinical studies in 10 families. J Urol 153:907–12, 1995.
33. Kiuru M, Launonen V, Hietala M et al: Familial cutaneous leiomyomatosis is a two-hit condition associated with renal cell cancer of characteristic histopathology. Am J Pathol 159:825–9, 2001.
34. Toro JR, Nickerson ML, Wei MH et al: Mutations in the fumarate hydratase gene cause hereditary leiomyomatosis and renal cell cancer in families in North America. Am J Hum Genet 73:95–106, 2003.
35. Zbar B, Alvord WG, Glenn G et al: Risk of renal and colonic neoplasms and spontaneous pneumothorax in the Birt–Hogg–Dube syndrome. Cancer Epidemiol Biomarkers Prev 11:393–400, 2002.
36. Russo P, Brady MS, Conlon K et al: Adult urological sarcoma. J Urol 147:1032–6; discussion 1036–7, 1992.
37. Levendoglu-Tugal O, Kroop S, Rozenblit GN, Weiss R: Primary renal lymphoma and hypercalcemia in a child. Leuk Lymphoma 43:1141–6, 2002.
38. Mills NE, Goldenberg AS, Liu D et al: B-cell lymphoma presenting as infiltrative renal disease. Am J Kidney Dis 19:181–4, 1992.

14

RENAL PARENCHYMAL TUMORS

Bladder cancer: superficial

Mark L Gonzalgo

SUMMARY

- Bladder cancer is the second most common genitourinary malignancy.
- Approximately 70% of bladder tumors are superficial.
- Only 10–20% of superficial bladder tumors will progress to muscle-invasive disease.
- Environmental exposures (i.e. tobacco smoke, aniline dyes) are strongly associated with development of bladder cancer.
- Gross, painless hematuria is the most common presenting symptom.
- Evaluation includes history and physical exam, urinalysis, urine culture and cytology, serum electrolytes and liver function tests, upper urinary tract imaging, and cystoscopy.
- Mainstay of treatment for superficial disease is transurethral resection of bladder tumor (TURBT) with or without adjuvant intravesical chemotherapy.
- Following initial transurethral resection, surveillance cystoscopy should be performed every 3 months during the first 2 years, every 6 months during the next 2 years, and once a year thereafter.
- Urinary tumor markers may be used as an adjunct to cystoscopy and urine cytology for diagnosis and/or surveillance.

EPIDEMIOLOGY

- Incidence of bladder cancer in the United States (2005) estimated to be 63 210 and the number of deaths from bladder cancer is approximately 13 180.[1]
- Male:female ratio is approximately 3:1.
- Incidence is higher in Caucasians compared with African-Americans.
- **Approximately 70% of bladder tumors are superficial.**
- **Chance of tumor recurrence is approximately 70 80%.**
- **Approximately 10–20% of superficial bladder tumors progress to muscle-invasive disease.**[2]
- Majority of superficial bladder tumors are non-invasive papillary cancers (stage Ta).
- Associations:
  - Aniline dyes
  - Cigarette smoking
  - Cyclophosphamide (acrolein)
  - Chronic infections (schistosomiasis, stones, indwelling catheter)
  - Ionizing radiation
  - Phenacetin
  - Dietary fat
  - Occupational exposure: painters, auto mechanics, dry cleaners, plumbers.

BIOLOGY

MAJOR CATEGORIES

Urothelial carcinoma (>90%)

- Derived from transitional epithelium of the bladder.
- Morphology:
  - Papillary: typically low-grade, non-invasive
  - Sessile: more likely to be invasive.
- *Carcinoma in situ* (CIS): a premalignant lesion associated with high likelihood of progression to invasive disease.[3]

Squamous cell carcinoma (5–7%)

- Associated with chronic infection, indwelling catheters, bladder calculi, and bilharzial infection (*Schistosoma haematobium*).
  - *S. haematobium*: medical management with praziquantel.

Adenocarcinoma (1–2%)

- Frequently associated with cystitis or metaplasia.
- Urachal adenocarcinomas arise from dome of bladder. Must rule out metastatic source (i.e. patients should have colonoscopy).

Undifferentiated carcinomas (<2%)

- No mature epithelial components.
- Small-cell type resembles small-cell cancer of the lung.

GRADE AND STAGE

- Almost all bladder cancer occurs sporadically.
- Tumor grade, stage, and presence of CIS increase risk for disease progression.[4]
- Genetic polymorphisms (variation) in detoxification pathways may alter risk of developing bladder cancer.
  - *N*-Acetyltransferase 2: slow vs rapid acetylation
  - Glutathione *S*-transferase M1: homozygous deletion
  - Cytochrome P450 1A2 enzyme induction.
- Molecular alterations in bladder cancer:
  - *Papillary tumors*: chromosome 9q, p15/16, p27
  - *CIS*: p53, pRB, p14, p21
  - Deletion of genetic material on chromosome 9 is one of the most common genetic alterations in bladder cancer
  - Deletions of chromosome 17p have been associated with tumor progression (*p53* gene).
- Histological grading of bladder cancer (2000 WHO/ISUP classification):[5]
  - *Grade 0*: papilloma (benign lesion)
  - *Grade 1*: papillary urothelial tumor of low malignant potential
  - *Grade 2*: low-grade urothelial carcinoma
  - *Grade 3*: high-grade urothelial carcinoma.
- Bladder cancer staging:
  - Ta: non-invasive papillary carcinoma
  - TIS (CIS): carcinoma in situ

- T1: tumor invasion into the lamina propria
- T2: muscle invasion (T2a, superficial; T2b, deep)
- T3: perivesical invasion (T3a, microscopic; T3b, macroscopic)
- T4: invasion into adjacent organs (T4a, prostate, uterus, vagina; T4b, pelvic or abdominal wall).

DIAGNOSIS

PRESENTATION

- **The most common presentation is gross, painless hematuria.**
- **Frequency, urgency, and dysuria are frequently associated with CIS.**
- Other presenting symptoms:
  - Microscopic hematuria (second most common symptom)
  - Irritative voiding symptoms
  - Incidental imaging findings.

EVALUATION

- History and physical examination.
- Urine culture.
- Urine cytology: highly specific.
- Serum electrolytes and liver function tests.
- Upper tract imaging if invasive lesion is suspected: abdominal computed tomography (CT), urogram/intravenous pyelogram (IVP), or magnetic resonance imaging (MRI).
  - Discontinue medications such as metformin 48 hours before IV contrast study to avoid potential acid–base imbalances
  - Obtain axial imaging (CT scan, MRI) *before* TURBT because of artifact produced by the procedure.
- Preoperative bone scan is generally unnecessary for patients with clinically organ-confined, muscle-invasive bladder cancer.
- Cystoscopy:
  - *5-aminolevulinic acid (5-ALA)*: a fluorescence-based technique that can be used to increase sensitivity for detecting urothelial abnormalities.[6]

TREATMENT

ENDOSCOPIC MANAGEMENT

- Entails examination under anesthesia (EUA), cystoscopy, and TURBT.
- Palpable mass after TURBT correlates with stage T3 disease and prognosis after treatment.
- Repeat TURBT is indicated, especially for high-grade T1 lesions when no detrusor muscle is identified on initial pathology.
- T1 lesions are often understaged on initial TUR and repeat resection may be of value prior to proceeding with definitive surgical therapy.[7]
- Lithotomy position (complications and prevention):
  - *Sciatic* nerve injury: inability to flex knee – avoid excessive external hip rotation
  - *Femoral nerve injury*: inability to flex hip or extend knee – avoid excessive external hip rotation

15

BLADDER CANCER: SUPERFICIAL

- *Common peroneal nerve*: foot drop – avoid compression of lateral knee at the fibular head
- *Obturator reflex*: stimulated by electrocautery, especially along lateral bladder wall.
- Bladder perforation:
  - Must distinguish between extraperitoneal (managed by catheter drainage) or intraperitoneal (may not respond to drainage alone and could require open repair).

INTRAVESICAL CHEMOTHERAPY

Bacille Calmette-Guérin (BCG)

- Therapeutic indications:
  - CIS, residual tumor, tumor prophylaxis
  - Primary form of adjuvant therapy for CIS.
- May reduce tumor recurrence by 30–40%.[8,9]
- Mechanism of action:
  - Unknown, but tumor contact with BCG is required and effects mediated by fibronectin and integrin receptors. Th1 (T-helper cell) response is important.[10]
- Cautions:
  - Gross hematuria and suspected bacterial infection are contraindications for BCG administration because toxicity is associated with intravascular inoculation
  - BCG treatment should be delayed for several days in the event of traumatic catheterization.
- Potential complications:
  - *BCGosis*: fever >38.5°C for more than 24 hours; fever >39.5°C. *Treatment*: 3 months of INH (300 mg daily)
  - *BCG sepsis*: from intravascular inoculation. *Treatment*: isoniazid, rifampin, ethambutol – or – ciprofloxacin, cycloserine, +/− steroids.
- Failure to respond to two 6-week courses of BCG therapy or early recurrence of high-risk disease indicates the need for more aggressive therapy (cystectomy) if the patient is clinically fit.

Mitomycin C

- Mechanism of action:
  - Cross-linking agent that inhibits DNA synthesis.
- Molecular weight is relatively large (334 kDa).
  - Therefore, lower risk of systemic absorption.
- May be used as *single-instillation* adjuvant therapy for preventing disease recurrence.
  - Most effective when used within 6 hours following TURBT
  - May decrease recurrence rates by as much as 50% and increase recurrence-free interval.[11]
- Potential complications:
  - Chemical cystitis, palmar desquamation, skin rash.

Thiotepa

- Mechanism of action:
  - An alkylating agent.
- Molecular weight is relatively small (189 kDa).
  - Therefore, higher risk of systemic absorption.
- Potential complications:
  - Leukopenia, thrombocytopenia, and irritiative voiding symptoms.

Doxorubicin

- Mechanism of action:
  - Inhibits topoisomerase II and protein synthesis.
- Molecular weight is relatively large (580 kDa).
  - Therefore, lower risk for systemic absorption.
- Potential complications:
  - Chemical cystitis.

Valrubicin

- Mechanism of action:
  - Synthetic analogue of doxorubicin.
- Lipophilic, with rapid uptake by cancer cells.

Cystectomy

- Although normally reserved for patients with invasive disease, cystectomy may also be appropriate for patients with high-risk, recurrent superficial bladder cancer (high-grade T1, multifocal, CIS) recalcitrant to intravesical chemotherapy.

SURVEILLANCE

- Most relapses occur within 2 years of initial TURBT.
- There is little evidence-based literature to support the most commonly practiced surveillance algorithms.
- Recommendations for surveillance cystoscopy for superficial disease after initial TURBT:[12,13]
  - Up to 2 years: every 3 months
  - 2–4 years: every 6 months
  - >4 years: once a year for life.
- Best prognostic factor: absence of disease recurrence at first 3-month cystoscopy.
- Obtain urine cytology during surveillance follow-up visits.
  - Excellent specificity (98–100%) and reasonable sensitivity for high-grade lesions and CIS.
  - Poor sensitivity for low-grade lesions (~25%).

URINARY TUMOR MARKERS

- May be used as an adjunct to cystoscopy and urine cytology.
  - However, routine use is not advocated for bladder cancer screening or disease surveillance at this time.

15

BLADDER CANCER: SUPERFICIAL

- Bladder tumor antigen (BTA) test:
  - Qualitative latex agglutination assay that detects specific proteolytic degradation complexes[14]
  - False-positive results may occur with infection and urinary calculi.
- Fluorescence in-situ hybridization (FISH):
  - Detects aneuploidy of chromosomes 3, 7, and 17, and loss of 9p21[15]
  - False-positive results may occur with infection, gross hematuria, and prostatitis.
- Microsatellite analysis:
  - Detects expansion, deletion, and loss of heterozygosity in repetitive DNA sequences
  - False-positive results may occur with cystitis and benign prostatic hyperplasia (BPH).[16]
- NMP22:
  - Uses monoclonal antibodies to detect two domains of the nuclear mitotic apparatus protein in voided urine specimens[17,18]
  - False-positive results may occur with infection, gross hematuria, and prostatitis.

REFERENCES

1. Jemal A, Murray T, Ward E et al: Cancer Statistics, 2005. CA Cancer J Clin 55:10–30, 2005.
2. Malkowicz SB: Management of superficial bladder cancer. In: Walsh PC, Retik AB, Vaughan ED, Wein AJ, eds. Campbell's Urology, 8th edn. Philadelphia: WB Saunders, 2002.
3. Hudson MA, Herr HW: Carcinoma in situ of the bladder. J Urol 153:664–72, 1995.
4. Zieger K, Wolf H, Olsen PR et al: Long-term follow-up of noninvasive bladder tumours (stage Ta): recurrence and progression. BJU Int 85:824–8, 2000.
5. Epstein JI, Amin MB, Reuter VR et al: The World Health Organization/International Society of Urological Pathology consensus classification of urothelial (transitional cell) neoplasms of the urinary bladder. Bladder Consensus Conference Committee. Am J Surg Pathol 22:1435–48, 1998.
6. Kriegmair M, Baumgartner R, Lumper W et al: Early clinical experience with 5-aminolevulinic acid for the photodynamic therapy of superficial bladder cancer. Br J Urol 77:667–71, 1996.
7. Dalbagni G, Herr HW, Reuter VE: Impact of a second transurethral resection on the staging of T1 bladder cancer. Urology 60:822–4, 2002.
8. Herr HW, Wartinger DD, Fair WR et al: Bacillus Calmette-Guerin therapy for superficial bladder cancer: a 10-year followup. J Urol 147:1020–3, 1992.
9. Jimenez-Cruz JF, Vera-Donoso CD, Leiva O et al: Intravesical immunoprophylaxis in recurrent superficial bladder cancer (Stage T1): multicenter trial comparing bacille Calmette-Guerin and interferon-alpha. Urology 50:529–35, 1997.
10. Ratliff TL, Kavoussi LR, Catalona WJ: Role of fibronectin in intravesical BCG therapy for superficial bladder cancer. J Urol 139:410–14, 1988.
11. Sylvester RJ, Oosterlinck W, van der Meijden AP: A single immediate postoperative instillation of chemotherapy decreases the risk of recurrence in patients with stage Ta T1 bladder cancer: a meta-analysis of published results of randomized clinical trials. J Urol 171:2186–90, 2004.
12. Evans CP: Follow-up surveillance strategies for genitourinary malignancies. Cancer 94:2892–905, 2002.
13. Morris SB, Gordon EM, Shearer RJ et al: Superficial bladder cancer: for how long should a tumour-free patient have check cystoscopies? Br J Urol 75:193–6, 1995.
14. Ianari A, Sternberg CN, Rossetti A et al: Results of Bard BTA test in monitoring patients with a history of transitional cell cancer of the bladder. Urology 49:786–9, 1997.

15. Sarosdy MF, Schellhammer P, Bokinsky G et al: Clinical evaluation of a multi-target fluorescent in situ hybridization assay for detection of bladder cancer. J Urol 168:1950–4, 2002.
16. Christensen M, Wolf H, Orntoft TF: Microsatellite alterations in urinary sediments from patients with cystitis and bladder cancer. Int J Cancer 85:614–17, 2000.
17. Soloway MS, Briggman V, Carpinito GA et al: Use of a new tumor marker, urinary NMP22, in the detection of occult or rapidly recurring transitional cell carcinoma of the urinary tract following surgical treatment. J Urol 156:363–7, 1996.
18. Carpinito GA, Stadler WM, Briggman JV et al: Urinary nuclear matrix protein as a marker for transitional cell carcinoma of the urinary tract. J Urol 156:1280–5, 1996.

Invasive bladder cancer and urinary diversion

Mark L Gonzalgo

SUMMARY

- Only 10–20% of superficial bladder tumors progress to muscle-invasive disease.
- Approximately 80% of patients with muscle-invasive bladder cancer initially present with muscle-invasive disease.
- Presence of a palpable mass after transurethral resection of bladder tumor (TURBT) correlates with stage T3 cancer.
- Hydronephrosis on intravenous pyelogram (IVP) or computed tomography (CT) urogram suggests the presence of advanced disease.
- Approximately 50% of patients with muscle-invasive bladder cancer will progress to metastatic disease despite aggressive local control with radiation or cystectomy.
- Median survival following diagnosis of metastatic bladder cancer is 2 years.
- Metabolic complications following cystectomy are specific to the bowel segment used for reconstruction.

BIOLOGY

- Majority of deaths from advanced disease are due to metastases.
- Common sites for metastases: lung, liver, bone.
- Late recurrences after surgery and chemotherapy can occur in CNS and peritoneum.
  - CNS recurrences are more common in patients who have been previously treated with systemic chemotherapy.
- Presence of lymphovascular invasion is an independent prognostic variable in patients with invasive bladder cancer.[1]
- AJCC-UICC lymph node and metastases staging:[2]
  - N0: nodes negative
  - N1: single lymph node ≤2 cm in diameter
  - N2: single lymph node >2 cm and ≤5 cm in diameter or multiple lymph nodes ≤5 cm
  - N3: lymph node(s) >5 cm in diameter
  - M0: no metastasis
  - M1: distant metastases present.
- Survival is related to extent of lymph node metastases present.
  - Lymph node density: number of positive nodes divided by the number of total nodes removed.[3,4]
- Molecular alterations in advanced disease:
  - *p53* gene mutation: altered in over half of invasive cancers. Independent predictor of prognosis[5]
  - Retinoblastoma (Rb) tumor suppressor gene: altered in ~50% of invasive bladder cancers. Inactivation of Rb is more frequent in high-grade and advanced-stage disease.[6]

DIAGNOSIS

STAGING

- Axial staging is recommended before TUR if an invasive lesion is suspected. Artifact from procedure may increase difficulty of radiological interpretation.[7]
- Presence of a palpable mass after TUR is correlated with stage T3 cancer and prognosis after treatment.[8]

CRITICAL COMPONENTS OF STAGING WORK-UP

- **Assess possibility of upper tract involvement, regional, and metastatic disease.**
  - Chest X-ray
  - CT scan of abdomen and pelvis
  - Upper tract imaging: IVP is good, CT urogram is better. Assess for filling defects in ureters or renal pelvices; may also identify patients with duplicated ureters. Bilateral hydronephrosis is associated with T3 disease[9]
  - Optional studies: CT scan of chest, bone scan, magnetic resonance imaging (MRI), positron emission tomography (PET).
- **Bimanual exam/exam under anesthesia.**[10]
  - Staging of mass based on palpable size and association with other pelvic structures:
    - T2a: non-palpable tumor
    - T2b: induration, but no palpable mass
    - T3: mobile, three-dimensional mass
    - T4a: invades adjacent structures
    - T4b: fixed, immobile.
- **TURBT with bladder biopsies.**
- **Bladder neck and/or urethral biopsies.**
  - Important to know pathology of prostatic urethra (via TURBT), especially in patients with multifocal carcinoma in situ (CIS)
  - In women: important to biopsy bladder neck when considering urethral preservation or orthotopic diversion.

TREATMENT

Radical cystectomy with pelvic lymphadenectomy remains the gold standard for treatment.

BLADDER-SPARING ALTERNATIVES TO CYSTECTOMY

- Radical TURBT – consider if this tumor is the initial, presenting lesion; in the absence of CIS; for size ≤3 cm; absence of palpable mass; absence of tumor in bladder dome or posterior wall. Recommend restaging TURBT at 3 months and lifelong surveillance.
- Partial cystectomy – consider if this tumor is the initial lesion; in the absence of CIS; if location is suitable for bladder preservation (i.e. dome). Bilateral pelvic lymphadenectomy should also be performed. Commonly used for patients with urachal adenocarcinoma of the bladder.

- External beam radiotherapy – consider for patients who are poor surgical candidates. Note that CIS is resistant to radiation.

INDICATIONS FOR URETHRECTOMY

- Male – diffuse CIS of prostatic urethra or ducts, invasion of prostatic stroma, or CIS or cancer present at apical margin.
- Female – CIS or cancer at the bladder neck or urethra or tumor involving the anterior vaginal wall.

CHEMOTHERAPY

- M-VAC [methotrexate, vinblastine, adriamycin (doxorubicin), cisplatin]: former gold standard combination chemotherapy regimen for advanced bladder cancer.
- Patients with neobladder reconstruction are at increased risk of reabsorption of methotrexate. Catheter should be placed during treatment to reduce excessive absorption.
- Gemcitabine, cisplatin: favored combination chemotherapy regimen. Similar efficacy as M-VAC with less toxicity.[11]

URINARY DIVERSION AND RECONSTRUCTION

GENERAL PRINCIPLES

- Principle for reconfiguration of bowel into spherical shape: Laplace's law:
  - Pressure – wall tension/radius.
- Detubularization of bowel is important to decrease peristalsis.
- Incontinent reservoir: conduit (ileum, transverse colon).
- Continent reservoir: requires manual dexterity (i.e. patient is able to self-catheterize) and normal renal function.
  - Catheterizable stoma: **Mitrofanoff principle uses appendix flap valve.** Can also use tapered ileal segment implanted into colon tinea or serosal lined rough. Monti is a short detubularized ileal segment rolled into a tube.
- Orthotopic diversion:
  - The bladder reconstruction is placed in the pelvis and attached to the distal urethra
  - May use different bowel segments in a variety of configurations. Suitable when apical/distal urethral margin is negative for cancer, motivated patient, normal external sphincter
  - Not ideal for patients with renal insufficiency (creatinine >2.0 mg/dl)
  - Nocturnal incontinence is a frequent complication.

INTESTINAL SEGMENTS FOR RECONSTRUCTION

Stomach

- Pedicle of stomach can be mobilized to pelvis on **gastroepiploic vessels.**
- Used more often for augmentation cystoplasty in children.
- Less permeable to urinary solutes, acidifies urine, net excretion of Cl^- and H^+ instead of absorption, less mucus production.

16

INVASIVE BLADDER CANCER AND URINARY DIVERSION

Jejunum

- Rarely used.
- May result in severe electrolyte imbalances.

Ileum

- Most commonly used segment.
- Simplest type of urinary diversion.
- Beware of nutritional deficiencies that may arise because of lack of vitamin B_{12} absorption.
- Not suitable for patients with short bowel syndrome, history of radiation, or inflammatory bowel disease.

COLON

- Transverse colon is suitable for use in patients with a history of pelvic irradiation.
- Use of ileocecal valve may result in diarrhea, malabsorption, fluid and bicarbonate loss.
- Cecum is the bowel segment associated with highest gastrointestinal potassium loss.
- Antirefluxing ureterointestinal anastomoses are easily performed via submucosal tunnels with colonic segments. May have higher incidence of ureteral obstruction with this technique compared with Kock pouch, which utilizes an intussuscepted nipple valve afferent limb to prevent reflux.
- Ureterosigmoidostomy involves direct anastomosis of the ureters to the sigmoid colon. Not commonly performed. May result in metabolic acidosis.

COMPLICATIONS

- For common metabolic complications, refer to Table 16.1.
- General:
  - Pyelonephritis, fistula, parastomal hernias, ureteroenteric strictures, stomal stenosis.

TABLE 16.1

METABOLIC COMPLICATIONS OR URINARY DIVERSION

Bowel segment	Electrolyte abnormalities	Comments
Stomach	Hypochloremic, hypokalemic metabolic alkalosis	Problematic in patients with renal failure because of impaired bicarbonate excretion. Hematuria-dysuria syndrome. Vitamin B_{12} malabsorption (intrinsic factor)
Jejunum	Hyperkalemic, hyponatremic, hypochloremic, metabolic acidosis	High incidence of complications from use of this segment. Jejunal conduit syndrome: nausea, emesis, fatigue. Cycle of Na^+ secretion and K^+ reabsorption activating the renin–angiotensin axis, leading to urine with a low Na^+ and high K^+. Secretion of K^+ in urine prevents adequate H^+ secretion. Treat with hydration and NaCl
Ileum and colon	Hyperchloremic, hypokalemic metabolic acidosis	Abnormalities result primarily from absorption of ammonium chloride in exchange for carbonic acid. Treat chronic acidosis with Polycitra, Bicitra, or $NaHCO_3$ +/− Ca^{2+} supplementation for osteomalacia

- 'Pipe-stem' deformity:
  - Ileal conduit narrowing, resulting from vascular insufficiency caused by inadequate mesenteric blood supply.
- Vitamin B_{12} deficiency:
  - May occur when longer segments of ileum are used for reconstruction.
- Urinary stones:
  - Fat malabsorption may increase risk of calcium, magnesium, and ammonium phosphate stone formation.
- Altered sensorium:
  - Results from magnesium deficiency or defective ammonia metabolism
  - Increased toxicity risk for drugs that are excreted unchanged by the kidney and undergo gastrointestinal absorption.
- Osteomalacia:
  - Most common in ureterosigmoidostomy diversion, but can occur with ileum and colon
  - May result from acidosis, renal calcium loss, and vitamin D resistance.
- Diarrhea:
  - Lack of bile salt reabsorption may contribute to diarrhea
  - Also seen when ileocecal valve is used for reconstruction.
- Malignancy:
  - Primarily seen with ureterosigmoidostomy, with increased risk of adenocarcinoma at the ureterocolonic anastomosis
  - Should perform intermittent colonoscopy for surveillance.
- Bowel obstruction:
  - 10% incidence of postoperative bowel obstruction requiring treatment when stomach or ileum is used compared with 5% incidence when colon is used for reconstruction.[12]

16

INVASIVE BLADDER CANCER AND URINARY DIVERSION

REFERENCES

1. Quek ML, Stein JP, Nichols PW et al: Prognostic significance of lymphovascular invasion of bladder cancer treated with radical cystectomy. J Urol 174:103–6, 2005.
2. Sobin LH, Wittekind C. International Union Against Cancer (UICC). Urinary bladder. In: TNM: Classification of Malignant Tumors. New York: Wiley-Liss, 1997, pp 187–90.
3. Herr HW: Superiority of ratio based lymph node staging for bladder cancer. J Urol 169:943–5, 2003.
4. Stein JP, Cai J, Groshen S et al: Risk factors for patients with pelvic lymph node metastases following radical cystectomy with en bloc pelvic lymphadenectomy: concept of lymph node density. J Urol 170:35–41, 2003.
5. Esrig D, Elmajian D, Groshen S et al: Accumulation of nuclear p53 and tumor progression in bladder cancer. New Engl J Med 331:1259–64, 1994.
6. Cordon-Cardo C, Wartinger D, Petrylak D et al: Altered expression of the retinoblastoma gene product: prognostic indicator in bladder cancer. J Natl Cancer Inst 84:1251–6, 1992.
7. Schoenberg MP: Management of invasive and metastatic bladder cancer. In: Walsh PC, Retik AB, Vaughan ED, Wein AJ, eds. Campbell's Urology, 8th edn. Philadelphia: WB Saunders , 2002.
8. Wijkstrom H, Lagerkvist M, Nilsson B et al: Evaluation of clinical staging before cystectomy in transitional cell bladder carcinoma: a long-term follow-up of 276 consecutive patients. Br J Urol 81:686–91, 1998.
9. Haleblian GE, Skinner EC, Dickinson MG: Hydronephrosis as a prognostic indicator in bladder cancer patients. J Urol 160:2011–14, 1998.

10. Marshall VF: The relation of the preoperative estimate to the pathologic demonstration of the extent of vesical neoplasms. J Urol 68:714–23, 1952.

11. von der Maase H, Sengelov L, Roberts JT et al: Long-term survival results of a randomized trial comparing gemcitabine plus cisplatin, with methotrexate, vinblastine, doxorubicin, plus cisplatin in patients with bladder cancer. J Clin Oncol 23:4602–8, 2005.

12. McDougal WS: Use of intestinal segments and urinary diversion. In: Walsh PC, Retik AB, Vaughan ED, Wein AJ, eds. Campbell's Urology, 8th edn. Philadelphia: WB Saunders, 2002.

Ureteral and renal pelvic tumors

Ioannis M Varkarakis

SUMMARY

- Ureteral and renal pelvic tumors are very rare, representing only a small fraction of all genitourinary and renal tumors.
- The majority are transitional cell carcinomas.
- Risk factors include smoking, aniline dyes, phenacetin abuse, Balkan nephropathy, and cyclophosphamide.
- The most common presenting symptoms are hematuria (75% of patients) and flank pain (30%).
- Evaluation includes history and physical exam, urinalysis, urine culture and cytology, serum electrolytes and liver function tests, upper urinary tract imaging, and cystoscopy. Some patients may also undergo ureteroscopy.
- Treatment options include radical nephroureterectomy with bladder cuff (open or laparoscopic), segmental ureterectomy (for ureteral lesions), and endoscopic resection.
- Tumor grade and stage are the most important variables that predict survival.
- Intensity of post-treatment surveillance should be tailored to the individual patient according to risk of disease progression.

17

EPIDEMIOLOGY AND NATURAL HISTORY

- Rare, accounting for approximately 1–2% of all genitourinary tumors and 5% of all urothelial tumors.[1,2]
  - There is some evidence to suggest that the frequency is increasing.[3]
- 90% are transitional cell carcinoma (TCC), 9% squamous cell carcinoma (SCC), 1% are adenocarcinomas, sarcomas or inverted papillomas.
- TCC of the renal pelvis is 3–4 times more frequent than TCC of the ureter.
- Males are affected 3–4 times more frequently than females.
- Caucasians are affected 2 times more frequently than Blacks.
- The incidence increases with age and peaks during the 6th to 7th decades.
- Recurrences are usually confined to the ipsilateral kidney and/or bladder and may occur in 30–50% of patients.[4,5]
- Recurrence in the contralateral kidney may occur in 1–5% of patients.
- Synchronous bilateral disease may occur in 2–4% of patients.
- 50% of ureteral tumors are multicentric.
- Tumors of the ureter tend to be less invasive and smaller than those of the renal pelvis.
- Risk factors are similar to bladder TCC and include:[4]
  - Smoking
  - Aniline dyes
  - Analgesic abuse, especially phenacetin: often associated with more aggressive disease
  - Balkan nephropathy: often bilateral and with multiple sites
  - Chronic infection with calculi and obstruction (usually associated with SCC)

- Cyclophosphamide (and its metabolite, acrolein): often associated with more aggressive disease.
- Occupations with increased risk include painters, leather workers, dry cleaners, dental technicians, beauticians, metal workers, truck drivers, and autoworkers.
- Potential genetic associations:
  - Low-grade tumors may have loss of *p15* and *p16*
  - High-grade tumors may have loss of *p53*.

DIAGNOSIS AND EVALUATION[6,7]

PRESENTATION

- The most common presenting symptoms are hematuria (up to 75% of patients) and flank pain (30%).
- Renal colic associated with obstruction caused by clot and/or tumor.
- Incidental finding during abdominal imaging for other indications (approximately 10% of patients).

HISTORY AND PHYSICAL EXAM

- If advanced disease present, may have cachexia and/or a palpable flank mass.

LABORATORY TESTING

- Urinalysis and urine culture.
- Voided urinary cytology.
- Selective renal pelvic cytology obtained from ureteral washings.
- Serum electrolytes and liver function tests.

COMPUTED TOMOGRAPHY (CT)/CT UROGRAM

- Particularly useful for the assessment of larger tumors and/or metastases; less accurate for smaller tumors.[8]
- Characteristic findings:
  - Luminal filling defect
  - Obstruction and/or non-visualization of the collecting system.

MAGNETIC RESONANCE IMAGING (MRI)

- MRI provides information similar to CT.

RETROGRADE PYELOGRAPHY

- Advantage: selective urinary cytology may be obtained at the same setting.

CYSTOSCOPY

- Indicated for the evaluation of potential bladder involvement.
- May also be useful for localizing a source of gross hematuria to one or both upper urinary tracts (i.e. bloody efflux observed emanating from the ureteral orifice).

URETEROSCOPY/RENOSCOPY

- Advantages:
  - Direct visualization of the tumor
  - Ability to perform biopsy (brush or cold cup) or endoscopic resection in the same setting.
- Biopsy is performed not for staging (since depth is difficult to access without perforation of the ureter or collecting system) but to determine tumor grade, which correlates with the final pathological grade approximately 92% of the time.[9]
- Tumor grade will correlate with stage approximately 96% of the time (i.e. higher-grade tumors tend to be higher stage).[10]
- Endoluminal ultrasound may help determine tumor size and invasion.

STAGING[11]

- Tx: primary tumor cannot be assessed.
- T0: no evidence of primary tumor.
- Ta: non-invasive papillary carcinoma.
- Tis: carcinoma in situ.
- T1: tumor invades subepithelial connective tissue.
- T2: tumor invades muscularis.
- T3: tumor invades beyond muscularis into peripelvic/periureteric fat or renal parenchyma.
- T4: tumor invades adjacent organs or through the kidney into perinephric fat.
- Nx: regional lymph nodes cannot be assessed.
- N0: no regional lymph node metastasis.
- N1: metastasis to single lymph node <2 cm in greatest dimension.
- N2: metastasis in a single lymph node >2 cm but <5 cm in greatest dimension, or multiple lymph nodes, none more than 5 cm in greatest dimension.
- N3: metastasis in a lymph node more than 5 cm in greatest dimension.
- Mx: distant metastasis cannot be assessed.
- M0: no distant metastasis.
- M1: distant metastasis.

TREATMENT

RADICAL NEPHROURETERECTOMY[3]

Open nephroureterectomy with bladder cuff

- Considered the gold standard therapy.
- Preferred for large high-grade invasive tumors or large multifocal or recurrent medium-grade non-invasive tumors.
- Can be performed with two incisions (flank and lower abdominal) or one large abdominal incision.
- It is important to keep the ureter in continuity with the kidney to avoid the risk of tumor spillage.
- Complete distal ureterectomy with part of a bladder cuff is very important since the risk of recurrence in a remaining ureteral stump is 30–75%.

- Regional lymphadenectomy is controversial and serves mostly for staging. It may be of benefit in some aggressive tumors.[12]

Laparoscopic-assisted radical nephroureterectomy[13]

- Same basic surgical principles as open procedure.
- Lower abdominal incision is used to remove the specimen and perform the distal ureterectomy.
- Less estimated blood loss (EBL), less analgesic requirement, less hospital stay, and faster recovery when compared with open procedure.
- Oncological outcomes are the same as with open procedures.

Total laparoscopic radical nephroureterectomy

- More technically demanding.
- A GIA stapler may be used to transect the distal ureter with the bladder cuff.
- Alternatively, the ureteral orifice may be resected endoscopically. This approach may not assure adequate removal of bladder cuff.[14]
- Isolated port site metastases have been reported but are very rare with proper technique.[15]
- May be done entirely retroperitoneal.[16]

OPEN SEGMENTAL URETERECTOMY[3,17]

- Consider for low-grade, non-invasive tumors located in the mid or distal ureter that are not amenable to complete ablation by endoscopic means due to size or multiplicity.
- May also consider for invasive disease if renal sparing is paramount.
- Reconstruction options include:
  - Segmental ureterectomy with ureteroureterostomy
  - Distal ureterectomy with direct neocystostomy
  - Ureteroneocystostomy with a psoas muscle hitch
  - Ureteroneocystostomy with Boari flap
  - Subtotal ureterectomy with ileal substitution.

ENDOSCOPIC TREATMENT

- Indications:
  - Solitary kidney
  - Marginal renal function
  - Bilateral disease
  - Substantial medical comorbidities precluding open surgery
  - Also consider in patients with low-grade tumors and no evidence of invasive disease on abdominal imaging.
- Biopsy (basket or cold cup) of the tumor before ablation is necessary.
- Local recurrence is 40% after endoscopic treatment of renal pelvic tumors and 25% after endoscopic treatment of ureteral tumors. Recurrences are also frequent in the bladder (39%).
  - Thus, close surveillance following the initial resection is important.
- Patients with low-grade disease have survivals similar to those that undergo radical nephroureterectomy.
- Patients with high-grade disease do poorly and are likely better served with more radical surgery.[18–20]

- **Ureteroscopic resection or ablation:**
  - Appropriate for smaller ureteral tumors[21–23]
  - Energy sources: electrocautery, Nd:YAG laser, or Ho:YAG laser[24]
  - Potential complications include ureteral perforation and stricture.
- **Percutaneous resection or ablation:**
  - Appropriate for larger tumors and for tumors located in the renal pelvis and proximal ureter[25–28]
  - Administration of adjuvant therapy in the form of BCG (bacille Calmette-Guérin) or mitomycin through the nephrostomy tract is possible, but outcomes data are limited[29–31]
  - Energy sources: electrocautery, Nd:YAG laser, and Ho:YAG laser
  - Potential complications include pneumothorax, hydrothorax, hemorrhage, and collecting system/ureteral stenosis
  - Nephrostomy tract seeding is possible but extremely rare.

OUTCOMES

- Survival strongly correlates with tumor stage and grade, regardless of the type of surgery performed.[32]
  - Patients with lower-grade, lower-stage tumors will generally do well with either conservative or radical surgery
  - Patients with high-grade, high-stage tumors often do poorly even with radical surgery.
- 5-year survival by stage:
  - Stage I: 80%
  - Stage II: 50%
  - Stages III and IV: <10%.
- Risk of ipsilateral recurrence after endoscopic resection of ureteral tumors is 33–55%.[3]

POST-TREATMENT SURVEILLANCE

GENERAL PRINCIPLES

- Post-treatment surveillance is important, especially for those treated with conservative therapy.
- Surveillance should begin after radical surgery or complete endoscopic resection.[3]
- There is little evidence-based literature to support current surveillance algorithms.

SURVEILLANCE RECOMMENDATIONS[3]

Standard protocol

- Physical exam and cystoscopy:
  - Year 1: every 3 months
  - Years 2–3: every 6 months
  - ≥Year 4: every 12 months.
- Upper urinary tract imaging (CT urogram or retrograde pyelogram):
  - Every 12 months.

17

URETERAL AND RENAL PELVIC TUMORS

Patients with high-grade disease

- Follow 'standard protocol' as above.
- In addition, obtain cytology at time of physical exam and cystoscopy.

Patients status post endoscopic/organ sparing therapy

- Follow 'standard protocol' as above.
- In addition, perform ipsilateral upper urinary tract endoscopy:
  - First several years: every 6 months
  - After first several years: every 12 months.

Patients at high risk of metastatic progression

- Includes patients with high-grade and/or invasive disease.
- Perform physical exam, cystoscopy, and cytology as per 'standard protocol'.
- Chest X-ray, metabolic panel, and liver enzymes:
  - Year 1: every 3 months
  - Years 2–3: every 6 months
  - Years 4–5: every 12 months.
- CT or MRI of abdomen and pelvis:
  - Years 1–2: every 6 months
  - Years 3–5: every 12 months.
- Bone scan:
  - Not routinely necessary
  - Perform only for elevated alkaline phosphatase or bone pain symptoms.

REFERENCES

1. Silverberg E. Cancer statistics. CA Cancer J Clin 34:7–23, 1984.
2. Messing EM. Urothelial tumors of the urinary tract. In: Walsh PC, Retik AB, Vaughan ED, Wein AJ, eds. Campbell's Urology, 8th edn. Philadelphia: WB Saunders, 2002, pp 2732–84.
3. Sagalowsky AI, Jarrett TW. Management of urothelial tumors of the renal pelvis and ureter. In: Walsh PC, Retik AB, Vaughan ED, Wein AJ, eds. Campbell's Urology, 8th edn. Philadelphia: WB Saunders, pp 2845–75.
4. Kang CH, Yu TJ, Hsieh HH et al: The development of bladder tumors and contralateral upper urinary tract tumors after primary transitional cell carcinoma of the upper urinary tract. Cancer 98:1620–6, 2003.
5. Oldbring J, Glifberg I, Mikulowski P, Hellsten S: Carcinoma of the renal pelvis and ureter following bladder carcinoma: frequency, risk factors, and clinicopathological findings. J Urol 141:1311–13, 1989.
6. McDonald MW, Zincke H: Urothelial tumors of the upper urinary tract. In: deKernion JR, Paulson DF, eds. Genitourinary Cancer Management, 1st edn. Philadelphia: Lea & Febiger, 1987, pp 1–39.
7. Gomella LG: Ureter and renal pelvis – transitional cell carcinoma. In: The 5-Minute Urology Consult, 1st edn. Philadelphia: Lippincott, Williams and Wilkins, 2000, pp 554–5.
8. Badalament RA, Bennett WF, Bova JG et al: Computed tomography for detection and staging of transitional cell carcinoma of upper urinary tracts. Urology 40:71–5, 1992.
9. Guarnizo E, Pavlovich CP, Seiba M et al: Ureteroscopic biopsy of upper tract urothelial carcinoma: improved diagnostic accuracy and histopathological considerations using a multi biopsy approach. J Urol 163:52–5, 2000.
10. Keeley FX, Kulp DA, Bibbo M et al: Diagnostic accuracy of ureteroscopic biopsy in upper tract transitional cell carcinoma. J Urol 157:33–7, 1997.

11. Fleming ID, Cooper JS, Henson DE et al (eds): AJCC Cancer Staging Manual, 5th edn. Philadelphia: Lippincott-Raven, 1997.
12. Skinner D. Technique of nephroureterectomy with regional lymph node dissection. Urol Clin North Am 5:253–60, 1978.
13. Shalhav AL, Dunn MD, Portis AJ et al: Laparoscopic nephroureterectomy for upper tract transitional cell cancer: the Washington University experience. J Urol 163:1100–4, 2000
14. Jarrett TW: Laparoscopic nephroureterectomy. In: Bishoff JT, Kavoussi LR eds. Atlas of Laparoscopic Retroperitoneal Surgery. Philadelphia: W Saunders, 2000, pp 105–20.
15. Ahmed I, Shaikh NA, Kapadia CR: Track recurrence of renal pelvic transitional cell carcinoma after laparoscopic nephrectomy. Br J Urol 81:319, 1998.
16. Gill IS, Sung GT, Hobart MG et al: Laparoscopic radical nephroureterectomy for upper tract transitional cell carcinoma: the Cleveland Clinic experience. J Urol 164:1513–22, 2000.
17. Pohar KS, Sheinfeld J: When is partial ureterectomy acceptable for transitional cell carcinoma of the ureter? J Endourol 15:405–8, 2001.
18. Daneshmand S, Quek ML, Huffman JL: Endoscopic management of upper urinary tract transitional cell carcinoma: long-term experience. Cancer 98:55–60, 2003.
19. Blute ML: Treatment of upper urinary tract transitional cell carcinoma. In: Smith AD, Badlani GH, Bagley DH et al, eds. Textbook of Endourology. 1st edn. St Louis: Quality Medical Publishing, 1996, pp 352–65.
20. Lee BR, Jabbour ME, Marshall FF, Smith AD, Jarrett TW: Thirteen-year survival comparison of percutaneous and open nephroureterectomy approaches for management of transitional cell carcinoma of renal collecting system: equivalent outcomes. J Endourol 13:289–94, 1999.
21. Chen GL, Bagley DH: Ureteroscopic management of upper tract transitional cell carcinoma in patients with normal contralateral kidneys. J Urol 164:1173–6, 2000.
22. Grossman HB, Schwartz SL, Konnak JW: Ureteroscopic treatment of urothelial carcinoma of the ureter and renal pelvis. J Urol 148:275–7, 1992.
23. Bagley DH: Ureteroscopic treatment of ureteral and renal pelvic tumors: extended follow-up. J Urol 149:492A, 1993.
24. Schmeller NT, Hofstetter AG: Laser treatment of ureteral tumors. J Urol 141:840–3, 1989.
25. Jarrett TW, Sweetser PM, Weiss GH, Smith AD: Percutaneous management of transitional cell carcinoma of the renal collecting system: 9-year experience. J Urol 154:1629–35, 1995.
26. Plancke HRF, Strijbos WEM, Delaere KPJ: Percutaneous treatment of urothelial tumors of the renal pelvis. Br J Urol 75:736–9, 1995.
27. Fulgsig S, Kraup T: Percutaneous nephroscopic resection of renal pelvic tumors Scand J Urol Nephrol 172:15–19, 1995.
28. Clark PE, Streem SB, Geisinger MA: Thirteen year experience with percutaneous treatment of transitional cell carcinoma. J Urol 161:772–5, 1999.
29. Studer UE, Casanova G, Kraft R, Zingg EJ: Percutaneous bacillus Calmette-Guerin perfusion of the upper urinary tract for carcinoma in situ. J Urol 142:975–7, 1989.
30. Eastham JA, Huffman JL: Technique of mitomycin C instillation in the treatment of upper urinary tract urothelial tumors. J Urol 150:324–5, 1993.
31. Herr HW: Long-term results of BCG therapy: concern about upper tract tumors. Semin Urol Oncol 16:13–16, 1998.
32. Huffman JL: Management of upper transitional cell carcinomas. In: Volgelzang NJ, Scardino PT, Shipley WU, Coffey DS, eds. Genitourinary Oncology, 2nd edn. Philadelphia: Lippincott, Williams and Wilkins, 2000, pp 367–83.

17

URETERAL AND RENAL PELVIC TUMORS

Testicular tumors

J Kellogg Parsons

SUMMARY

- Testicular cancer is the most common solid cancer among men 15–34 years old.
- It is associated with cryptorchidism and testicular trauma.
- The most common types are seminoma and non-seminoma.
- Initial evaluation should include scrotal ultrasound, chest CT, abdominal CT, serum AFP and β-HCG, CBC, electrolytes, and liver function tests.
- Postorchiectomy treatments for seminoma include observation, radiation therapy, and chemotherapy.
- Postorchiectomy treatments for non-seminoma include observation, retroperitoneal lymph node dissection (RPLND), and chemotherapy.

18

GENERAL PRINCIPLES

Epidemiology

- Most common solid tumor in males aged 15–34 years.[1]
- Lifetime risk 1 in 500.[2,3]
- In the United States, the incidence of germ cell from 1994–1998 was 4.8 per 100 000.[1] In 1999, there were 7400 new cases.[4]
- Incidence in the Western world increased in the latter half of the 20th century for unknown reasons.[1,5]
- In the United States, rates are 5-fold greater among Whites than Blacks.[1]
- Tumors are bilateral in 2–5% of cases and may occur simultaneously or successively.[6,7] Right-sided tumors are more common.
- Associations include:
  - **Cryptorchidism** (7–10% of cases, relative risk 3–14). If unilateral, the normal testis is also at risk. It is generally believed that orchidopexy does *not* decrease the risk of subsequent cancer in either testicle but does facilitate cancer surveillance[5]
  - **Testicular trauma**.[8,9] No known causal relationship
  - Testicular microlithiasis on scrotal ultrasound. Controversial, and data are conflicting[10,11]
  - Exogenous estrogen exposure in utero[12,13]
  - Mumps orchitis[14]
  - Early onset of puberty and frequent sexual activity at a young age.[15,16]

BIOLOGY AND DEFINITIONS

Classifications

- There are two main types of testicular cancer:
  - Non-germ cell (3%): derived from non-reproductive testicular cells
  - Germ cell (97%): derived from primordial reproductive cells.

- There are two main types of germ cell cancer:
  - Seminoma
  - Non-seminoma.
- The most common type of testicular tumor in children and infants is yolk sac tumor.

Seminoma

- The most common kind of testicular cancer (60%).
- Peak incidence is at ages 35–39 years.

Non-seminoma

- Less common and more aggressive.
- There are five histologic subtypes:
  - Embryonal, teratocarcinoma, teratoma, yolk sac, and choriocarcinoma.

Etiology

- Etiology is unknown.
- One theory is that testicular atrophy may induce malignant transformation of germ cells.[8]
- The relative risk for germ cell cancer is higher among sons and brothers of affected individuals.[16,17]

Metastases

- The most common sites of metastases are retroperitoneal lymph nodes, lungs, mediastinum, and abdominal viscera.
- Initial sites for retroperitoneal metastases are called *landing zones*:
  - Right-sided landing zones: interaortocaval, precaval, and preaortic nodes
  - Left-sided landing zones: para-aortic, preaortic, and interaortocaval nodes
  - Right-sided tumors may metastasize to left-sided nodes.

Intratubular germ cell neoplasia (ITGCN)

- Formerly known as carcinoma in situ (CIS).
- A histological lesion thought to be a cancer precursor.
- 5–6% of patients with germ cell tumors will have ITGCN in the contralateral testicle on biopsy.
  - Of these, 50% will progress to invasive disease within 5 years.[18,19]
- Treatment of ITGCN is controversial.
  - Radiation will prevent subsequent cancer but may induce sterility[20]
  - Orchiectomy is curative but may lead to anorchia.

DIAGNOSIS

- Most common presentation is a palpable, painless nodule and/or painless swelling of the affected testicle (50–60%).[21]
- Other presenting symptoms:[5,21]
  - Dull ache or heavy sensation in the affected testicle (30–40%)
  - Acute testicular pain (10%)
  - Metastatic symptoms (10%)
  - Gynecomastia (5%).

- Initial evaluation:
  - Scrotal ultrasound
  - Chest X-ray *or* chest CT
  - Abdominal CT with IV contrast
  - CBC
  - Serum electrolytes and liver function tests
  - Serum tumor markers.
- Serum tumor markers:
  - After orchiectomy, elevated markers should fall to normal, commensurate with their serum half-life
  - If markers remain elevated, residual disease should be suspected
  - The two most important markers are β-HCG and AFP
  - 70% of all patients and 90% of non-seminoma patients will have an elevation in one or both of these markers.[22,23]
- *β-HCG (human chorionic gonadotropin):*
  - *Half-life = 24–36 hours*
  - Elevated in 40–60% of all testicular cancers and 10% of all seminomas[5]
  - Shares homology with luteinizing hormone (LH) and may be falsely elevated in conditions that produce elevated LH (e.g. hypogonadism).
- *AFP (α-fetoprotein):*
  - *Half-life = 5–7 days*
  - Elevated in 50–70% of all testicular tumors[5]
  - *Never elevated in pure seminoma or choriocarcinoma*
  - Normally elevated in children <1 year of age.
- Other markers:
  - LDH (lactate dehydrogenase) is a non-specific marker for testicular tumors[24]
  - PLAP (placental alkaline phosphatase) is usually expressed in fetal and infant germ cells and is rarely used clinically.[24]

INITIAL TREATMENT OF TESTICULAR TUMORS

Radical Orchiectomy

- Key surgical principles include:
  - Inguinal approach (avoids risk of scrotal violation)
  - Identification and preservation of the ilioinguinal nerve
  - Spermatic cord ligation 1–2 cm proximal to the internal ring with a permanent suture (i.e. silk) for subsequent identification during retroperitoneal lymph node dissection (RPLND).
- If the scrotum is inadvertently violated, the following treatment protocol may be followed:[25]
  - For stages I or II seminoma treated with radiation therapy (XRT), extend the radiated field to include the inguinal nodes and scrotum
  - For stages II or III seminoma treated with chemotherapy, no further treatment is required
  - For stage I non-seminoma treated with observation, resect the scrotal scar
  - For stages I–II non-seminoma treated with RPLND, resect the scrotal scar and spermatic cord

- For stages II–III non-seminoma treated with chemotherapy, no further treatment is required.

PARTIAL ORCHIECTOMY

- Partial orchiectomy to preserve testicular tissue in select patients (bilateral tumors or a solitary testicle) is an option if the tumor is small (<25 mm).[26]
- Disease-free survival may be comparable to radical orchiectomy in carefully selected patients.[27,28]

TREATMENT AND PROGNOSIS OF GERM CELL TESTICULAR TUMORS

GENERAL PRINCIPLES

- Type of treatment after orchiectomy depends upon:
  - *Tumor stage*
  - *Histology* (seminoma vs non-seminoma).
- Staging for testicular tumors (adapted from the staging system of the American Joint Committee on Cancer and the International Union Against Cancer) is given in Table 18.1.

TREATMENT AND PROGNOSIS OF SEMINOMA

- Recommendations for initial treatment for seminoma by stage are given in Table 18.2 (see also Figure 18.1).[5,29]
- 75% of seminoma patients present with stage I.
- If tumor recurs after primary XRT performed for stages I, IIA or IIB, then chemotherapy should be performed.
- If tumor recurs after primary chemotherapy, then RPLND should be performed.

TABLE 18.1

STAGING FOR TESTICULAR CANCERS

Stage	Description
Stage I	Confined to the testicle, spermatic cord, or scrotum, with or without vascular invasion
Stage IIA	Lymph node mass ≤2 cm, or multiple lymph node masses all ≤2 cm
Stage IIB	Lymph node mass >2 cm and ≤5 cm, or multiple lymph node masses with any one mass >2 cm and ≤5 cm
Stage IIC	Lymph node mass >5 cm
Stage III	Non-regional nodal, pulmonary, or visceral metastases

TABLE 18.2

INITIAL TREATMENT FOR SEMINOMA

Seminoma stage	Treatment
Stage I	Surveillance or XRT
Stage IIA	XRT
Stage IIB	XRT
Stage IIC	Chemotherapy
Stage III	Chemotherapy

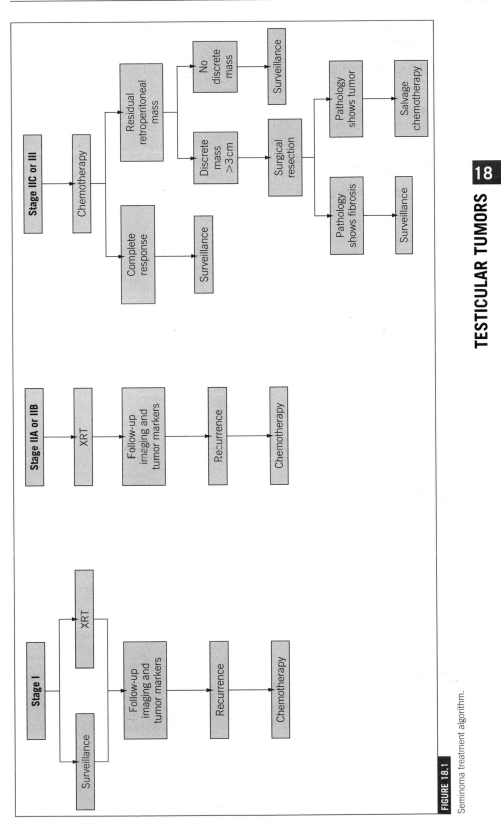

FIGURE 18.1

Seminoma treatment algorithm.

- Disease-free and cancer-specific survival rates for seminoma by treatment are given in Table 18.3.

TREATMENT AND PROGNOSIS OF NON-SEMINOMA

- Recommendations for initial treatment for non-seminoma by stage in the United States are given in Table 18.4 (see also Figure 18.2).[5,29,30]
- Disease-free and cancer-specific survival rates for non-seminoma by treatment are given in Table 18.5.[5,30]
- 30% of stage I patients treated with surveillance will relapse, >95% within 2 years of orchiectomy.[31]
- The risk for relapse in stage I patients is increased by four pathological characteristics. *If any are present, RPLND is recommended:*[32]
  - *Vascular invasion*
  - *Lymphatic invasion*
  - *Lack of yolk sac tumor*
  - *Embryonal cell carcinoma.*

TABLE 18.3

RESULTS OF SEMINOMA TREATMENT

Seminoma stage	Treatment	Disease-free survival	Cancer-specific survival
Stage I	Surveillance	84%	99%
Stage I	XRT	97%	99%
Stage IIA/B	XRT	91%	95%
Stage IIC	Chemotherapy	75–90%	>85%
Stage III	Chemotherapy	75–90%	>85%

TABLE 18.4

INITIAL TREATMENT FOR NON-SEMINOMA

Non-seminoma stage	Treatment
Stage I	Surveillance or RPLND
Stage IIA	RPLND
Stage IIB	RPLND or chemotherapy
Stage IIC	Chemotherapy
Stage III	Chemotherapy

TABLE 18.5

RESULTS OF NON-SEMINOMA TREATMENT

Non-seminoma stage	Treatment	Disease-free survival*	Cancer-specific survival
Stage I	Surveillance	65–75%	>95%
Stage I	RPLND	99%	99%
Stage IIA/B	RPLND	75%	98%
Stage IIC	Chemotherapy	>90%	70%
Stage III	Chemotherapy	50–90%	60–70%

*Includes treatment with salvage therapy if relapse occurs.

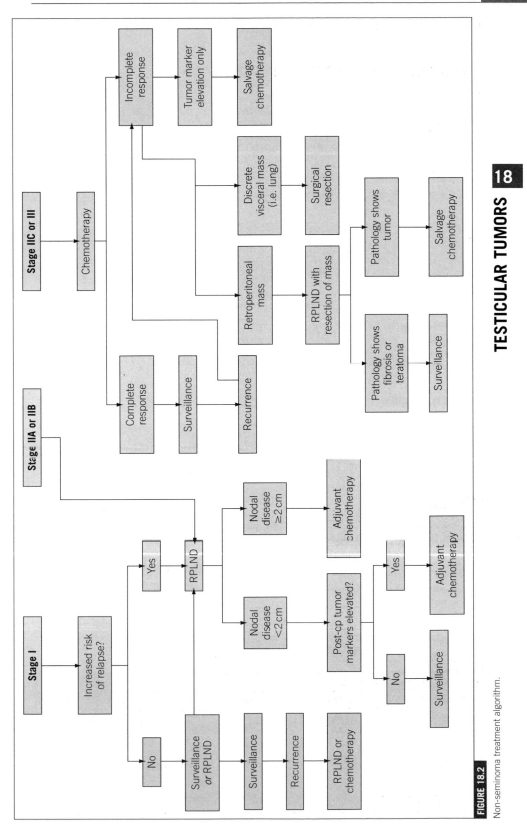

18

TESTICULAR TUMORS

FIGURE 18.2

Non-seminoma treatment algorithm.

RETROPERITONEAL LYMPH NODE DISSECTION

- Therapeutic surgery to remove metastases from the retroperitoneal lymph nodes.
- Traditionally performed through a thoracoabdominal or midline (xyphoid-to-pubis) incision.
- Key principles include:
  - 'Split and role' technique: the inferior vena cava and aorta are mobilized by splitting anterior tissue and ligating dorsal vessels
  - Nerve-sparing techniques that spare the paravertebral sympathetic chains, postganglionic efferent sympathetic nerves, and hypogastric plexus and preserve ejaculatory function in >95% of patients[5,32]
  - Removal of lymphatic tissue from the renal hila caudal to the bifurcations of the great vessels.
- Complications (13%):
  - Small bowel obstruction
  - Lymphocele
  - Wound dehiscence.
- Laparoscopic RPLND:
  - Usually performed through three midline ports
  - Morbidity and hospital stay are substantially diminished
  - Efficacy at achieving survival rates comparable to open RPLND has yet to be proven.

CHEMOTHERAPY

- Indicated as initial treatment for stages IIC and III seminoma and non-seminoma.
- First-line treatment: 2–3 cycles of bleomycin, etoposide (VP-16), and platinum (BEP). Salvage regimen includes ifosfamide and carboplatin.
- Select toxicities:
  - Bleomycin: pulmonary fibrosis
  - Carboplatin: bone marrow suppression
  - Ifosfamide: hemorrhagic cystitis.
- In the United States, primary chemotherapy for stages I, IIA, or IIB seminoma or non-seminoma remains investigational.[5]
- Adjuvant chemotherapy after RPLND for stages I, IIA, or IIB non-seminoma is recommended for patients with node-positive disease >2 cm or with persistently elevated postoperative markers.
- A retroperitoneal mass >3 cm remaining after chemotherapy most often represents desmoplastic fibrosis and/or teratoma.

TREATMENT AND PROGNOSIS OF NON-GERM CELL TESTICULAR TUMORS

SEX CORD/STROMAL TUMORS

- Sertoli cell tumor.
- Approximately 1% of all testicular tumors.[33]
- 90% are benign.
- For these, radical orchiectomy is curative.

- 10% will metastasize (retroperitoneal nodes, lung, bone).
- RPLND is indicated for nodal metastases.

LEYDIG CELL TUMOR

- May present as precocious puberty in young boys (increased testosterone).
- 90% are benign.
- For these, radical orchiectomy is curative.[5]
- 10% will metastasize (retroperitoneal or supradiaphragmatic nodes, lung, liver).
- RPLND is indicated for retroperitoneal metastases.

GRANULOSA CELL TUMOR

- Rare and similar to ovarian tumors.[33,34]
- Normally benign, but may occasionally be malignant in adults.

GONADOBLASTOMA

- Constitute 0.5% of all testicular tumors.
- Occur almost exclusively in patients with gonadal dysgenesis.[5]
- 80% of patients are phenotypic females.
- Gonadectomy is curative.
- 50% are bilateral, so bilateral gonadectomy is recommended.
- If germ cell elements present, treat per germ cell protocols.

CARCINOID

- Rare (60 case reports) and histologically identical to gastrointestinal carcinoid.
- Present with a painless testicular mass without the typical carcinoid prodrome.
- Radical orchiectomy is usually curative. Approximately 10% will metastasize.[35]

EPIDERMOID CYST

- Typical age of onset is early twenties.
- Benign.[5]
- Ultrasound shows a well-circumscribed lesion with a hyperechoic central core.
- Surgery is curative.

ADENOCARCINOMA OF THE RETE TESTIS

- Occurs in older men (peak incidence at 70 years).
- Rare (<60 case reports).
- Aggressive.
- 54% present with metastases at diagnosis.
- 1-year cancer-specific survival is <50%.
- Radical orchiectomy is indicated. The efficacy of adjuvant chemotherapy or radiation is unproven.[36]

18

TESTICULAR TUMORS

LYMPHOMA

- The most frequent testicular tumor in men >50 years old (median age at diagnosis = 60 years).[5]
- Presents as painless, diffuse testicular enlargement.
- Treatment is radical orchiectomy followed by combination chemotherapy.[37]

METASTATIC TUMORS

- Rare (approximately 200 case reports).
- Primary sources are prostate, lung, gastrointestinal tract, melanoma, and kidney.[5]

TREATMENT AND PROGNOSIS OF EXTRATESTICULAR TUMORS

These tumors originate from the epididymis, spermatic cord, or testicular tunicae and usually present as a painless scrotal mass.

ADENOMATOID TUMOR

- Most common type of paratesticular tumor.
- Incidence peaks in the 4th decade.[38]
- Benign.
- Surgery is curative.[38]

RHABDOMYOSARCOMA

- Occurs primarily in children and adolescents (80% <21 years at diagnosis).[38]
- Treatment is radical orchiectomy and chemotherapy. RPLND and radiation remain controversial.
- 5-year disease-specific survival is 58–80%.[38]

MESOTHELIOMA

- Usually presents as a painless, firm scrotal mass in association with a hydrocele.
- Most common in men aged 55–75 years.
- Associated with asbestos exposure.
- Treatment is radical orchiectomy.
- 50% of patients will develop metastases or local recurrence. Disease-specific survival is 60%.[38]

CYSTADENOMA

- Usually originates from the epididymis.
- Benign.
- Associated with von Hippel–Lindau disease.[38]
- Surgery is curative.

REFERENCES

1. McGlynn KA, Devesa SS, Sigurdson AJ et al: Trends in the incidence of testicular germ cell tumors in the United States. Cancer 97:63–70, 2003.
2. Moller H: Clues to the aetiology of testicular germ cell tumours from descriptive epidemiology. Eur Urol 23:8–15, 1993.
3. Davies JM: Testicular cancer in England and Wales; some epidemiological aspects. Lancet 2:928, 1981.
4. Steele GS, Kantoff PW, Richie JP: Staging and imaging of testis cancer. In: Vogelzang NJ, Scardino PT, Shipley WU, Coffey DS, eds. Genitourinary Oncology. Philadelphia: Lippincott, Williams and Wilkins, 2000, pp 939–49.
5. Richie JP, Steele GG: Neoplasms of the testis. In: Walsh PC, Retik AB, Vaughan ED, Wein AJ, eds. Campbell's Urology, 8th edn. Philadelphia: WB Saunders, 2002, pp 2876–919.
6. Sokal M, Peckham MJ, Hendry WF: Bilateral germ cell tumors of the testis. Br J Urol 52:158–62, 1980.
7. Dieckmann KP, Broeckmann W, Brosig W, Jonas D, Bauer HW: Bilateral testicular germ cell tumors. Report of nine cases and review of the literature. Cancer 57:1254, 1986.
8. Oliver RTD: Epidemiology of testis cancer: a clinical perspective. In: Vogelzang NJ, Scardino PT, Shipley WU, Coffey DS, eds. Genitourinary Oncology. Philadelphia: Lippincott, Williams and Wilkins, 2000, pp 880–90.
9. Merzenich H, Ahrens W, Stang A et al: Sorting the hype from the facts in testicular cancer: is testicular cancer related to trauma? J Urol 164:2143–4, 2000.
10. Otite U, Webb JA, Oliver RT, Badenoch DF, Nargund VH: Testicular microlithiasis: is it a benign condition with malignant potential? Eur Urol 40:538–42, 2001.
11. Derogee M, Bevers RF, Prins HJ et al: Testicular microlithiasis: prevalence, histopathologic findings, and relation to testicular tumor. Urology 57:1133–7, 2001.
12. Depue RH, Pke MC, Henderson BE: Estrogen exposure during gestation and risk of cancer of the testis. J Natl Cancer Inst 71:1151–5, 1983.
13. Schottenfeld D, Warshauer ME, Sherlock S et al: The epidemiology of testicular cancer in young adults. Am J Epidemiol 112:232–46, 1980.
14. Swerdlow AJ, Huttly SR, Smith PG: Testicular cancer and antecedent diseases. Br J Cancer 55:97–103, 1987.
15. Group UTCS: Social, behavioral, and medical factors in the aetiology of testicular cancer: results from the UK study. Br J Cancer 70:513–20, 1994.
16. Forman D, Chilvers C, Oliver R, Pike M: The aetiology of testicular cancer: association with congenital abnormalities, age at puberty, infertility and exercise. BMJ 308:1393–9, 1994.
17. Heimdal K, Olsson H, Trelli S et al: Familial testicular cancer in Norway and southern Sweden. Br J Cancer 73:964–9, 1996.
18. von der Maase H, Rorth M, Walbom-Jorgensen S et al: Carcinoma in situ of contralateral testis in patients with testicular germ cell cancer: study of 27 cases in 500 patients. BMJ 293:1398–401, 1986.
19. Berthelsen JG, Skakkebaek NE, von der Maase H, Sorensen BL, Mogensen P: Screening for carcinoma in situ of the contralateral testis in patients with germinal testicular cancer. BMJ 1982:1683–6, 1982.
20. Meyts ERD, Giwercman A, Skakkebaek NE: Carcinoma in situ of the testis – a precursor of testicular germ cell cancer: biological and clinical aspects. In: Vogelzang NJ, Scardino PT, Shipley WU, Coffey DS, eds. Genitourinary Oncology. Philadelphia: Lippincott, Williams and Wilkins, 2000, pp 897–908.
21. Kennedy BJ. Testis cancer: clinical signs and symptoms. In: Vogelzang NJ, Scardino PT, Shipley WU, Coffey DS, eds. Genitourinary Oncology. Philadelphia: Lippincott, Williams and Wilkins, 2000, pp 877–9.
22. Barzell WE, Whitmore WF: Clinical significance of biologic markers: Memorial Hospital experience. Semin Oncol 6:48–52, 1979.
23. Fraley EE, Lange PH, Kennedy BJ: Germ-cell testicular cancer in adults. New Engl J Med 301:1370–7, 1979.

18

TESTICULAR TUMORS

24. Bower M, Rustin GJS: Serum tumor markers and their role in monitoring germ cell cancers of the testis. In: Vogelzang NJ, Scardino PT, Shipley WU, Coffey DS, eds. Genitourinary Oncology. Philadelphia: Lippincott, Williams and Wilkins, 2000, p 931.
25. Sheinfeld J, McKiernan J, Bosl GJ: Surgery of testicular tumors. In: Walsh PC, Retik AB, Vaughan ED, Wein AJ, eds. Campbell's Urology, 8th edn. Philadelphia: WB Saunders, 2002, pp 2920–44.
26. Heidenreich A, Holtl W, Albrecht W, Pont J, Engelmann UH: Testis-preserving surgery in bilateral testicular germ cell tumors. Br J Urol 79:253–7, 1997.
27. Maneschg C, Rogatsch H, Neururer R, Bartsch G, Hobisch A: Follow-up of organ preserving tumor enucleation in testicular tumors. J Urol 163(4 Suppl):144, 2000.
28. van der Schyff S, Heidenreich A, Weissbach L, Hohlt W: Organ preserving surgery in testicular cancer – long-term results. J Urol 163(4 Suppl):145, 2000.
29. Bosl GJ, Motzer RJ: Testicular germ-cell cancer. New Engl J Med 337(4):242–53, 1997.
30. Kondagunta GV, Sheinfeld J, Mazumdar M et al: Relapse-free and overall survival in patients with pathologic stage II nonseminomatous germ cell cancer treated with etoposide and cisplatin adjuvant chemotherapy. J Clin Oncol 22(3):464–7, 2004.
31. Daugaard G, Roerth M: Observation and expectant management for low-stage seminoma and nonseminoma. In: Vogelzang NJ, Scardino PT, Shipley WU, Coffey DS, eds. Genitourinary Oncology. Philadelphia: Lippincott, Williams and Wilkins, 2000, p 976.
32. Chang SS, Sheinfeld J: Clinical Stage I Nonseminomatous Germ Cell Tumors: Treatment Options. American Urological Association Update Series 20(5):34–39, 2001.
33. Mostofi FK, Sesterhenn IA, Davis CJ. Anatomy and pathology of testis cancer. In: Vogelzang NJ, Scardino PT, Shipley WU, Coffey DS, eds. Genitourinary Oncology. Philadelphia: Lippincott Williams and Wilkins; 2000, p 909.
34. Lawrence WD, Young RH, Scully RE. Juvenile granulosa cell tumor of the infantile testis: a report of 14 cases. Am J Surg Pathol 9:87–94, 1985.
35. Singer AJ, Anders KH. Primary carcinoid of the testis 25 years after contralateral testicular seminoma. Urology 57(3):554–5, 2001.
36. Spataro V, Caldiera S, Rusca T, Sessa C, Cavalli F. Adenocarcinoma of the rete testis. J Urol 164(4):1307–8, 2000.
37. Colevas AD, Kantoff PW, DeWolf WC, Canellos GP. Malignant lymphoma of the genitourinary tract. In: Vogelzang NJ, Scardino PT, Shipley WU, Coffey DS, eds. Genitourinary Oncology. Philadelphia: Lippincott Williams and Wilkins; 2000. pp 1120–6.
38. Khoubehi B, Mishra V, Ali M, Motiwala H, Karim O. Adult paratesticular tumours. BJU Int 90(7):707–15, 2002.

Penile and urethral cancer

Craig Rogers

SUMMARY

- >95% of penile cancers are squamous cell carcinoma.
- Circumcision virtually eliminates the risk of penile cancer. Other factors associated with increased risk include HPV, smoking, and poor hygiene.
- Evaluation of a penile tumor includes physical exam (particularly of inguinal lymph nodes), biopsy, and abdominal–pelvic CT or MRI.
- Treatment of penile cancer is based on T stage, size, and proximal extent of tumor. Surgical treatment options range from circumcision and local excision to anterior exenteration.
- Inguinal lymph nodes are the most common site for metastases.
- Patients presenting with adenopathy should receive a 6-week course of antibiotics. If adenopathy persists after treatment, lymphadenectomy is indicated.

19

CANCER OF THE PENIS

EPIDEMIOLOGY

- >95% are squamous cell carcinoma.
- Incidence:[1]
  - Thought to be decreasing
  - 0.3–0.6% of all genitourinary cancers in US males
  - Up to 10% of male malignancies in some uncircumcised populations of Asia and Africa.
- Associations:
  - Phimosis: newborn circumcision virtually eliminates the risk of penile cancer, whereas circumcision after puberty is not protective[2]
  - HPV 16, 18, 31, 33
  - Smoking
  - Smegma (chronic irritation/inflammation)
  - Poor hygiene
  - No proven associations with race, substance abuse, occupation.[3]

STAGING (AMERICAN JOINT COMMITTEE ON CANCER 1997)[4]

- Tumor:
  - Tis: carcinoma in situ
  - T0: no evidence of primary tumor
  - Ta: non-invasive verrucous carcinoma
  - T1: tumor invasion into subepithelial connective tissue
  - T2: tumor invasion into corpus spongiosum or cavernosum
  - T3: tumor invasion into urethra or prostate
  - T4: tumor invasion into other structures.
- Node:
  - Nx: regional nodes cannot be assessed

- NO: no evidence of regional lymph node metastases
- N1: metastasis in a single regional lymph node
- N2: metastases in multiple or bilateral superficial inguinal lymph nodes
- N3: Metastases in deep inguinal or pelvic lymph nodes, unilateral or bilateral.
- Metastasis:
  - Mx: distant metastasis cannot be assessed
  - M0: no distant metastasis
  - M1: distant metastasis.

DIAGNOSIS

Presentation

- Generally diagnosed in older men (mean age 58 years).
- Delayed presentation relatively common owing to reluctance of patients to seek medical care.
- Presentation:
  - Most common: painless lesion that occasionally may itch or burn
  - Less common: paraneoplastic syndrome (i.e. hypercalcemia).
- Location:
  - Glans more common than prepuce more common than shaft.

Evaluation

- Physical exam:
  - Primary lesion may appear nodular, ulcerative, or fungating
  - Important to assess for inguinal lymphadenopathy.
- Biopsy:
  - Normally indicated for tissue diagnosis primary to definitive management; however, if there is high clinical suspicion, may consider performing an intraoperative frozen section to confirm diagnosis prior to penectomy
  - Include normal-appearing adjacent tissue for comparison
  - May need dorsal slit for exposure
  - Topical acetic acid 5% may help delineate extent of the lesion.
- Imaging:
  - Assessment of the primary lesion with CT, MRI, or ultrasound usually adds little information, especially for small-volume, distal lesions
  - However, pelvic and abdominal CT or MRI is useful for assessing lymph node involvement and distant metastases, or for guiding fine needle aspiration of suspicious lymph nodes.

MANAGEMENT OF PRIMARY TUMOR

Tis, Ta, T1

- Local excision/circumcision.
- Laser excision:
  - Appropriate for small, superficial, distal tumors
  - CO_2 or Nd:YAG.
- Mohs' micrographic surgery:
  - Remove layer by layer (zinc chloride fixation vs fresh tissue technique) under microscopic guidance until negative margin is achieved

- Best for small lesions of the glans
- Potential complications: meatal stenosis and glanular disfigurement.
- Topical 5-FU (5-fluorouracil):
  - May cause topical dermatitis, which may be difficult to distinguish from progression.
- Radiation therapy (XRT):
  - Rarely indicated
  - Occasionally appropriate for small, distal, superficial lesions in patients refusing surgery
  - Good response in select patients but may later require partial penectomy for local complications, including fistula, stricture, stenosis, and penile necrosis.[5]
- Inguinal lymph node management:
  - Risk of inguinal lymph node disease is small (<10%)
  - Therefore, lymphadenectomy is not indicated.

T2–T4

- Partial penectomy:
  - Appropriate for smaller, more distal tumors
  - 2 cm proximal margin is required
  - Goal if possible is to preserve ≥3 cm of penile shaft, which should preserve the ability to stand while urinating and maintain some sexual function.
- Total penectomy.
  - Appropriate for larger, more proximal tumors
  - Perineal urethrostomy allows patient to sit and void.
- Anterior exenteration:
  - Appropriate for tumors involving the scrotum or pubis or for those with extensive, fixed inguinal lymph nodes
  - May involve scrotectomy, orchiectomy, resection of lower abdominal wall, and/or resection of the pubic symphysis.
- Inguinal lymph node (LN) management if non-palpable:
  - Up to 2/3 of lymph nodes positive even if non-palpable. Prophylactic inguinal LN dissection acceptable.[6]

MANAGEMENT OF INGUINAL LYMPH NODES

General principles

- Most common metastatic site.
- Lymph node drainage from penis is as follows: superficial inguinal to deep inguinal to pelvic.
- Complications associated with advanced inguinal lymph node disease: skin necrosis, infection, sepsis, and hemorrhage from erosion of femoral vessels.
- Lymph node management of penile cancer continues to evolve.

Treatment of lymphadenopathy

- Inguinal lymphadenopathy is due to inflammation – not metastatic tumor – in up to 50% of cases.
- Therefore, for patients presenting with lymphadenopathy, a 6-week course of antibiotics following complete resection of the primary tumor is indicated.

19

PENILE AND URETHRAL CANCER

- If adenopathy remains after antibiotic treatment, lymphadenectomy is indicated.
- For unilateral palpable adenopathy, consider superficial lymph node dissection of the contralateral side with frozen section analysis followed by deep dissection if tumor present:
  - If delayed presentation of unilateral palpable lymph nodes after management of primary lesion, consider unilateral dissection only.

Inguinal lymph node dissection

- Anatomical boundaries: femoral triangle (sartorius, inguinal ligament, adductor longus) lies over iliopsoas and pectineus under fascia lata.
- Superficial and deep lymph nodes are separated by the fascia lata.
- Recommended if high risk for progression: ≥T2, palpable LN after resection of primary lesion and antibiotics or with prior history of penile cancer, biopsy-proven positive LN, high-grade tumors (low-grade, non-invasive tumors have low potential for inguinal metastases), or lymphovascular invasion.
- Sartorius flap can be used to cover femoral vessels.
- Surgical principles – 'modified' LN dissection:[7] smaller skin incision, limited LN dissection with boundaries of adductor longus (medial), femoral artery (lateral), spermatic cord (superiorly), fossa ovalis (inferiorly). Dissection lateral to femoral artery and caudal to fossa ovalis omitted. Preserves saphenous vein. No transposition of sartorius.

Radiation

- Less effective and more morbid compared with lymphadenectomy.
- Consider as palliative option for patients with advanced disease who want penile preservation.

Management of metastatic disease

- ≤10% of patients will present with distant metastases.
- Most common sites (in order from most to least common): lung, liver, bone, and brain.
- Chemotherapy:
  - Bleomycin, methotrexate, cisplatin, and vincristine have been used
  - Response is usually partial and of short duration.
- Neoadjuvant chemotherapy potentially may have role in down-staging prior to resection.

PROGNOSIS

- Adverse prognostic factors:
  - Positive lymph nodes
  - High stage
  - High grade.
- 95% of untreated patients with inguinal lymph node involvement will die within 2–3 years.[8]
- 5-year disease-specific survival:[9]
  - Negative lymph nodes: 73% (range 46–100%)
  - Positive inguinal nodes: 60% (0–86%)
  - Positive pelvic nodes: <10%.

OTHER NEOPLASTIC LESIONS OF THE PENIS

CARCINOMA IN SITU (CIS)

- Premalignant lesion.
- <10% will progress to invasive squamous cell carcinoma.
- Gross appearance: a red, velvety, well-marginated lesion.
- CIS lesions are classically referred to by two different terms, depending on the location of the lesion:
  - Distal (prepuce, glans, or shaft): *erythroplasia of Queyrat*
  - Proximal (remainder of genitalia/perineum): *Bowen's disease.*
- Treatment:
  - As above (under Tis).

CUTANEOUS HORN

- Overgrowth of epithelium, usually over a pre-existing skin lesion.
- May evolve to carcinoma or develop as a reaction to underlying carcinoma.[10]

BALANITIS XEROTICA OBLITERANS (BXO)

- A genital form of lichen sclerosus et atrophicus.
- Usually presents as white patches of the glans/prepuce; often involves the meatus and urethra.
  - May cause distal urethral obstruction secondary to meatal and/or urethral obstruction.
- Associated with urethral strictures and squamous cell carcinoma.[11]
- Treatment:
  - Steroids (topical vs injectable), meatoplasty, meatal/urethral dilation, excision
  - Consider biopsy if recurrent or rapidly progressive.

CONDYLOMA ACUMINATUM

- Rare before puberty, usually on glans, shaft, or prepuce.
- Associated with human papillomavirus (HPV) and squamous cell carcinoma.[12]
- Approximately 5% will involve the urethra.
- Diagnosis: 5% acetic acid helps detect subclinical disease (turns involved area 'aceto-white' to direct biopsy).
- Treatment:
  - Podophyllin (since it may induce atypical histological changes, consider biopsy prior to use)
  - Laser ablation
  - 5-FU for intraurethral lesions.

BOWENOID PAPULOSIS

- Histologically identical to CIS but benign clinical course.[13]

LEUKOPLAKIA

- Presents as white plaques, often causing irritation.
- May involve the meatus.

- Malignant transformation may occur in up to 10–20%.
- Associated with squamous cell carcinoma and verrucous carcinoma.[14,15]
- Treatment:
  - Biopsy/local excision.

VERRUCOUS CARCINOMA (BUSCHKE–LÖWENSTEIN TUMOR)

- Presents clinically as an exophytic, cauliflower-like lesion.
- Similar to squamous cell carcinoma but does not metastasize.
  - Is locally invasive: displaces, invades, and destroys adjacent structures by compression.
- Can have concomitant squamous cell carcinoma.
- Treatment:
  - Complete excision: will recur if excision is incomplete.

KAPOSI'S SARCOMA[16]

- A vascular lesion associated with AIDS and immunosuppression.
- Presents as raised, blue papules or ulcers that may bleed.
- Associated with HHV-8 (human herpesvirus).[17]
- Treatment:
  - Local radiation
  - Laser ablation
  - May consider perineal urethrostomy for severe, recalcitrant disease with urinary obstruction.

METASTASES[18]

- Rare.
- Most common primary sites: bladder, prostate, and rectum.
  - May also occur with leukemia.
- Most common symptom: priapism.
  - Other symptoms: edema, pain, penile nodules, ulceration, and urinary obstruction.
- Usually portends a poor prognosis, with survival often less than 1 year.

CARCINOMA OF THE URETHRA

EPIDEMIOLOGY[19,20]

- Very rare, representing <1% of all genitourinary (GU) cancers.
- The only GU cancer that occurs more frequently in females than males (4:1).
- Associations:
  - Sexually transmitted diseases (STDs), including HPV
  - Urethral stricture disease.
- Age range at presentation: 13–91 years (mean 50 years).

LOCATION AND HISTOLOGY[21]

- Location and histology vary by gender.

Women

- Frequency by location:
  - 35–50%: anterior (distal 1/3 of the urethra)
  - 50–65%: posterior (proximal 2/3).
- Pathology (typical location):
  - 50–70%: squamous cell carcinoma (anterior)
  - 12–15%: transitional cell carcinoma (posterior)
  - 15–35%: adenocarcinoma (posterior urethral; urethral diverticula; Cowper's glands).

Men

- Frequency by location:
  - 20–30%: anterior (penile urethra)
  - 70–80%: posterior (bulbomembranous and prostatic urethra).
- Pathology (typical location):
  - 60–80%: squamous cell carcinoma (anterior)
  - 15–20%: transitional cell carcinoma (posterior)
  - <5%: adenocarcinoma (membranous).

STAGING (TNM STAGING SYSTEM)[22]

- Tumor:
  - Tx: primary tumor cannot be assessed
  - T0: no evidence of primary tumor
  - Ta: non-invasive papillary, polypoid, or verrucous carcinoma
  - Tis: carcinoma in situ
  - T1: tumor invasion into subepithelial connective tissue
  - T2: tumor invasion into any of the following: corpus spongiosum, prostate, or periurethral muscle
  - T3: tumor invasion into any of the following: corpus cavernosum, beyond prostatic capsule, anterior vagina, or bladder neck
  - T4: tumor invasion into adjacent organs.
- Node:
  - Nx: regional nodes cannot be assessed
  - N0: no evidence of regional lymph node metastases
  - N1: metastasis in a single lymph node, ≤2 cm
  - N2: metastases in a single lymph node >2 cm and ≤5 cm or in multiple nodes ≤5 cm
  - N3: metastases in any lymph node >5 cm.
- Metastasis:
  - Mx: distant metastasis cannot be assessed
  - M0: no distant metastasis
  - M1: distant metastasis.

DIAGNOSIS

Presentation

- Ulceration, fistula, urethral stricture, urinary obstruction, palpable urethral mass, frequency, urethral bleeding, and/or discharge.
  - More proximal lesions tend to be diagnosed at more advanced stages.

19

PENILE AND URETHRAL CANCER

Evaluation

- Cystourethroscopy with biopsy.
- Imaging:
  - Retrograde urethrogram: may be useful for localizing tumor prior to cystoscopy
  - CT or MRI useful for staging (i.e. assessing direct pelvic extension and lymph node involvement).

SURGICAL THERAPY

Women

- Anterior:
  - Transurethral resection (for superficial tumors only)
  - Partial urethrectomy.
- Posterior:
  - Anterior exenteration.

Men

- Anterior:
  - Transurethral resection (for superficial tumors only)
  - Partial or total penectomy.
- Posterior
  - Radical cystoprostatectomy
  - Anterior exenteration.

RADIATION THERAPY

- A therapeutic option primarily for women.
- May be used alone or in combination with surgery.
- Most effective for small, early-stage, distal lesions.[23]

ADVANCED DISEASE

- Locally aggressive:
  - Combinations of radiation, chemotherapy, and surgery have been used (multimodality therapy).
- Distant metastases:
  - Chemotherapy: regimens include MMC (mitomycin C)/5-FU and MVAC (methotrexate, vinblastine, Adriamycin, cyclophosphamide)
  - Palliative radiation.

LYMPH NODES[21]

- Anterior urethra drains to the inguinal lymph nodes.
- Posterior urethra drains to the pelvic lymph nodes.
  - Pelvic lymph node disease portends an extremely poor prognosis.
- Palpable inguinal nodes at time of presentation are usually involved with cancer and should be removed with lymphadenectomy.
  - Unlike penile cancer, antibiotics are not given.
- Prophylactic inguinal lymphadenectomy has no proven benefit.

PROGNOSIS

- Depends on tumor location and stage.
- Unlike penile cancer, grade is *not* a prognostic factor.
- Anterior urethral tumors are more amenable to surgery and generally have better prognoses.
- Posterior tumors are more likely to have extensive local involvement and distant metastasis with poorer prognosis.[24]

SPECIAL CASE: THE RETAINED URETHRA AFTER RADICAL CYSTECTOMY

- 10% risk of urethral recurrence after radical cystectomy for transitional cell carcinoma.
- Risk is increased with invasion of prostatic ducts (15%), prostatic stroma (23%), bladder neck, or with positive urethral margin.
- Recommendations for post-op surveillance:
  - Urethral wash cytology and urethroscopy (with biopsy if indicated) every 4–6 months.[25]
- Treatment for recurrence: urethrectomy.
  - Although biopsy-proven recurrence is the strongest indication, also consider urethrectomy for positive urethral wash cytology or persistent bloody urethral discharge[26]
  - Urethrectomy may adversely affect potency.

19

PENILE AND URETHRAL CANCER

REFERENCES

1. Gloeckler-Ries LA, Hankey BF, Edwards BK: Cancer Statistics Review. National Cancer Institute, National Institutes of Health Publication No. 90–2789. Bethesda: National Institutes of Health, 1990.
2. Maden C, Sherman KJ, Beckmann AM et al: History of circumcision, medical conditions, and sexual activity and risk of penile cancer. J Natl Cancer Inst 85:19–24, 1993.
3. Lynch DF, Pettaway CA: Tumors of the penis. In: Walsh PC, Retik AB, Vaughan ED, Wein AJ, eds. Campbell's Urology, 8th edn. Philadelphia: WB Saunders, 2002, pp 2945–81.
4. Fleming ID, Cooper JS, Henson DE: Penis. AJCC Cancer Staging Manual/American Joint Committee on Cancer. Philadelphia: Lippincott-Raven, 1977, pp 215–17.
5. Duncan W, Jackson SM: The treatment of early cancer of the penis with megavoltage x-rays. Clin Radiol 23:246–8, 1972.
6. Cabanas RM: An approach for the treatment of penile carcinoma. Cancer 39: 456–66, 1977.
7. Catalona WJ: Modified inguinal lymphadenectomy for carcinoma of the penis with preservation of saphenous veins: technique and preliminary results. J Urol 140:306–10, 1988.
8. Derrick FC Jr, Lynch KM Jr, Kretkowski RC, Yarbrough WJ: Epidermoid carcinoma of the penis: computer analysis of 87 cases. J Urol 110:303–5, 1973.
9. Ravi R: Correlation between the extent of nodal involvement and survival following groin dissection for carcinoma of the penis. Br J Urol 72:817–19, 1993.
10. Hassan AA, Orteza AM, Milam DF: Penile horn: review of literature with 3 case reports. J Urol 97:315–17, 1967.
11. Simonart T, Noel JC, De Dobbeleer G, Simonart JM: Carcinoma of the glans penis arising 20 years after lichen sclerosus. Dermatology 196:337–8, 1998.
12. Dawson DF, Duckworth JK, Bernhardt H, Young JM: Giant condyloma and verrucous carcinoma of the genital area. Arch Pathol 79:225–31, 1965.
13. Su CK, Shipley WU: Bowenoid papulosis: a benign lesion of the shaft of the penis misdiagnosed as squamous carcinoma. J Urol 157:1361–2, 1997.

14. Hanash KA, Furlow WL, Utz DC, Harrison EG Jr: Carcinoma of the penis: a clinicopathologic study. J Urol 104:291–7, 1970.
15. Reece RW, Koontz WW Jr: Leukoplakia of the urinary tract: a review. J Urol 114:165–71, 1975.
16. Braun M: Classics in oncology. Idiopathic multiple pigmented sarcoma of the skin by Kaposi. CA Cancer J Clin 32:340–7, 1982.
17. Jaffe HW, Pellett PE: Human herpesvirus 8 and Kaposi's sarcoma – some answers, more questions. New Engl J Med 340:1912–13, 1999.
18. Robey EL, Schellhammer PF: Four cases of metastases to the penis and a review of the literature. J Urol 132:992–4, 1984.
19. Dalbagni G, Zhang ZF, Lacombe L, Herr HW: Male urethral carcinoma: analysis of treatment outcome. Urology 53:1126–32, 1999.
20. Donat SM, Cozzi PJ, Herr HW: Surgery of penile and urethral carcinoma. In: Walsh PC, Retik AB, Vaughan ED, Wein AJ, eds. Campbell's Urology, 8th edn. Philadelphia: WB Saunders, 2002, pp 2983–99.
21. Grisby PW, Herr HW: Urethral tumors. In: Vogelzang N, Scardino PT, Shipley WU, eds. Comprehensive Textbook of Genitourinary Oncology. Baltimore: Williams and Wilkins, 2000, pp 1133–9.
22. Donat SM, Cozzi PJ, Herr HW: Surgery of penile and urethral carcinoma. In: Walsh PC, Retik AB, Vaughan ED, Wein AW, eds. Campbell's Urology, 8th edn. Philadelphia: WB Saunders, 2002, pp 2983–99.
23. Sailer SL, Shipley WU, Wang CC: Carcinoma of the female urethra: a review of results with radiation therapy. J Urol 140:1–5, 1988.
24. Zeidman EJ, Desmond P, Thompson IM: Surgical treatment of carcinoma of the male urethra. Urol Clin North Am 19:359–72, 1992.
25. Schellhammer PF, Whitmore WF Jr: Urethral meatal carcinoma following cystourethrectomy for bladder carcinoma. J Urol 115:61–4, 1976.
26. Hermansen DK, Badalament RA, Whitmore WF Jr, Fair WR, Melamed MR: Detection of carcinoma in the post-cystectomy urethral remnant by flow cytometric analysis. J Urol 139:304–7, 1988.

Diseases of the adrenal gland

J Kellogg Parsons

SUMMARY

- Conn's syndrome is autonomous secretion of aldosterone, resulting in hyperaldosteronism. The two primary causes are adrenal adenoma and bilateral adrenal hyperplasia. Treatment for adenoma is surgery; treatment for hyperplasia is spironolactone.
- Pheochromocytoma is a catecholamine-secreting tumor. Classic presentation is headache, tachycardia, diaphoresis, and hypertension. Treatment is surgery.
- Adrenal cortical carcinoma is a rare, aggressive malignancy. Up to 80% are functional and may secrete cortisol and/or androgens. Treatment is surgery. Prognosis is poor.
- Cancers that most commonly metastasize to the adrenals include kidney, melanoma, breast, and lung.
- Cushing's syndrome is caused by an excess of circulating glucocorticoids and presents with hypertension, glucose intolerance, muscle wasting, thin skin, hirsutism, moon facies, buffalo hump, and easy bruisability. It may be ACTH-independent or -dependent. Treatment depends upon etiology.
- Acute adrenal insufficiency requires urgent intervention.
- Adrenal incidentaloma is a mass detected in a patient who undergoes abdominal imaging for reasons unrelated to the adrenal. Approximately 80% of incidentalomas are non-functioning adenomas.

20

ADRENAL ANATOMY

CORTEX

- Outermost layer.
- 85–90% of adrenal tissue.
- Little to no innervation.
- Contains three distinct zones (Table 20.1).

TABLE 20.1

ADRENAL ANATOMY

	Zone	Hormones
Superficial	Zona glomerulosa	Aldosterone (and other mineralocorticoids)
↓	Zona fasciculata	Cortisol
Deep	Zona reticularis	Sex steroid hormones

MEDULLA

- Innermost layer, surrounded by the cortex.
- 10–15% of adrenal tissue.
- Innervation is primarily sympathetic.
- Composed of chromaffin cells derived from neuroectoderm tissue.
- Secretes catecholamines (epinephrine, norepinephrine, and dopamine).

PRIMARY HYPERALDOSTERONISM: (CONN'S SYNDROME)

GENERAL INFORMATION

- Autonomous secretion of aldosterone independent of the normal angiotensin–renin axis.
- Caused by cortical adenoma (75%) or bilateral adrenal hyperplasia (25%).[1]
- The overabundance of aldosterone results in sodium retention, potassium wasting, and hypertension.
- Typically affects whites 30–60 years of age.
- Prevalence:[2]
  - ~ 0.5–1% of patients with essential hypertension and hypokalemia
  - ~ 5–13% of patients with essential hypertension.

DIAGNOSIS

Presentation

- Usually asymptomatic.
  - May have muscle weakness, polydipsia, headache, urinary frequency, and nocturia.
- Essential hypertension.

Evaluation

- Hypokalemia (<3.0 mEq/dl):
  - Worsened by diuretics.
- May have mild metabolic alkalosis and hypernatremia.
- Increased plasma aldosterone (>15 ng/dl).
- Decreased plasma renin (<2 ng/ml).
- Increased plasma aldosterone:renin (>20:1).
- Sodium restriction will reduce potassium wasting and will decrease symptoms; sodium load will worsen potassium wasting.
- Administration of high sodium diet × 3 days (>200 mEq/day).
- 24-hour urine aldosterone >14 μg and potassium >30 mEq.
- Distinguishing adenoma from bilateral hyperplasia:
  - Abdominal CT showing cortical mass
  - Potassium <3.0 ng/ml
  - Increased plasma 18-hydroxycorticosterone
  - Increased urine 18-hydroxycortisol
  - Adrenal vein sampling of aldosterone.

TREATMENT

- Adenoma:
  - Initial treatment is antihypertensive (spironolactone) and repletion of potassium
  - Definitive treatment is adrenalectomy (laparoscopic or open)
  - Outcomes: 35% cured, 56% improved, 9% no improvement.
- Bilateral hyperplasia.

PHEOCHROMOCYTOMA

GENERAL INFORMATION

- Tumor which secretes catecholamines (primarily epinephrine and norepinephrine).
- Responsible for 0.2% of cases of hypertension.
- Most often adrenal in origin, but may occur anywhere in the paraganglion system.
- 'Rule of 10's':
  - 10% bilateral
  - 10% familial
  - 10% pediatric
  - 10% malignant
  - 10% extra-adrenal.
- Associations:
  - Multiple endocrine neoplasia (IIA and IIB)
  - Von Recklinghausen's neurofibromatosis
  - Von Hippel–Lindau disease.

DIAGNOSIS

Presentation

- Classic triad:
  - Headache, tachycardia, and diaphoresis.
- ~90% are hypertensive.
  - ~10% are normotensive.

Evaluation[3]

- Elevated plasma-free metanephrines:
  - Most sensitive test.
- Elevated 24-hour urinary catecholamines.
- Elevated 24-hour urinary metanephrines:
  - Total metanephrines
  - Vanillylmandelic acid (VMA).
- Clonidine suppression test:
  - Positive test: no suppression of hypertension 3 hours after administration of clonidine 0.3 mg PO.
- Imaging:
  - CT
  - MRI
  - MIBG.

20

DISEASES OF THE ADRENAL GLAND

TREATMENT

Standard treatment is adrenalectomy.

PREOPERATIVE MANAGEMENT

- Obtain anesthesiology and endocrinology consultations.
- Treat hypertension with:
  - Calcium channel blockers
  - Selective alpha-1 blocker: prazosin
  - Non-selective alpha blocker: phenoxybenzamine
  - Beta blocker: use only after alpha blocker has been started; usually used to treat associated cardiac arrhythmias.

Surgery

- Laparoscopic or open.

Perioperative management

- Monitor/control intraoperative hypertension.
  - May have postexcision hypotension.
- Postoperative hypotension usually associated with hypovolemia.
- Postoperative hypertension may be secondary to temporarily elevated catecholamine levels or retained tissue.

Outcomes

- 5% will have benign recurrence.
- 10% will have malignant recurrence.
- 20-year cause survival is 80%.

ADRENAL CORTICAL CARCINOMA

GENERAL INFORMATION[4]

- Rare, malignant tumor of the adrenal cortex.
- Incidence: 1 per 1.7 million per year.
- Accounts for only 0.02% of cancers.
- Up to 80% are functional.
  - May secrete multiple hormones
  - Cortisol and androgen are most common.
- Aggressive.
- Most common sites of metastases are lymph nodes, lung, and liver.

DIAGNOSIS

Presentation

- Asymptomatic (i.e. incidentaloma).
- Constitutional symptoms:
  - Fevers, weight loss, malaise.
- Endocrine symptoms:
  - Increased cortisol: Cushing's disease (see below)
  - Increased androgens: virilization in females
  - Increased estrogens: oligomenorrhea in females and feminization in males.

Evaluation

- Imaging:
  - Diagnosis is typically made on CT or MRI
  - Most are >6 cm
  - Typically have an irregular, heterogeneous appearance
  - Will appear bright on T-2 weighted MRI (benign adenoma will not).
- Endocrine evaluation.

STAGING

- Tumor:
  - T1: <5 cm, no invasion of adjacent structures
  - T2: >5 cm, no invasion of adjacent structures
  - T3: local invasion only
  - T4: invasion into adjacent organs.
- Node:
  - Nx: regional nodes cannot be assessed
  - N0: no evidence of regional lymph node metastases
  - N1: involvement of regional lymph nodes.
- Metastasis:
  - Mx: distant metastasis cannot be assessed
  - M0: no distant metastasis
  - M1: distant metastasis.

TREATMENT

- Surgery:
  - Adrenalectomy with regional lymphadenectomy and excision of involved adjacent organs.
- Metastases:
  - Mitotane.
- Outcomes:
  - Generally poor
  - 5-year survival is 15–60%[4,5]
  - Overall mean survival is 18 months
  - Median survival for metastatic disease is 6.5 months.

ADRENAL METASTASES

GENERAL INFORMATION[6,7]

- Autopsy series show that 8–38% of patients with extra-adrenal cancers will have adrenal metastases.
- Organs that most commonly metastasize to the adrenal gland are kidney, melanoma, breast, and lung.
- Among patients with a known primary cancer, an adrenal mass will be a metastasis ~50% of the time.

20

DISEASES OF THE ADRENAL GLAND

DIAGNOSIS

Presentation

- Commonly presents as an adrenal mass in the setting of a known extra-adrenal primary cancer.
- May also present as an incidentaloma.

Evaluation

- Imaging:
  - CT: irregular, heterogeneous appearance
  - MRI: Bright on T-2 weighted MRI.
- If there are no other sites of metastasis present, perform same evaluation as for incidentaloma (see below).
- Consider CT-guided fine needle aspiration.
- Rule out pheochromocytoma first.

TREATMENT

- Depending on type of primary cancer and patient status, adrenalectomy may be considered for treatment of a solitary adrenal metastasis.

CUSHING'S SYNDROME

GENERAL INFORMATION

- Definition: the clinical syndrome caused by an excess of circulating glucocorticoids.
  - *Cushing's disease*: an excess of circulating glucocorticoids caused by hypersecretion of adrenocorticotropic hormone (ACTH) by the anterior pituitary
  - *Pseudo-Cushing's syndrome*: excess cortisol caused by an exogenous source (i.e. medication), major depression, alcoholism, obesity, or diabetes.[8]
- Incidence is 2–13 per million per year.[9,10]
- 0.2% of patients with hypertension.
- Causes of Cushing's syndrome are generally classified as ACTH-dependent and ACTH-independent (Table 20.2).[2,8–10]

TABLE 20.2

CAUSES OF CUSHING'S SYNDROME

Cause	Proportion (%)
ACTH-dependent:	
Pituitary hypersecretion of ACTH	70
Ectopic ACTH production	12
ACTH-independent:	
Adrenal adenoma	8
Adrenal cortical carcinoma	6
Bilateral adrenal hyperplasia	4

DIAGNOSIS

Presentation

- Obesity (especially truncal), hypertension, glucose intolerance/diabetes, muscle wasting, thin skin, hirsutism, amenorrhea, moon facies, buffalo hump, easy bruisability, and impaired wound healing.

Evaluation[2]

- First, rule out pseudo-Cushing's syndrome.
- Secondly, perform 24-hour urinary free cortisol:
  - >100 mg is diagnostic for Cushing's syndrome.
- If urinary free cortisol result is equivocal, perform low-dose dexamethasone suppression test:
  - Late p.m.: administer dexamethasone 1 mg PO × 1
  - Early next a.m.: check plasma cortisol
  - If a.m. cortisol <5 ng/ml, then patient is suppressing cortisol appropriately and does *not* have Cushing's syndrome
  - Sensitivity is 78–86% and specificity is 92–93%.[11]
- If urinary cortisol or dexamethasone suppression test suggest Cushing's disease, check serum ACTH:
  - ACTH >15 pg/ml indicates ACTH dependence: perform high-dose dexamethasone suppression test (see below)
  - ACTH <5 pg/ml indicates ACTH independence: perform abdominal CT or MRI.
- If ACTH is elevated, perform high-dose dexamethasone suppression:
  - Late p.m.: administer dexamethasone 8 mg PO × 1
  - Early next a.m.: check plasma cortisol
  - If a.m. cortisol level reduced <50%: ectopic ACTH
  - If a.m. cortisol level reduced >50%: pituitary tumor.

TREATMENT

Depends upon etiology.

Pituitary tumor

- Trans-sphenoidal hypophysectomy.
- If fails, consider radiotherapy vs bilateral adrenalectomy.

Ectopic ACTH production

- Surgical therapy:
  - Excise source if possible.
- Medical therapy:
  - Adrenolytic agents including metyrapone, ketoconazole, mitotane, or aminoglutethimide.

Adrenal adenoma or cortical carcinoma

- Unilateral adrenalectomy.

Bilateral adrenal hyperplasia

- Bilateral adrenalectomy:
  - *Nelson's syndrome* = Caused by ACTH-secreting pituitary adenoma
  - Occurs in 10–20% of patients postoperatively; may occur years later
  - Characterized by vision changes, headache, and hyperpigmentation.

ADRENAL INSUFFICIENCY

GENERAL INFORMATION

- Definition: deterioration of adrenal mineralocorticoid and glucocorticoid function.
- May be acute or chronic.
  - Acute also called adrenal crisis.
- Etiologies include surgical removal, abrupt removal of an exogenous steroid source (i.e. medication), pituitary disease, autoimmune and infectious adrenalitis, adrenal hemorrhage, metastatic disease, and hypoperfusion (typically in a critically ill patient).
- Prevalence is 1 in 4500 to 1 in 6250 hospitalized patients.

DIAGNOSIS

Presentation

- Acute:
  - Severe hypotension, lethargy/weakness, fevers, and nausea/vomiting.
- Chronic:
  - Weight loss
  - Chronic fatigue
  - Nausea/vomiting.
- *A common clinical presentation is in a hospitalized patient after surgery and/or in the ICU.*

Evaluation

- Hyperkalemia, hyponatremia, and hypoglycemia.[3]
- 15–20% may have eosinophilia.
- Check serum cortisol and ACTH levels.
- Cosyntropin stimulation test.[3]
  - 0.25 mg cosyntropin IV × 1
  - Check serum cortisol 60 minutes later – if cortisol remains low, then diagnosis of adrenal insufficiency is made.

TREATMENT

- *A common clinical presentation is in a hospitalized patient after surgery and/or in the ICU in adrenal crisis with severe hypotension. Treatment in these patients should be implemented urgently.*
- Acute treatment: dexamethasone 4 mg IV every 8 hours.
- Diagnosis will be confirmed if clinical improvement and with serum cortisol drawn at 60 minutes – check dexamethasone suppression test.

- Follow-up treatment (after diagnosis confirmed):
  - Mineralocorticoid replacement with fludrocortisone
  - Identify and treat primary etiology.

APPROACH TO THE PATIENT WITH AN INCIDENTAL ADRENAL MASS

GENERAL INFORMATION

- Incidentaloma: an adrenal mass detected in a patient who undergoes abdominal imaging for reasons unrelated to the adrenal and who has no symptoms associated with adrenal disease.
- Detected in ~0.35–4.4% of abdominal CTs performed.
- Autopsy prevalence of incidentalomas ~1 to 8.7%.
- Characterization of masses (Table 20.3).[12]

EVALUATION[2]

- First, rule-out occult malignancy from an extra-adrenal site.
- Secondly, evaluate incidentaloma size:
  - If ≥6 cm, plan for surgical excision
  - If <6 cm, assess for function.
- Thirdly, evaluate incidentaloma function:
  - No consensus on protocol which should be followed
  - Potential tests (all discussed previously) include serum K; plasma aldosterone and renin and aldosterone:renin; dexamethasone suppression; plasma metanephrines; and urinary free cortisol
  - In planning tests, consider history and physical exam.
- Fourthly, if mass is indeterminate, may consider additional imaging to determine whether mass is adenoma or carcinoma:
  - No consensus on protocol – criteria are evolving
  - Modalities include MRI (T1 and T2), chemical-shift MRI, and nuclear scintigraphy.

TREATMENT

- If ≥6 cm: adrenalectomy.
- If <6 cm and functional: adrenalectomy.
- If <3 cm and non-functional: observation.
- If imaging suggests malignancy: adrenalectomy.

TABLE 20.3

CHARACTERIZATION OF ADRENAL MASSES

Type of mass	Proportion (%)
Non-functioning adenoma	76–81
Pheochromocytoma	5–10
Cushing's syndrome	5
Adrenal cortical carcinoma	5
Adrenal metastasis	3
Aldosteronoma	1

20

DISEASES OF THE ADRENAL GLAND

- If between 3 cm and 6 cm and non-functional: no consensus on treatment. Some have recommended age cut-offs to limit follow-up/radiation exposure in younger individuals:
  - 3–5 cm and age <50 years: adrenalectomy
  - 3–5 cm and age ≥50 years: observation.

OBSERVATION

- Problem: biological significance and natural history of small, non-functioning adenomas is not well understood.
- Observational protocols vary, but generally follow a similar pattern:[1]
  - CT scan every 6–12 months
  - Endocrine evaluation every 12 months
  - Surgery indicated for substantial growth of mass and/or development of endocrine function
  - Consider increasing interval between exams if no growth or endocrine function development within.
- Up to 25% will increase in size during observation and up to 10% will develop hormonal function within 10 years.[1]

PRINCIPLES OF ADRENALECTOMY

- Left adrenal vein empties into left renal vein; right adrenal vein directly into IVC.
- For pheochromocytoma, ligate the adrenal vein first to prevent intraoperative surge of catecholamines.
- For adrenal cortical carcinoma, consider open approach.

APPROACHES

- Open:
  - Anterior: chevron or subcostal incision
  - Flank
  - Posterior: lumbotomy.
- Thoracoabdominal.
- Laparoscopic:
  - Transperitoneal
  - Retroperitoneal.

REFERENCES

1. Shen WT, Sturgeon C, Duh QY: From incidentaloma to adrenocortical carcinoma: the surgical management of adrenal tumors. J Surg Oncol 89:186–92, 2005.
2. Lin DD, Loughlin KR: Diagnosis and management of surgical adrenal diseases. Urology 66:476–83, 2005.
3. Vaughan ED, Blumenfeld JD, Del Pizzo J, Schichman SJ, Sosa RE: The adrenals. In: Walsh PC, Retik AB, Vaughan ED, Wein AJ, eds. Campbell's Urology, 8th edn. Philadelphia: WB Saunders, 2002, pp 3507–69.
4. Dackiw AP, Lee JE, Gagel RF, Evans DB: Adrenal cortical carcinoma. World J Surg 25:914–26, 2001.
5. Acosta E, Pantoja JP, Gamino R, Rull JA, Herrera MF: Laparoscopic versus open adrenalectomy in Cushing's syndrome and disease. Surgery 126:1111–16, 1999.
6. Sarela AI, Murphy I, Coit DG, Conlon KC: Metastasis to the adrenal gland: the emerging role of laparoscopic surgery. Ann Surg Oncol 10:1191–6, 2003.

7. Kim SH, Brennan MF, Russo P, Burt ME, Coit DG: The role of surgery in the treatment of clinically isolated adrenal metastasis. Cancer 82:389–94, 1998.
8. Orth DN: Cushing's syndrome. New Engl J Med 332:791–803, 1995.
9. Tsigos C, Chrousos GP: Differential diagnosis and management of Cushing's syndrome. Annu Rev Med 47:443–61, 1996.
10. Yanovski JA, Cutler GB Jr: Glucocorticoid action and the clinical features of Cushing's syndrome. Endocrinol Metab Clin North Am 23:487–509, 1994.
11. Ashcraft MW, Van Herle AJ, Vener SL, Geffner DL: Serum cortisol levels in Cushing's syndrome after low- and high-dose dexamethasone suppression. Ann Intern Med 97:21–6, 1982.
12. Sturgeon C, Kebebew E: Laparoscopic adrenalectomy for malignancy. Surg Clin North Am 84:755–74, 2004.

DISEASES OF THE ADRENAL GLAND

Obstructing congenital anomalies of the urinary tract: ureteropelvic junction obstruction, ureterocele, megaureter, and posterior urethral valves

Caleb P Nelson

SUMMARY

- Congenital obstruction of the urinary tract can result in renal insufficiency and renal failure, permanent renal injury, oliguria or anuria, skeletal and soft tissue malformation, and pulmonary hypoplasia.
- Urinary tract dilatation is suggestive of, but not equivalent to, obstruction.
- Many of these conditions now present antenatally due to screening with ultrasonographic imaging. The role of antenatal intervention based on such findings remains controversial.
- In many cases of congenital urinary tract dilatation, conservative management via observation and serial imaging is adequate, as the dilatation may be stable or may diminish over time.
- Intervention is usually reserved for cases in which ongoing renal injury is believed to be occurring.

ANTENATAL HYDRONEPHROSIS

GENERAL INFORMATION

- Observed in 0.1–2.0% of maternal ultrasound examinations.
  - False-positive results in 9–22%
  - 66–75% of postpartum studies confirm dilatation.
- Commonly defined as AP renal pelvic diameter of >10 mm.
- Associated diagnoses: ureteropelvic junction (UPJ) obstruction, renal cysts, multicystic dysplastic kidney, vesicoureteral reflux (VUR), ureterovesical junction obstruction, ureterocele with or without duplication, prune belly syndrome, bladder outlet obstruction.

ASSOCIATED BLADDER FINDINGS

- Dilated, thick-walled bladder suggests bladder outlet obstruction.
- Empty bladder suggests decreased urine production.
- Inability to identify the bladder on repeated studies is concerning for bladder exstrophy.

POSTNATAL STUDIES

- Renal and bladder ultrasound:
  - For bilateral hydronephrosis: scan on first day of life, repeat negative study at 1–2 weeks

- For unilateral hydronephrosis: scan at 2–6 weeks (or at least after 48–72 hours of life, to avoid underdiagnosis due to neonatal dehydration and oliguria).
- Voiding cystourethrogram (VCUG):
  - For infants with significant dilatation.
- Functional renal scintigraphy:
  - Timing controversial
  - Ideally wait until 3 months of age to allow kidney maturation and improved handling of radiotracer.

URETEROPELVIC JUNCTION OBSTRUCTION

EPIDEMIOLOGY

- Bimodal peak of incidence:
  - Antenatal hydronephrosis
  - Adolescents or adults with flank or abdominal pain, hypertension, hematuria, stones, and/or infections.
- The most common condition diagnosed postnatally among newborns with a history of antenatal hydronephrosis (~50%).
- Is more common:
  - Among males
  - On the left.
- Bilateral in 10–40% of cases.
- Occurs in 15% of horseshoe kidneys.

PATHOPHYSIOLOGY

- Urine flow from renal pelvis into proximal ureter is impeded.
  - Results in dilation of the collecting system, decreased glomerular filtration rate (GFR), and potential injury to renal parenchyma
  - Increased duration of obstruction correlates with increased injury
  - Neonatal kidneys may be more susceptible to injury than adult kidneys, with impaired renal growth and renal dysplasia.
- Intrinsic:
  - The most common cause of UPJ obstruction among neonates
  - Likely caused by segment of hypoplastic, adynamic, proximal ureter. Associated with excess collagen and attenuated, separated muscle fibers
  - Rarely, obstruction may be caused by mucosal folds or benign fibroepithelial polyps.
- Extrinsic:
  - Most common cause is aberrant lower pole renal arteries. Unclear whether they cause obstruction or are simply associated with intrinsic lesions
  - Other proposed causes: ureteral kinking (sometimes associated with high-grade VUR), adhesions, and periureteral fibrosis.

DIAGNOSIS

Intravenous urography (IVP)

- Historically, the primary method of diagnosis.
- Now rarely used in initial work-up for children.

Renal ultrasonography

- Identifies renal pelvic and ureteral dilation and/or duplication and abnormalities of renal parenchyma.
- Serial ultrasounds monitor changes in abnormalities and renal growth.
- Renal resistive index (RI) >0.66–0.77 correlates with obstructive pattern on functional renal scintigraphy:
  - RI = (peak systolic velocity − low diastolic velocity) ÷ peak systolic velocity.

Functional renal scintigraphy

- Intravenous administration of radiotracer agent, with renal uptake and excretion of the agent measured by a gamma camera, followed by diuretic administration to observe washout of tracer from collecting system.
- Patients should be well-hydrated with bladder catheter in place to ensure drainage. Conscious sedation as needed to minimize movement.
- Best performed after 3 months of age.
- Two most common tests: DPTA and MAG-3.
- Technetium (Tc) 99m diethylenetriamine pentaacetic acid (DPTA):
  - Excreted only by glomerular filtration so can be used to estimate GFR.
- Tc 99m mercuroacetyltriglycine (MAG-3):
  - Currently the agent of choice at most centers
  - Excreted primarily by secretion, with some filtration
  - A better study in the neonatal period since it is less dependent on GFR.
- Tracer agent is injected, followed by furosemide 15–20 minutes later.
- Normal tracer activity curves show 3 phases:
  - Rapid initial rise during renal uptake
  - Peak activity during cortical transfer
  - Rapid decline during excretion into collecting system.
- Lack of tracer decline suggests either obstruction or non-obstructive dilatation.
  - Rapid washout after furosemide suggests dilatation without obstruction.
- Diagnosis based on time required to achieve 50% reduction in tracer activity as measured at time of furosemide injection ($T^{1/2}$):
  - $T^{1/2}$ >20 minutes = obstruction
  - $T^{1/2}$ <15 minutes = no obstruction
  - $T^{1/2}$ = 15–20 minutes = equivocal.

Pressure–flow studies

- Also called the Whitaker test.
- Not commonly used.
- Involves antegrade saline perfusion (with or without contrast) through a percutaneous nephrostomy tube with measurement of renal pelvic pressures:
  - Pressures >15 cmH$_2$O suggest obstruction
  - Perfusion rates need to be adjusted for patient size and GFR
  - Optimal perfusion rates and pressure cutoffs for obstruction are unclear.

21

OBSTRUCTING CONGENITAL ANOMALIES OF THE URINARY TRACT

Magnetic resonance and computed tomographic urography

- Protocols vary and are under development.

Voiding cystourethrogram

- Useful for ruling out VUR and/or posterior urethral valves.

TREATMENT

Surgery

- Reconstruction of the ureteropelvic junction to facilitate drainage.
- Unclear as to which patients will benefit.
- Indications:
  - Symptomatic patients with clear evidence of obstruction
  - Newborns with severe bilateral obstruction (nephrostomy tube drainage may temporize, although technically difficult in small neonates).
- Open surgery:
  - Success rates ≥90%
  - Dismembered pyeloplasty (Anderson–Hynes): excision of the stenotic segment with reanastomosis of the renal pelvis and proximal ureter to form a widely patent channel. The 'gold standard' for repair
  - YV plasty: incision across the stenotic segment, with interposition of a V-flap from the renal pelvis, creating a widely patent channel
  - Anastomoses can be stented or unstented.
- Laparoscopy:
  - Replicates open surgery
  - Utilized with success in older children, adolescents, and adults.
- Endoscopy:
  - Technically difficult in small children and infants
  - Full-thickness incision (retrograde more common) made across the hypoplastic segment using cold knife, laser, or cautery. Balloon dilation also described
  - Cut is made *laterally* to avoid medial vessels
  - Success rates = 63–90% in absence of crossing vessels; less effective in presence of crossing vessels.
- Complications:
  - Reobstruction. Rare after open repair, 10–20% after endoscopy
  - Urine leak. Usually resolves. Consider placement of a ureteral stent if persists >10 days
  - Ureteral ischemia, scarring, and fibrosis. May result in complete obstruction. Reoperation with extensive mobilization of ureter and kidney is necessary; rarely, ureterocalycostomy or bowl interposition may be needed.

Observation

- Most newborns with unilateral UPJ obstruction and a normal contralateral kidney can be observed.
  - Intervention is recommended for infection or if the involved kidney shows evidence of decreased function/worsening obstruction
  - Unclear if intervention improves long-term outcomes, since ~50% of patients will not recover lost function after surgery.

- Newborns with bilateral UPJ obstruction can be observed if:
  - Hydronephrosis is mild to moderate
  - Renal function is stable
  - No infections on prophylactic antibiotics.

MEGAURETER

DEFINITION AND EPIDEMIOLOGY

- Ureteral diameter >7 mm (normal <5 mm).
- Classification:
  - Obstructing
  - Refluxing
  - Both
  - Neither.
- In newborns, most are nonobstructing.
- Cause 20–25% of cases of neonatal hydroureteronephrosis.
- More common:
  - In males
  - On left side.
- Contralateral renal agenesis occurs in 9%.

PATHOPHYSIOLOGY

Primary

- Likely due to localized defect in ureteral muscle, resulting in an adynamic segment.

Secondary

- Due to bladder or bladder outlet abnormalities that prevent normal urine transit, including:
  - Neurogenic bladder (or non-neurogenic voiding dysfunction)
  - Posterior urethral valves
  - Mechanical obstruction by a thickened bladder wall due to inflammation, scarring, or other anatomical problems (e.g. bladder diverticulum).
- Refluxing megaureter:
  - Equivalent to grade V VUR.
- Non-obstructive, non-refluxing megaureter:
  - Most common of megaureters detected in newborns
  - Proposed mechanisms include: transient prenatal obstruction, peristalsis abnormalities, and abnormal ureteral elasticity/compliance.

DIAGNOSIS

- Ultrasound:
  - Best location to visualize the dilated distal ureter is transverse view through the bladder
  - Echogenic or severely thinned parenchyma suggestive of obstruction.
- Voiding cystourethrogram:
  - Important to evaluate for VUR, bladder function, and urethra.

21

OBSTRUCTING CONGENITAL ANOMALIES OF THE URINARY TRACT

- Functional renal scintigraphy:
  - Delayed drainage from a large dilated system can make interpretation difficult.
- Pressure–flow studies:
  - Can demonstrate obstruction, but invasive and technically challenging.

TREATMENT: OBSTRUCTING

Issues

- Definitive diagnosis is difficult.
- Timing of treatment is controversial.
- Surgery is technically challenging in small infants.

Options

- Observation with prophylactic antibiotics:
  - Improvement often occurs
  - Also allows time for bladder growth prior to definitive surgery.
- Diverting ureterostomy:
  - Good option for newborns with massive dilatation and evidence of renal impairment
  - May improve ureteral tone and function
  - Allows recovery/stabilization of renal function
  - Performed through extraperitoneal low inguinal approach.
- Ureteral reimplantation with excision of the adynamic segment and reconstruction of the dilated distal ureter:
  - Generally reserved for cases with mild–moderate dilatation
  - Involves imbrication (folding of the distal ureter on itself lengthwise to reduce luminal diameter).
- Ureteral reimplantation with excisional tapering:
  - Useful for massively dilated ureters for which imbrication would be difficult
  - Involves excision of redundant tissue and reconstruction of a new lumen of normal caliber.

TREATMENT: REFLUXING

- Generally managed as grade V VUR.
- See Chapter 24 for details.

TREATMENT: NON-OBSTRUCTIVE, NON-REFLUXING

- Observation with antibiotic prophylaxis:
  - 80–90% will have improvement in dilatation without decrease in renal function.
- If dilatation is severe and persistent, or if clinical deterioration, consider surgery as above.

URETEROCELE

EPIDEMIOLOGY

- Incidence: 1/500–1/4000.
- More common:
  - Among whites
  - Females (4–7 times compared with males)
  - On left.
- 10% bilateral.
- 60–80% are ectopic.
- 80% are associated with the upper pole of a duplex kidney.
- Single-system ectopic ureterocele associated with cardiac and genital anomalies.

BIOLOGY

- Definition: cystic dilatation of the terminal ureter.
- Etiology unclear:
  - Possibly related to persistent membrane between ureteral bud and urogenital sinus or abnormal muscular development of the ureterovesical junction.

CLINICAL SEQUELAE

- Urinary tract infection (UTI).
- Contralateral renal obstruction:
  - Large ureterocele may block contralateral ureteral orifice.
- Urinary retention:
  - Prolapsing ureterocele can block the bladder outlet.
- Incontinence:
  - May hinder sphincteric function and/or cause bladder neck dysfunction.

DIAGNOSIS

Clinical manifestations

- Palpable abdominal mass.
- Bladder outlet obstruction.
- UTI.
- Incontinence.
- Urolithiasis.

Exam

- In girls, a prolapsing ureterocele may present as an interlabial mass:
  - Has smooth, round surface and congested appearance
  - Urethral lumen usually lies anterior, allowing for catheterization.
- In small infants, palpable bladder or kidney may be present.

Ultrasound

- Hydronephrosis or intravesical cystic dilatation.
- Can identify duplicated system.
- Note that bladder filling may compress, evert, and conceal the ureterocele.

Intravenous urography

- Provides useful anatomical details.
- Findings with a single-system intravesical ureterocele:
  - 'Cobra head' or 'spring onion': opacified urine in distal ureter surrounded by lucent halo resulting from the wall of the ureterocele.
- Findings with a duplex system:
  - 'Drooping lily': the non-visualized, non-functioning upper pole pushes the well-visualized lower pole laterally and inferiorly
  - The lower pole ureter may be laterally deviated, notched, and serpiginous.

Voiding cystourethrogram

- Typical finding: smooth-walled, radiolucent filling defect.
- With a duplex system, reflux into lower pole observed in 50–65% of cases.
- Imaging during early filling recommended to minimize ureterocele eversion and concealment.

Cystoscopy

- May help diagnosis.
- If needed, contrast can be injected into ureterocele through endoscopically placed needle to delineate side of origin.

Renal scintigraphy

- Estimates renal function and drainage.

TREATMENT

Principles

- Treatment should be individualized.
- Goals include:
  - Prevent UTI
  - Preserve renal function
  - Maintain continence
  - Manage any associated VUR
  - Minimize treatment morbidity.
- Factors to consider in planning treatment:
  - Renal function
  - Intravesical or ectopic ureterocele
  - Patient age and clinical status
  - Associated VUR
  - Involvement of bladder neck
  - Single vs duplex system.
- Newborns may need to be temporized with endoscopic incision or ureterostomy.

Options

- Endoscopic incision:
  - Urgently indicated for urosepsis
  - Low morbidity

- An option for primary elective treatment for neonates, intravesical or single-system ureteroceles, or duplex systems with good upper pole function
  - Incision is made with cautery on the front wall of the intravesical portion
  - New reflux is seen after incision in 18–44% of cases
  - Rarely effective as sole treatment for ectopic ureteroceles.
- Open excision, reimplantation, and bladder reconstruction:
  - Challenging in newborns
  - Best performed before toilet training
  - Dissection of ureterocele distal to bladder neck should proceed cautiously to avoid injury to external sphincter
  - Reflux into lower pole of duplex system may be corrected concomitantly.
- Open ureteroureterostomy and ureteropyelostomy:
  - Allows decompression of ureterocele and permanent drainage without excision of renal parenchyma
  - End-to-side anastomosis allows flow of urine from upper pole into lower pole system
  - Upper pole ureter should be dissected to the iliac vessels: if no reflux, distal stump can be left open; if reflux, stump should be ligated.
- Upper pole nephrectomy and partial ureterectomy:
  - Indicated when upper pole demonstrates no significant function
  - Can be performed laparoscopically
  - Good option when reflux to lower pole is minimal.

POSTERIOR URETHRAL VALVES (PUV)

DEFINITION AND PATHOPHYSIOLOGY

- Rare condition characterized by congenital obstruction of the posterior urethra in males.
  - Obstruction leads to oliguria, impaired renal function, and lower urinary tract dysfunction.
- Renal function:
  - Severe bilateral hydronephrosis and renal dysplasia are typical
  - Impaired renal tubular function is often irreversible and results in reduced concentrating ability and polyuria.
- Vesicoureteral reflux (VUR):
  - Seen in 33–50% of cases
  - Resolves in up to 33% after treatment
  - Has been associated with poor prognosis: mortality rate increased from 10% with no VUR to 50–60% with bilateral VUR
  - Unilateral VUR with renal dysplasia on the refluxing side may have protective effect on contralateral kidney due to pressure 'pop-off' effect – the VURD (**V**alves, **U**nilateral **R**eflux, and renal **D**ysplasia) syndrome.
- Bladder function:
  - Impaired due to thick-walled bladder with poor compliance and reduced sensation
  - May present as incontinence, UTI, and/or lower urinary tract symptoms
  - Infants undergoing early valve ablation appear to have better long-term bladder function than patients who undergo supravesical diversion
  - Dysfunction may persist after treatment.

- Pulmonary hypoplasia:
  - Associated with severe obstruction
  - Likely caused by oligohydramnios, which leads to impaired pulmonary development
  - May need aggressive supportive care postnatally, including mechanical ventilation or extracorporeal membrane oxygenation. Mortality approaches 50%.

DIAGNOSIS

Antenatal

- Common: constitute ~10% of cases of antenatally detected congenital obstructive uropathy.
- Ultrasonography (U/S) performed at <24 weeks may miss up to 50% of cases.
- Oligohydramnios and echogenic renal parenchyma are associated with poor prognosis.
- Patients with antenatal findings suggestive of valves should undergo ultrasound soon after birth.

Newborns

- May present with oliguria and renal failure, abdominal distension, patent urachus, UTI, respiratory distress, and failure to thrive.
- U/S during first 48 hours of life may miss mild–moderate dilatation due to neonatal dehydration, but severe obstruction will likely be visualized even in dehydrated infants. Negative studies should be repeated at 1–2 weeks of age.
- Voiding cystourethrogram should be performed in all infants with abnormal U/S:
  - Oblique view of posterior urethra should be obtained
  - Dilated, elongated prostatic urethra (due to elevation of bladder neck) is classic finding.

Children and adolescents

- Typically present with UTIs and/or voiding dysfunction.
- Often have renal insufficiency (35%), but may have better prognosis than those presenting as infants.

TREATMENT

Antenatal

- Several centers have attempted antenatal procedures to divert urine. Most have involved placement of percutaneous vesicoamniotic shunt.
  - Hypothesis is that early decompression of collecting system will prevent further deterioration of renal and bladder function.
- Improved postnatal outcomes have not yet been demonstrated.
  - Renal dysplasia probably develops early in gestation, prior to earliest point at which obstruction can be diagnosed (i.e. damage is already done).

- Technical problems with placement and retention of shunt devices are common.
- Serious adverse events to mother and fetus have occurred.

Newborns

- Initial management: Foley catheter drainage (may need to verify position with imaging), antibiotics, hydration, and correction of electrolytes.
- Obtain serial creatinine measurements over 7–10 days to establish nadir creatinine.
- If nadir creatinine <1.0 mg/dl (i.e. normal renal function), proceed with endoscopic valve ablation:
  - Cold-knife hook, Bugbee ball electrode, cautery loops and hooks, neodymium:YAG laser, KTP laser, catheter balloons, and valvulotomes have been used
  - Valve is incised at 4–5, 7–8, and 12 o'clock to release valve leaflets and relieve obstruction
  - Credé's maneuver may facilitate incision
  - Catheter left in place for several days post-op.
- If nadir creatinine >1.0 mg/dl (i.e. persistent renal insufficiency):
  - Management is controversial. Diversion may worsen bladder dysfunction (possibly due to decreased bladder cycling). Moreover, it is not clear that diversion improves long-term renal function
  - If VUR is not present, loop ureterostomy is primary option
  - It VUR is present, vesicostomy is primary option
  - Many experts now reserve diversion for infants with severe renal impairment (nadir creatinine >2.0 mg/dl).

Bladder dysfunction in children and adolescents

- Obtain history and physical, voiding diary, and urodynamics.
- For detrusor hyperreflexia:
  - Timed voiding, anticholinergic medications, and clean intermittent catheterization (CIC).
- For high-pressure, low-compliance bladder:
  - Anticholinergic medications, CIC, and – in severe cases – bladder augmentation.
- For hypocontractile bladders:
  - Timed voiding and CIC to keep residual volumes low.
- Polyuria may exacerbate problems by worsening bladder dilation.
  - Consider CIC and/or nocturnal indwelling catheterization.

FURTHER READING

GENERAL

Carr MC: Prenatal management of urogenital disorders. Urol Clin North Am 31:389–97, vii, 2004.

Elder JS: Antenatal hydronephrosis. Fetal and neonatal management. Pediatr Clin North Am 44:1299–321, 1997.

Peters CA: Perinatal urology: In: Walsh PC, Retik AB, Vaughan EB, Wein AJ, eds. Campbell's Urology, 8th edn. Philadelphia: WB Saunders, 2002, pp 1781–811.

Pope JC, Brock JW III, Adams MC, Stephens FD, Ichikawa I: How they begin and how they end: classic and new theories for the development and deterioration of congenital anomalies of the kidney and urinary tract, CAKUT. J Am Soc Nephrol 10:2018–28, 1999.

Swana HS, Sutherland RS, Baskin L: Prenatal intervention for urinary obstruction and myelomeningocele. Int Braz J Urol 30:40–8, 2004.

Woodward M, Frank D: Postnatal management of antenatal hydronephrosis. BJU Int 89:149–56, 2002.

UPJ OBSTRUCTION

Carr MC: Anomalies and surgery of the ureteropelvic junction in children. In: Walsh PC, Retik AB, Vaughan EB, Wein AJ, eds. Campbell's Urology, 8th edn. Philadelphia: WB Saunders, 2002, pp 1995–2006.

Churchill BM, Feng WC: Ureteropelvic junction anomalies: congenital UPJ problems in children. In: Gearhart JP, Rink RC, Mouriquand PDE, eds. Pediatric Urology. Philadelphia: WB Saunders, 2001, pp 318–46.

DiSandro MJ, Kogan BA: Neonatal management. Role for early intervention. Urol Clin North Am 25:187–97, 1998.

Eskild-Jensen A, Gordon I, Piepsz A, Frokiaer J: Interpretation of the renogram: problems and pitfalls in hydronephrosis in children. BJU Int 94:887–92, 2004.

Hanna MK: Antenatal hydronephrosis and ureteropelvic junction obstruction: the case for early intervention. Urology 55:612–15, 2000.

Josephson S: Antenatally detected, unilateral dilatation of the renal pelvis: a critical review. 1. Postnatal non-operative treatment 20 years on – is it safe? Scand J Urol Nephrol 36:243–50, 2002.

Josephson S: Antenatally detected, unilateral dilatation of the renal pelvis: a critical review. 2. Postnatal non-operative treatment – long-term hazards, urgent research. Scand J Urol Nephrol 36:251–9, 2002.

Park JM, Bloom DA: The pathophysiology of UPJ obstruction. Current concepts. Urol Clin North Am 25:161–9, 1998.

Sfakianakis GN, Sfakianaki E: Renal scintigraphy in infants and children. Urology 57:1167–77, 2001.

MEGAURETER

Atala A, Keating MA: Vesicoureteral reflux and megaureter. In: Walsh PC, Retik AB, Vaughan ED, Wein AJ, eds. Campbell's Urology, 8th edn. Philadelphia: WB Saunders, 2002, pp 2053–116.

Joseph DB: Ureterovesical junction anomalies – megaureters. In: Gearhart JP, Rink RC, Mouriquand PDE, eds. Pediatric Urology. Philadelphia: WB Saunders, 2001, pp 347–58.

Meyer JS, Lebowitz RL: Primary megaureter in infants and children: a review. Urol Radiol 14:296–305, 1992.

Shokeir AA, Nijman RJ: Primary megaureter: current trends in diagnosis and treatment. BJU Int 86:861–8, 2000.

Wilcox D, Mouriquand P: Management of megaureter in children. Eur Urol 34:73–8, 1998.

URETEROCELE

Cooper CS, Snyder HM III: Ureteral duplication, ectopy, and ureteroceles. In: Gearhart JP, Rink RC, Mouriquand PDE, eds. Pediatric Urology. Philadelphia: WB Saunders, 2001, pp 430–49.

Coplen DE: Management of the neonatal ureterocele. Curr Urol Rep 2:102–5, 2001.

Coplen DE, Barthold JS: Controversies in the management of ectopic ureteroceles. Urology 56:665–8, 2000.

Schlussel RN, Retik AB: Ectopic ureter, ureterocele, and other anomalies of the ureter. In: Walsh PC, Retik AB, Vaughan ED, Wein AJ, eds. Campbell's Urology, 8th edn. Philadelphia: WB Saunders, 2002, pp 2007–52.

Shokeir AA, Nijman RJ: Ureterocele: an ongoing challenge in infancy and childhood. BJU Int 90:777–83, 2002.

POSTERIOR URETHRAL VALVES

Close CE, Mitchell ME: Posterior urethral valves. In: Gearhart JP, Rink RC, Mouriquand PDE, eds. Pediatric Urology. Philadelphia: WB Saunders, 2001, pp 595–605.

Fernbach SK, Feinstein KA, Schmidt MB: Pediatric voiding cystourethrography: a pictorial guide. Radiographics 20:155–68, 2000.

Glassberg KI: The valve bladder syndrome: 20 years later. J Urol 166:1406–14, 2001.

Gonzales ET Jr: Alternatives in the management of posterior urethral valves. Urol Clin North Am 17:335–42, 1990.

Gonzales ET Jr: Posterior urethral valves and other urethral anomalies. In: Walsh PC, Retik AB, Vaughan ED, Wein AJ, eds. Campbell's Urology, 8th edn. Philadelphia: WB Saunders, 2002, pp 2207–30.

Karmarkar SJ: Long-term results of surgery for posterior urethral valves: a review. Pediatr Surg Int 17:8–10, 2001.

Manzoni C, Valentini AL: Posterior urethral valves. Rays 27:131–4, 2002.

Strand WR: Initial management of complex pediatric disorders: prunebelly syndrome, posterior urethral valves. Urol Clin North Am 31:399–415, vii, 2004.

21

OBSTRUCTING CONGENITAL ANOMALIES OF THE URINARY TRACT

Developmental abnormalities of the genitalia: intersex, hypospadias, and cryptorchidism

Jennifer Miles-Thomas

22

SUMMARY

- There are four types of intersex disorders: female pseudohermaphroditism (genetic female with masculinized phenotype), male pseudohermaphroditism (genetic male with feminized phenotype), true hermaphroditism, and gonadal dysgenesis.
- The most common intersex disorder is congenital adrenal hyperplasia.
- Treatments for intersex disorders depend upon the type of the disorder and the severity of the disease.
- Hypospadias is a developmental anomaly of the penis associated with ventral curvature of the shaft, a ventral opening of the urethral meatus, and abnormal distribution of the foreskin. Treatment is reconstructive surgery.
- Cryptorchidism is failure of one or both testes to descend into the scrotum. Undescended testicles are associated with increased risks of infertility and cancer. Treatment is surgical placement of the affected testicle into the scrotum or hormonal therapy to induce testicular descent.
- Other congenital scrotal abnormalities include inguinal hernia and hydrocele.

INTERSEX

NORMAL SEXUAL DEVELOPMENT[1]

- The default pathway for sexual development *in utero* is female.
- Male development requires the presence and normal expression of the testis-determining factor (TDF), located on the sex-determining region of the Y chromosome (SRY).
  - TDF initiates development of male structures
  - Female structures will regress during development of male structures (Figure 22.1).
- Embryological remnants in adults are given in Table 22.1.

TABLE 22.1

EMBRYOLOGICAL REMNANTS IN ADULTS

	Müllerian duct	Wolffian duct
Male	Appendix testis	Appendix epididymis
	Prostatic utricle	Paradidymis
Female		Epoöphoron
		Paroöphoron
		Gartner's duct cysts

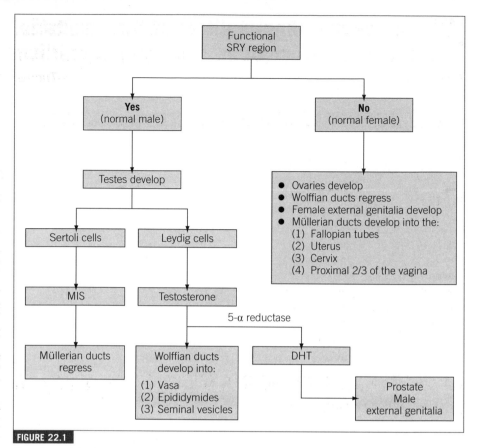

FIGURE 22.1

Normal sexual development.

PRESENTATION[2,3]

- Intersex conditions typically present as ambiguous genitalia in the neonate.
- There are four main types of intersex conditions (see below).
- Possible phenotypes include:
  - Male phenotype (i.e. phallic-appearing structure) with non-palpable gonads
  - Female phenotype with palpable gonads
  - Cliteromegaly
  - Hypospadias with non-palpable testis.

EVALUATION

- History:
  - Maternal exposures (i.e. androgens, finasteride, etc.)
  - Prior intersex in family
  - Infertility
  - Prior infant deaths in family.

EXAM

- Phallus:
  - Note size, structure (i.e. chordee), and position of urethral meatus.
- Appearance of labia/scrotum:
  - Note presence of labioscrotal fusion.
- Palpable gonads:
  - Hypospadias and unilateral non-palpable gonad is intersex until proven otherwise.
- Hyperpigmentation:
  - Characteristic of adrenal hyperplasia.

WORK-UP

- Initially may include:
  - Karyotype
  - Serum electrolytes
  - Urinary and serum androgens/adrenal steroid levels
  - Urogenitogram
  - Pelvic ultrasound or MRI.
- More extensive work-up may include:
  - Endoscopy of the genitourinary tract
  - Laparoscopy.

FEMALE PSEUDOHERMAPHRODITISM

GENERAL INFORMATION

- Definition: genetic female with masculinized phenotype (46 XX with ovaries)
- Exam:
  - Non-palpable gonads
  - Varying amounts of virilization with masculinized external genitalia.
- Pelvic ultrasound will show uterus.
- Etiology is prenatal exposure to increased androgens:
  - Exogenous source: highly unlikely
  - Endogenous source: congenital adrenal hyperplasia.

CONGENITAL ADRENAL HYPERPLASIA (CAH)

- Autosomal recessive.
- Most common intersex disorder (60%).
- Incidence is 1:40 000 live births.
- Caused by enzyme defects in cortisol synthesis, which increases adrenocorticotropic hormone (ACTH) – lack of feedback inhibition – and increases shunting of cholesterol to androgen synthesis pathways.
- Hyperpigmentation associated with increased levels of ACTH.

TYPES OF CAH[2]

- 21-hydroxylase deficiency:
  - Most common type (causes 95% of CAH cases)
  - Incidence is 1 in 50 000 live births

- 50–70% are salt wasting due to aldosterone deficiency[3]
- Presentation: failure to thrive, vomiting, dehydration, adrenal crisis, hyperpigmentation, and virilization
- Diagnosis: will have elevated plasma level of 17-hydroxyprogesterone and progesterone.
- 11β-hydroxylase deficiency:
  - <5% of CAH
  - Not salt wasting (i.e. no mineralocorticoid deficiency)
  - Presentation: hypertension, hyperpigmentation, virilization (and precocious puberty in males)
  - Diagnosis: will have elevated serum levels of 11-deoxycortisol and 11-deoxycorticosterone.
- 3β-hydroxysteroid dehydrogenase:
  - Rare
  - Salt wasting
  - Inhibition of synthesis of aldosterone, cortisol, and sex steroids
  - May also have ambiguous genitalia in genetic males.[3]

TREATMENT OF CAH

- Medical: cortisol and mineralocorticoid replacement:
  - For salt wasting, treat with hydrocortisone and fludrocortisone
  - For non-salt wasting, treat with hydrocortisone alone.
- Surgical:
  - Genitoplasty.
- Prenatal:
  - Diagnosis: elevated amniotic 17-hydroxyprogesterone[4]
  - May consider treatment with dexamethasone, which will inhibit ACTH.

MALE PSEUDOHERMAPHRODITISM

GENERAL INFORMATION

- Definition: genetic male with feminized phenotype (46 XY with testes).
- Caused by defects in the normal pathway of male development.
- There are four main causes.[3]

TESTOSTERONE BIOSYNTHESIS DISORDERS

- Rare defect in any of five enzymes responsible for testosterone biosynthesis.
- May have concomitant problems with glucocorticoid and/or mineralocorticoid production.
- Typically are sterile.

ANDROGEN INSENSITIVITY

- Androgen production is normal, but the androgen receptor is defective.
- Complete androgen insensitivity:[2]
  - Incidence is 1 in 20 000 to 40 000 live births
  - Have normal female phenotype with short vagina and undescended, undeveloped testes
  - Are infertile

- Presentation: primary amenorrhea and/or bilateral inguinal hernias
- Management: gonadectomy (risk of seminoma or gonadoblastoma in undeveloped testes 2–5%).
- **Incomplete androgen insensitivity (Reifenstein syndrome):[5]**
  - X-linked disorder
  - Associated with decreased androgen receptor binding affinity or decreased overall number of receptors[6]
  - Presentation: varying degrees of feminization
  - Management is individualized.

5α-REDUCTASE DEFICIENCY

- Autosomal recessive disorder:
  - Mutation in the type II 5α-reductase gene.
- Results in decreased levels of dihydrotestosterone, which causes abnormal development of the external genitalia.
- Presentation: newborns with feminized phenotype:
  - Penoscrotal hypospadias
  - Microphallus.
- May also present at puberty as sudden masculinization secondary to increased serum androgen levels.
- Management: assignment of male gender favored with surgical genitoplasty.
- Fertility has been reported in adult individuals.

MÜLLERIAN-INHIBITING SUBSTANCE DEFICIENCY

- Also known as hernia uteri inguinalis.
- Condition caused by deficiency of Müllerian-inhibiting substance (MIS), resulting in persistence of Müllerian structures.
- Presentation: phenotypically normal males with retained internal Müllerian structures – fallopian tubes, uterus, and/or proximal vagina contiguous with the prostatic utricle – and cryptorchidism.
- Normal fertility.
- Management: orchidopexy and excision of Müllerian remnants if necessary.
  - If uterus present, partial hysterectomy should be performed to preserve vasa.

TRUE HERMAPHRODITISM

GENERAL INFORMATION

- Condition in which both female and male sexual tissue is present in an affected individual.
- Autosomal recessive.
- Genotype is variable, but 67% of affected individuals are 46 XX.
- Ovatestis or separate ovary and testis.

PRESENTATION

- Variable.
- External genitalia are usually ambiguous.

22

DEVELOPMENTAL ABNORMALITIES OF THE GENITALIA

MANAGEMENT

- Gonadal biopsy, gender assignment, and removal of discordant tissues.
  - If female, fertility is possible
  - If male, consider gonadectomy, since fertility is unlikely and there is 4–10% risk of malignancy.

GONADAL DYSGENESIS

MIXED GONADAL DYSGENESIS

- Genotype is 45 XO/46 XY.
- The second most common cause of ambiguous genitalia.[2]
- A unilateral testis secretes testosterone but lacks germinal elements.
- A contralateral 'streak' gonad is present.
- Increased risk of Wilms' tumor (Denys–Drash syndrome).
- Infertile.
- Presentation:
  - Masculinized male external genitalia
  - Retained Müllerian structures.
- Management:[2]
  - Gender assignment (historically female).
  - Gonadectomy or orchidopexy.
  - Screening for Wilms' tumor.

PURE GONADAL DYSGENESIS[2]

- Bilateral dysgenetic gonads with variable genotype and phenotype.
- 46 XX:
  - Female phenotype with normal external genitalia and internal Müllerian structures
  - Bilateral streak gonads
  - Treatment: cyclic hormone replacement with estrogen and progesterone.
- 46 XY or 45 X/46 XY:
  - Bilateral dysgenetic testes
  - Treatment: gonadectomy secondary to risk of malignancy (46%).

TURNER'S SYNDROME

- 45 XO (95–98%):[2]
  - Female phenotype with bilateral streak gonads
  - Appearance: short stature, broad chest, webbed neck, no secondary sex characteristics
  - 33–60% will have coarctation of aorta and/or renal abnormalities (horseshoe kidney, duplication, agenesis, or malrotation)
  - Treatment: consider ± gonadectomy, ultrasound screening for renal and cardiac abnormalities, human growth hormone to achieve adult height.
- 45 XO/46 XY (2–5%):
  - Require excision of streak gonad secondary to risk of gonadoblastoma (~30%).[7]

KLINEFELTER'S SYNDROME

- One Y with $\geq 2 \times$ chromosomes (XXY, XXXY, etc.).[2]
- Male phenotype with poorly developed secondary sex characteristics.
- Gynecomastia common.
- Increased risk of breast cancer (8 times compared with other males).[8]
- Infertility secondary to azoospermia.
  - Histopathology of testicle will show degenerated seminiferous tubules replaced with hyaline.
- Low–normal serum testosterone with increased serum follicle-stimulating hormone/luteinizing hormone (FSH/LH).
- Management:
  - Androgen supplementation
  - Reduction mammoplasty as needed.

HYPOSPADIAS

GENERAL INFORMATION AND EPIDEMIOLOGY

- Definition: developmental anomaly of the penis associated with ventral curvature of the shaft, a ventral opening of the urethral meatus, and abnormal distribution of the foreskin.
- Caused by arrested development between 8 and 12 weeks of age.[3]
- Incidence is 1 in 250 live births.
- Of affected individuals:
  - 6–8% have affected fathers
  - 14% have affected male siblings.
- Abnormal karyotype (i.e. intersex condition) often seen in patients with severe hypospadias.
- Circumcision should *not* be performed so as to preserve skin for later reconstruction.

TREATMENT

- Treatment is surgical correction to prevent difficulties with urination and/or sexual function.
  - Best time for repair is between 6 and 12 months of age.
- Preoperative hormones: some support using β-HCG (β-human chorionic gonadotropin), testosterone, or DHT (dihydrotestosterone) therapy prior to surgical repair in order to increase penile size
  - Testosterone enathate IM (2 mg/kg) 5 and 2 weeks before surgery has been shown to cause 50% increase in penile size, vascularity, and penile skin
  - DHT topical cream increases penile circumference and length 50%.
- Surgery should be individualized according to the severity of the defect. Correction may require more than operation (i.e. staged approach). General principles of repair include:
  - Correction of penile curvature (orthoplasty)
  - Urethroplasty
  - Skin coverage.

DEVELOPMENTAL ABNORMALITIES OF THE GENITALIA

22

- Orthoplasty:[3]
  - Options include dorsal plication (Nesbit), rotation of corporal bodies, dermal or tunica vaginalis grafting, and total penile disassembly.
- Urethroplasty:
  - Options include meatoplasty/glanuloplasty, meatal advancement and glanuloplasty (MAGPI), urethral plate incision and tubularization (Snodgrass), tissue flaps (including Onlay), and grafts.
- Skin coverage:
  - Foreskin reconstruction and ventral transfer of redundant preputial skin.
- Complications:
  - Bleeding
  - Fistula: should wait 6 months before repairing
  - Urethral stricture and/or diverticulum
  - Wound dehiscence.

CRYPTORCHIDISM

GENERAL INFORMATION

- Definition: a developmental defect in which there is a failure of the testis to descend into the scrotum.[9]
  - *Non-palpable testis:* testis cannot be detected on physical exam and therefore is intra-abdominal, absent, or ectopic
  - *Retractile testis:* testis may retract out of scrotum but may easily be brought down into position and remains in place once let go
  - *Vanishing testis:* absent testis with blind-ending spermatic vessels proximal to internal ring.
- Incidence: occurs in 3% of term males.[10]
- Embryology:
  - Descent of testes based upon the differential growth of lumbar vertebral column and pelvis; migration begins ~23rd week and is complete between 30 and 32 weeks
  - Spontaneous descent should be complete by 6 months of age.

RATIONALE FOR TREATMENT[3,11]

- Infertility:
  - ~7% in normal men
  - ~10% with unilateral cryptorchidism
  - ~33% with bilateral cryptorchidism
  - Orchidopexy prior to puberty improves long-term fertility.
- Risk of testicular cancer:
  - Three to 14 times increased risk compared with the general population
  - If only one side is undescended, risk is also increased in the contralateral (i.e. normally descended) testicle
  - It is generally believed that orchidopexy does not decrease the risk of subsequent cancer in either testicle but does facilitate cancer surveillance
  - Most common tumor type is seminoma.
- Cosmesis.

EVALUATION

- History:
  - Duration (i.e. when was the non-palpable testis first noted? Was the involved testis ever palpable?)
  - Prenatal and maternal history of exposures
  - Family history.
- Exam:
  - Note presence of other congenital defects, genitourinary or otherwise
  - Note any asymmetries or abnormalities of the scrotal structure.

ENDOCRINE STUDIES

- May consider in patients with bilateral cryptorchidism.
- Müllerian-inhibiting substance (MIS), inhibin B, and FSH levels:
  - Increased FSH in a prepubescent boy suggests anorchia.

TREATMENT

- Treatment should be initiated if no testicular descent by 1 year old.
- The lower the pretreatment position of the testis, the higher the likelihood of successful treatment.[9,12]

HORMONAL THERAPY WITH β-HCG OR GNRH

- Overall efficacy ~20%.
- β-HCG has a similar structure to LH and will induce testicular Leydig cells to produce testosterone.
- Gonadotropin-releasing hormone (GnRH) will induce pituitary secretion of LH.
- Subsequent testosterone levels are generally higher with β-HCG than with GnRH:
  - β-HCG dose: 1500 IU/m^2 IM twice a week × 4 weeks
  - GnRH dose: 1.2 mg/day nasal spray × 4 weeks.[12]

SURGERY

- Gold standard.
- Requires mobilization sufficient to achieve adequate spermatic cord length to place testicle into scrotum without tension.
- If adequate length cannot be achieved, the following maneuvers may be performed:
  - Retroperitoneal dissection with enlargement of the inguinal ring
  - Division of the inferior epigastrics with medial placement of the cord (Prentiss maneuver)
  - Ligation of the testicular vessels with preservation of the blood supply from the deferential artery and cremasteric arteries (Fowler–Stevens; may be performed in 1 or 2 stages).
- Laparoscopy:
  - Effective for management of non-palpable testes
  - Management is dependent upon intraoperative findings

- If blind-ending vessels identified, no further treatment necessary
- If a spermatic cord entering inguinal ring is identified, inguinal exploration is performed
- If an intra-abdominal testis is identified, laparoscopic orchidopexy may be performed using the same surgical principles as open surgery.

ASSOCIATED ABNORMALITIES

Direct inguinal hernia[13]

- Definition: the presence of abdominal contents within a patent processus vaginalis.
- Incidence: 3–5% of term male children.
- Majority occur within the first year of life.
- Occur more frequently on right.
- Treatment is surgery.
  - Involves identification and isolation of hernia sac, followed by ligation at the internal ring.

Hydrocele[3]

- Definition: a collection of fluid within the tunica vaginalis.
  - *Communicating hydroceles* are associated with a patent processus vaginalis.
- A common finding in newborn males; most resolve spontaneously.
- History:
  - Fluctuations in size suggest a communicating hydrocele.
- Exam:
  - Transillumination of the sac fluid is a classic finding.

Treatment

- Observation for:
  - Non-symptomatic, stable hydroceles
  - Communicating hydroceles in infants.
- Surgery for:
  - Enlarging hydroceles or persistent hydroceles in older children
  - New onset of a communicating hydrocele.
- Same surgical principles as for hernia repair.

REFERENCES

1. Schafer AJ: Sex determination and its pathology in man. Adv Genet 33:294, 1995.
2. Diamond D: Sexual differentiation: normal and abnormal. In: Walsh PC, Retik AB, Vaughan ED, Wein AJ, eds. Campbell's Urology, 8th edn. Philadelphia: WB Saunders, 2002, pp 2395–423.
3. Snodgrass W: Intersex, hypospadias, cryptorchidism, hernias and hydroceles, epispadias and exstrophy. AUA Annual Review Course, 97–157, 2005.
4. Laue L, Rennert OM: Congenital adrenal hyperplasia: molecular genetics and alternative approaches to treatment. Adv Pediatr 42:113–43, 1995.
5. Griffin JE: Androgen resistance: the clinical and molecular spectrum. New Engl J Med 326:611–18, 1992.
6. Griffin JE, Durrant JL: Qualitative receptor defects in families with androgen resistance: failure of stabilization of the fibroblast cytosol androgen receptor. J Clin Endocrinol Metab 55:465–74, 1982.

7. Hall JG, Gilchrist DM: Turner syndrome and its variants. Pediatr Clin North Am 37:1421–41, 1990.
8. Harnden DG, Maclean N, Langlands AO: Carcinoma of the breast and Klinefelter's syndrome. J Med Genet 8:460–1, 1971.
9. Schneck FX, Bellinger MF: Abnormalities of the testes and scrotum and their surgical management. In: Walsh PC, Retik AB, Vaughan ED, Wein AJ, eds. Campbell's Urology, 8th edn. Philadelphia: WB Saunders, 2002, pp 2353–89.
10. Scorer CG, Farrington GH: Congenital Deformities of the Testis and Epididymis. New York: Appleton-Century-Crofts, 1971.
11. Richie JP, Steele GG: Neoplasms of the testis. In: Walsh PC, Retik AB, Vaughan ED, Wein AJ, eds. Campbell's Urology. 8th edn. Philadelphia: WB Saunders; 2002, pp 2876–919.
12. Rajfer J, Handelsman DJ, Swerdloff RS et al: Hormonal therapy of cryptorchidism: a randomized, double-blind study comparing human chorionic gonadotropin and gonadotropin-releasing hormone. New Engl J Med 314:466–70, 1986.
13. Holder TM, Ashcraft KW: Groin hernias and hydroceles. In: Holder TM, Ashcraft KW, eds. Pediatric Surgery. Philadelphia: WB Saunders, 1980, pp 594–608.

22

DEVELOPMENTAL ABNORMALITIES OF THE GENITALIA

Pediatric urinary infections, vesicoureteral reflux, and voiding dysfunction

Benjamin H Lowentritt

SUMMARY

- During the first year of life, males have more urinary tract infections than females. Uncircumcised males are at greater risk.
- After the first year of life, females have more urinary tract infections than males (10:1 risk compared with males).
- Most common pathogen is *E. coli*.
- Pediatric urinary tract infection requires further evaluation in the following situations: children <5 years, fever, family history of vesicoureteral reflux, and school-age girls with recurrent infections.
- Commonly used antibiotics include trimethoprim–sulfamethoxazole, nitrofurantoin, and amoxicillin.
- Vesicoureteral reflux affects up to 1–5% of children. It may be primary (due to abnormal implantation of ureter into bladder) or secondary (due to increased intravesical pressure). It is generally diagnosed on voiding cystourethrogram. Treatment is medical (antibiotic prophylaxis) or surgical (reimplantation of ureters into bladder or transurethral injection of bulking agents into ureter).
- Voiding dysfunction disorders in children include urinary incontinence, dysfunctional elimination syndrome, and nocturnal enuresis.
- Treatments for nocturnal enuresis include behavioral modification, DDAVP (desmopressin), and imipramine.

PEDIATRIC URINARY TRACT INFECTIONS (UTIs)

CLASSIFICATION[1]

- Cystitis – bladder involvement only.
- Clinical pyelonephritis – fever, abdominal/flank pain, and infection.
- Acute pyelonephritis – Renal parenchymal involvement, seen on DMSA, CT, or ultrasound.
- Asymptomatic bacteriuria – not usually seen in children.
- Recurrent UTI – not an adequately descriptive term
- Unresolved bacteriuria – infection not adequately treated.
- Persistent UTI – same bacterial etiology after documented infection-free period; need to investigate for foreign bodies, calculi, or anatomical abnormalities.
- Reinfection – new infection with different bacteria.

EPIDEMIOLOGY

- Males have more UTIs than females during the first year of life.
  - Circumcised boys have 1% incidence, uncircumcised 5–20 times increased risk.[2]

- After 1 year, females predominate.
  - 10:1 risk compared with males.
- First infection often manifests at toilet training.
- Girls have 60–80% chance of reinfection within 5 years of initial infection.[3]

BIOLOGY

Bacteriology

- *Escherichia coli* most common, followed by other Enterobacteriaceae (*Klebsiella, Enterobacter, Proteus*).
- Rare causes: *Staphylococcus, Enterococcus, Haemophilus influenzae,* and non-bacterial.
- Most will have $>10^6$ counts in urine.
- Symptomatic children with $>10^5$ should be considered infected.

Virulence factors

- Type I fimbriae (mannose sensitive) – found in most *E. coli*, attaches to D-mannosyl residue.
- Type II fimbrae (P-fimbriae, mannose resistant) – present in most *E. coli* that cause pyelonephritis, attaches to glycosphingolipid on red blood cells of P1 blood group and urothelial cells.[4]
- Hemolysin – causes damage to renal tubular cells.
- K antigen – capsular polysaccharide that shields bacteria from phagocytosis.

Host factors

- Foreskin increases risk in boys.[2]
- Vesicoureteral reflux is most important host factor, allowing less virulent pathogens to cause pyelonephritis.
- Adequate emptying of bladder dramatically reduces likelihood of UTI; voiding dysfunction often manifests with incomplete or infrequent emptying, causing UTI.
- Non-secretors (Lewis antibody b−) have increased incidence of UTI compared with secretors (Lewis antibody b+).[5]
- Number of receptors for P fimbriae is inherited.
- African-American children have less UTI, reflux, and pyelonephritis.

RENAL SCARRING

- Occurs in as many as 60% of patients with UTI and vesicoureteral reflux (higher-grade reflux yields more scarring).
- Immune/inflammatory response activated by endotoxin during pyelonephritis.
- Byproducts of inflammation cause ischemia and direct tissue injury.
- Sterile reflux does not cause scarring (after birth).
- If no scarring by age 4–5, risk is markedly decreased, even with pyelonephritis.
- Pyelonephritic scarring is most common cause of pediatric hypertension.[6]

DIAGNOSIS

Signs/symptoms

- Often can be vague – irritability, poor feeding, etc.
- Older children may have urinary frequency, dysuria, pain, or new-onset/ worsening incontinence.
- Fevers suggest pyelonephritis (1/2–2/3 of febrile UTIs will show acute pyelonephritis on DMSA scan).

Urine evaluation

- Urine bags yield high levels of contamination.
- Catheterized urine is reliable, but traumatic; suprapubic aspirate is gold standard but also traumatic.
- Voided samples in toilet-trained children can be adequate, especially in circumcised males.
- Urine should be centrifuged and evaluated with microscopy for pyuria and bacteria.
- Nitrate and leukocyte esterase can be helpful adjuncts but can have false negatives.

RADIOLOGICAL EVALUATION: GENERAL PRINCIPLES

- Who needs to be evaluated?
  - Children <5 years with documented UTI
  - Any child with a febrile UTI
  - Any child with UTI and a family history of vesicoureteral reflux
  - School-age girls with multiple UTIs.
- Initial work-up includes renal ultrasound and VCUG.
  - School-age boys with one episode of cystitis or school-age girls with two episodes of cystitis can be evaluated with ultrasound only, with further imaging as needed.

IMAGING MODALITIES

- Ultrasound:
  - Shows renal size, cortical thickness, hydronephrosis, duplication
  - Less sensitive for vesicoureteral reflux, scarring, acute pyelonephritis.
- Intravenous pyelogram (IVP):
  - Shows scars well
  - Disadvantage: associated with radiation/contrast dosing.
- Tc 99m dimercaptosuccinic acid (DMSA) scan:
  - Gold standard for diagnosis of acute pyelonephritis and renal scarring
  - Scarring can often be demonstrated within 6 months after acute pyelonephritis
  - Role in acute pyelonephritis debatable since it rarely changes management.
- Voiding cystourethrogram (VCUG):
  - Necessary to diagnose reflux and document grade
  - Important to have filling and voiding phases of study, as some patients only reflux with contraction.

23

URINARY INFECTIONS, VESICOURETERAL REFLUX, AND VOIDING DYSFUNCTION

TREATMENT PRINCIPLES

General principles

- For first infection, use antibiotic prophylaxis until VCUG performed.
- If patient septic, poorly compliant, or unable to tolerate PO, may require hospitalization for IV antibiotics.
- Recheck cultures after 2 weeks.

Duration

- Pyelonephritis: 10–14 days; oral medications acceptable.[7]
- Cystitis: 3–5 days.[8]
- Asymptomatic bacteriuria: treatment not recommended.

Antibiotics

- Trimethoprim–sulfamethoxazole (8 mg trimethoprim/kg/day divided bid):
  - Block bacterial folate pathways
  - Trimethoprim concentrates in vaginal secretions
  - Rarely associated with Stevens–Johnson syndrome
  - Avoid in first 2 months of life: can cause neonatal hyperbilirubinemia and kernicterus.
- Nitrofurantoin (5 mg/kg/day divided qid):
  - Blocks bacterial Krebs cycle
  - Concentrated in urine but not in tissue
  - Nausea and vomiting common with liquid form
  - Avoid in patients with G6PD (glucose-6-phosphate dehydrogenase) deficiency and in infants in first 2 months of life because of risk of hemolytic anemia.
- Amoxicillin (40 mg/kg/day divided tid):
  - Safe at all ages.
- Fluoroquinolones:
  - Currently not approved in children
  - Potentially may cause tendon rupture or abnormal bone development.

VESICOURETERAL REFLUX (VUR)

CLASSIFICATION AND GENERAL INFORMATION

- Primary.
- Secondary – associated with the following:
  - Voiding dysfunction
  - Neuropathic bladder
  - Ectopic ureterocele
  - Posterior urethral valves
  - Prune belly
  - Posterior urethral valves
  - Exstrophy.
- International grading system:
  - One: ureter visible; 5% risk of renal scarring
  - Two: entire ureter and normal-appearing collecting system visible; 10% risk of scarring

- Three: mild dilation of ureter, pelvis, and calyces, with minimal blunting of fornices; 20% risk of scarring
- Four: dilated ureter and marked calyceal distortion; 40% risk of scarring
- Five: tortuous ureter with 'blown-out' calyces; 60% risk of scarring.
- Antenatal reflux (congenital reflux nephropathy):
  - More common in boys
  - Can cause renal damage in absence of infection.

EPIDEMIOLOGY

- Affects 1–5% of all children.[9]
- Age at onset correlates to age at toilet training.
- 32% of siblings of refluxing patients found to have VUR.[10]
- 50% of children of refluxing mothers will have VUR.[11]
- 4:1 female to male ratio in those diagnosed after UTI.
  - However, of those screened for antenatal hydronephrosis, males are more common.[12]
- 40% of children with pyelonephritis will have VUR.[13]

BIOLOGY

Primary reflux

- Secondary to abnormal implantation of ureter into bladder.
- Refluxing ureter comes in at a straighter, less oblique angle than a normal ureter and has a shorter submucosal tunnel length (normal = 5 × greater than ureteral diameter).[14]

Secondary reflux

- Caused by increased intravesical pressure.
- Therapy includes identifying the underlying cause.

DIAGNOSIS

History

- Voiding pattern. If patient is already toilet trained, dysfunctional voiding may be present.
- Frequency and severity of UTIs.
- Family history.
- Bowel habits. Constipation is commonly present and can affect treatment.

Physical exam

- Signs of chronic renal scarring include below average height/weight and high blood pressure.
- Signs of unrecognized neurological disease include sacral depression and abnormal perineal sensation/reflexes.
- Abdominal masses.

Laboratory

- Urinalysis (U/A) and cuture consistent with UTI.
- Creatinine increases are rare.

Radiological evaluation

- VCUG:
  - Requires bladder filling and voiding phases
  - May reveal signs of ureteral duplication ('drooping lily') or dysfunctional voiding ('spinning top urethra' in girls).
- Ultrasound:
  - Useful for screening (i.e. small kidney size and/or abnormal collecting system).
- DMSA scan:
  - Not necessary for low-grade (I–II) reflux with normal ultrasound
  - Useful for: baseline in high-grade VUR, evaluating for renal scars 3–6 months after febrile UTI, and determining kidney function.
- IVP:
  - Not commonly used or recommended.
- Diuretic renogram (technetiumTc 99m mercaptoacetyltriglycine [MAG-3] or technetium Tc 99m diethylenetriamine pentaacetic acid [DTPA]):
  - Useful in determining if obstruction is present
  - Important to have well-hydrated patient with Foley catheter in place for accurate test.
- Nuclear cystogram:
  - Very sensitivite for detecting reflux, but not useful for grading reflux
  - Not used for initial evaluation, but can be used to follow VUR patients.

TREATMENT

Basic principles

- Prevent infection and renal scarring.
- If reflux is secondary, treat the VUR *and* the underlying condition.[12]

Medical therapy

- Basic principle: most cases of reflux will resolve spontaneously and renal injury occurs only with active infection.
- Basic components:
  - Daily antibiotic prophylaxis: usually with trimethoprim–sulfamethoxazole
  - Treatment of concomitant voiding dysfunction and constipation
  - Annual VCUG or nuclear cystogram
  - Urinalysis and culture for *any* febrile illness (optional: U/A in asymptomatic patients every 3–6 months).
- Medical therapy continues until the VUR resolves, breakthrough infections and/or renal scarring occur, growth is delayed, or VUR continues >5 years after diagnosis.
- Outcomes are listed in Table 23.1.[9]

TABLE 23.1

REFLUX RESOLUTION WITH MEDICAL THERAPY OVER 5 YEARS[9]

| Grade, laterality, age (months) | Percent chance of resolution | | | | |
	1 year	2 years	3 years	4 years	5 years
I, any laterality/age	39.3	63.1	77.6	86.4	91.8
II, any laterality/age	28	48.1	62.7	73.1	80.6
III, unilateral, age 0–24	21.4	38.2	51.5	61.9	70
III, unilateral, age 25–60	13.4	25	35.1	43.8	51.3
III, unilateral, age 61–120	10.8	20.5	29.1	36.7	43.6
III, bilateral, age 0–24	12.7	23.8	33.5	41.9	49.3
III, bilateral, age 25–60	7	13.5	19.6	25.2	30.5
III, bilateral, age 61–120	2.6	5.2	7.7	10.1	12.5
IV, unilateral*	16.1	29.7	41	50.5	58.5
IV, bilateral*	4.5	6.4	7.8	8.9	9.9

*Not age-specific; grade V reflux not included in this meta-analysis.

Surgical therapy (ureteral reimplantation)

- Basic principle: eliminates need for antibiotic prophylaxis and prevents renal scarring.[15]
- Goal is to re-establish 5:1 ratio of submucosal tunnel length to ureteral diameter.
- Surgical approaches include open intravesical, open extravesical, and laparoscopic.[16]
- Common intravesical approaches include:
  - Politano–Leadbetter: new tunnel created through new hiatus in posterior wall of bladder
  - Cohen transtrigonal: advancement of orifice to opposite side of trigone.
- Common extravesical approaches include:
  - Lich–Gregoir – ureteral orifice left intact, new tunnel of bladder muscle created and ureter buried within.
- Surgery successful in 96–98% of cases of grades I–IV and 80% of grade V.[9,17]
  - Half of failures are due to persistent dysfunctional voiding.
- Unilateral surgical repair results in contralateral reflux in 1–5% of cases.[9]

Endoscopic therapy

- Principle is to bulk the back of the distal ureter and enable coaptation during filling and contraction.
- Commonly used agents:
  - Teflon
  - Collagen: volume often decreases with time
  - Silicone microspheres
  - Deflux (dextranomer/hyaluronic acid) – has resulted in 75–85% success rate in improving/eliminating reflux.[18]

Outcomes: medical vs surgical

- Risk of cystitis:
  - Same.

23

URINARY INFECTIONS, VESICOURETERAL REFLUX, AND VOIDING DYSFUNCTION

- Risk of pyelonephritis:
  - 2.5 times higher in patients on medical therapy.
- No difference in renal scarring, renal growth, renal function, overall growth, or incidence of hypertension.[13]

Current treatment recommendations[9]

- Antibiotic prophylaxis recommended for:
  - Grades I–IV if 0–5 years old
  - Grade V if <1 year old
  - Unilateral grade V if 1–5 years old and no renal scarring.
- Surgery recommended for:
  - Grades III–V if ≥6 years old at initial presentation
  - Grade V if renal scarring present
  - Grades III–V if no resolution after 5 years of antibiotic therapy.
- Breakthrough infections or scarring may justify surgery.

VOIDING DYSFUNCTION

NORMAL VOIDING DEVELOPMENT

Prenatal voiding

- Reflex – full bladder starts signal via S2–S4 pathway to pons, which coordinates parasympathetic signals back to bladder via pelvic plexus.[19]
- During storage, sympathetic tone and pudendal nerve inhibit detrusor muscle and keep bladder neck and sphincter closed.

Postnatal voiding

- Normal voiding 15–20 times per day via reflex.
- Bladder grows at predictable pace:
  - *Normal bladder capacity (ounces) = Age in years +2*
- Toilet training usually started between ages 2 and 4.
- By 5 years 90–95% are dry during day, 80–85% dry at night.[20]

PEDIATRIC URINARY INCONTINENCE

Evaluation

- By 12 years old, 99% of children are dry day and night.
- Incontinence may be sign of UTI, stress at home, abuse, or dysfunctional elimination syndrome.
- History:
  - Patterns of incontinence (urge, stress, mixed, or continuous)
  - Constipation
  - Age at toilet training
  - Associated bowel and/or neurological disease.[21]
- Physical exam:
  - Neurological evaluation: perineal sensation and/or sacral defects.[22]
- Additional work-up:
  - U/A and culture: if UTI, initiate appropriate work-up (see above)
  - Consider urodynamics
  - For dysuria-hematuria: consider hypercalciuria and obtain 24-hour urine.

Treatment

- Aimed at reinforcing normal voiding habits.
- Continous incontinence in girls: consider ectopic ureter.
- Post-voiding incontinence in girls: consider labial adhesions.
  - Can result in vaginal voiding and post-voiding incontinence
  - Treat adhesions with 2 weeks of estrogen cream.
- Giggle incontinence:
  - Cause unknown
  - Usually resolves spontaneously
  - Timed voiding and anticholinergics are treatment options.

DYSFUNCTIONAL ELIMINATION SYNDROME

Several different conditions that were previously treated as separate diseases are now felt to be part of a spectrum of conditions of varying severity involving the urinary and gastrointestinal tracts.

NON-NEUROGENIC NEUROGENIC BLADDER (HINMAN'S SYNDROME, VOLUNTARY DETRUSOR-SPHINCTER DYSSYNERGIA)

- Severe end of spectrum.
- Possibly a learned behavior.[23]
- Urodynamics may show overactive bladder contractions without overt neurological dysfunction.[24]
- Radiological studies can show large 'dumbbell-shaped' bladder, hydronephrosis wth secondary reflux, or 'spinning-top urethra.'
- Constipation, poor intake of liquids, and UTIs may occur.
- Treatment:
  - Biofeedback to help relax pelvic floor
  - Timed voiding
  - Antibiotics for reflux
  - Management of constipation
  - Anticholinergics and/or clean intermittent catheterization if necessary.[25]

UNSTABLE BLADDER

- Child struggles to prevent incontinence by constricting the sphincter.
- 'Vincent's curtsy' may be seen as children try to prevent leaking with urge by squatting.
- Can lead to small, contracted bladder.
- Treatment similar to Hinman's syndrome.
- May take years to resolve.[26]

INFREQUENT VOIDING

- More frequently affects girls.
- Can present with overflow incontinence, retention, or UTIs.
- May void only 2–3 times per day.
- Urodynamics usually normal except for large-capacity bladder.
- Often associated with constipation.

- Management includes timed voiding and management of constipation.
  - Clean intermittent catheterization rarely necessary.

NOCTURNAL ENURESIS (NE)

Incidence

- Affects 15–20% of 5 year olds; decreases spontaneously at rate of 15% per year such that only 1% of 15 year olds are affected.[27]
- Primary enuresis (never were dry): 75% of enuretics.
- Diurnal incontinence occurs in 25%.
- Risk markedly elevated in children of affected parents: 1 parent = 44% risk, both parents = 77% risk.[28]

Pathogenesis

- Unknown: may be associated with developmental delay, sleep disorder, or psychological stress.[28]
- May be associated with lower serum vasopressin levels.

Evaluation

- History and exam.
- Radiological studies usually not indicated unless treatment fails.

Treatment

- Behavioral:
  - Include motivational techniques and alarms
  - Generally work better in older children.[29]
- DDAVP (desmopressin):
  - Desmopressin 10–40 µg nasal spray or 10–30 mg tablets
  - Functions by decreasing urine output and increasing urine osmolality at night
  - More effective in nasal preparation; pills need to be taken several hours before bedtime
  - Successful in 60%; success may be increased if combined with behavioral therapies.[30]
- Imipramine:
  - 25–75 mg qhs
  - Only for children >6 years
  - May work through several effects: anticholinergic, altered sleep pattern, reduction of nocturnal urine volume.

REFERENCES

1. Chon CH, Lai FC, Shortliffe LM: Pediatric urinary tract infections. Pediatr Clin North Am 48(6):1441–59, 2001.
2. Circumcision policy statement: American Academy of Pediatrics. Task Force on Circumcision. Pediatrics 103(3):686–93, 1999.
3. Rushton HG: Urinary tract infections in children. Epidemiology, evaluation, and management. Pediatr Clin North Am 44(5):1133–69, 1997.
4. Majd M, Rushton HG, Jantausch B, Wiedermann BL: Relationship among vesicoureteral reflux, P-fimbriated Escherichia coli, and acute pyelonephritis in children with febrile urinary tract infection. J Pediatr 119(4):578–85, 1991.

5. Sheinfeld J, Schaeffer AJ, Cordon-Cardo C, Rogatko A, Fair WR: Association of the Lewis blood-group phenotype with recurrent urinary tract infections in women. New Engl J Med 320(12):773–7, 1989.

6. Dillon MJ: Recent advances in evaluation and management of childhood hypertension. Eur J Pediatr 132(3):133–9, 1979.

7. Malhotra SM, Kennedy WA: Urinary tract infections in children: treatment. Urol Clin North Am 31(3):527–34, 2004.

8. Shapiro E, Elder JS: The office management of recurrent urinary tract infection and vesicoureteral reflux in children. Urol Clin North Am 25(4):725–34, 1998.

9. Elder JS, Peters CA, Arant BS Jr et al: Pediatric Vesicoureteral Reflux Guidelines Panel summary report on the management of primary vesicoureteral reflux in children. J Urol 157(5):1846–51, 1997.

10. Hollowell JG, Greenfield SP: Screening siblings for vesicoureteral reflux. J Urol 168(5):2138–41, 2002.

11. Noe HN, Wyatt RJ, Peeden JN Jr, Rivas ML: The transmission of vesicoureteral reflux from parent to child. J Urol 148(6):1869–71, 1992.

12. Farhat W, McLorie G, Geary D et al: The natural history of neonatal vesicoureteral reflux associated with antenatal hydronephrosis. J Urol 164(3 Pt 2):1057–60, 2000.

13. Fanos V, Cataldi L: Antibiotics or surgery for vesicoureteric reflux in children. Lancet 364(9446):1720–2, 2004.

14. Paquin AJ Jr: Ureterovesical anastomosis: the description and evaluation of a technique. J Urol 82:573–83, 1959.

15. Cooper CS, Austin JC: Vesicoureteral reflux: who benefits from surgery? Urol Clin North Am 31(3):535–41, 2004.

16. Austin JC, Cooper CS: Vesicoureteral reflux: surgical approaches. Urol Clin North Am 31(3):543–57, 2004.

17. Marshall S, Guthrie T, Jeffs R, Politano V, Lyon RP: Ureterovesicoplasty: selection of patients, incidence and avoidance of complications. A review of 3,527 cases. J Urol 118(5):829–31, 1977.

18. Lackgren G, Wahlin N, Skoldenberg E, Stenberg A: Long-term followup of children treated with dextranomer/hyaluronic acid copolymer for vesicoureteral reflux. J Urol 166(5):1887–92, 2001.

19. Yeung CK, Godley ML, Duffy PG, Ransley PG: Natural filling cystometry in infants and children. Br J Urol 75(4):531–7, 1995.

20. Fergusson DM, Horwood LJ, Shannon FT: Factors related to the age of attainment of nocturnal bladder control: an 8-year longitudinal study. Pediatrics 78(5):884–90. 1986.

21. Bloom DA, Faerber G, Bomalaski MD: Urinary incontinence in girls. Evaluation, treatment, and its place in the standard model of voiding dysfunctions in children. Urol Clin North Am 22(3):521–38, 1995.

22. Feng WC, Churchill BM: Dysfunctional elimination syndrome in children without obvious spinal cord diseases. Pediatr Clin North Am 48(6):1489–504, 2001.

23. Wan J, Kaplinsky R, Greenfield S: Toilet habits of children evaluated for urinary tract infection. J Urol 154(2 Pt 2):797–9, 1995.

24. Parekh DJ, Pope JC, Adams MC, Brock JW III: The use of radiography, urodynamic studies and cystoscopy in the evaluation of voiding dysfunction. J Urol 165(1):215–18, 2001.

25. Schulman SL: Voiding dysfunction in children. Urol Clin North Am 31(3):481–90, ix, 2004.

26. Asnes RS, Mones RL: Extraordinary urinary frequency. Pediatrics 87(6):953, 1991.

27. Forsythe WI, Redmond A: Enuresis and spontaneous cure rate. Study of 1129 enuretis. Arch Dis Child 49(4):259–63, 1974.

28. Bakwin H: Enuresis in twins. Am J Dis Child 121(3):222–5, 1971.

29. Blum NJ: Nocturnal enuresis: behavioral treatments. Urol Clin North Am 31(3):499–507, ix, 2004.

30. Mammen AA, Ferrer FA: Nocturnal enuresis: medical management. Urol Clin North Am 31(3):491–8, ix, 2004.

URINARY INFECTIONS, VESICOURETERAL REFLUX, AND VOIDING DYSFUNCTION

Pediatric genitourinary oncology

Jennifer Miles-Thomas, Matthew E Nielsen, and Caleb P Nelson

SUMMARY

- Wilms' tumor of the kidney is the most common malignant tumor of the genitourinary (GU) tract. Peak incidence is at ages 3–4 years. Typical presentation is an abdominal mass in a healthy-appearing child. Treatment combines surgery, chemotherapy, and radiation. Prognosis depends upon stage.
- Congenital mesoblastic nephroma is the most common renal tumor in infants. Clear cell sarcoma is associated with bone metastases.
- Neuroblastoma arises from neural crest cells and is the second most common solid tumor of childhood. It may occur in the adrenals/retroperitoneum. Primary therapy is surgery; chemotherapy and radiation may also be used in unfavorable disease.
- Yolk sac tumor is the most common prepubertal testicular tumor. Typical presentation is a scrotal mass. Treatment is radical orchiectomy.
- Leydig cell tumors of the testes produce testosterone. Typical presentation is painless testicular mass with precocious puberty. Treatment is radical orchiectomy.
- Rhabdomyosarcoma is the most common soft tissue sarcoma of childhood and may involve the bladder, prostate, paratesticular tissue, vagina, vulva, or uterus. Treatment typically combines surgery with chemotherapy and/or radiation.

24

TUMORS OF THE KIDNEY

WILMS' TUMOR (NEPHROBLASTOMA)

Epidemiology

- Most common malignant tumor of the GU tract:
  - 80% of GU tumors in children <5 years.[1]
- ~350 new cases/year in the United States.
- 75% <5 years; 90% <7 years.
- Peak incidence: ages 3–4 years.
- Males and females affected equally.
- More common in blacks compared with whites compared with Asians.
- 12% are multifocal.

Types

- Classic Wilms' tumor:
  - Most common.
- Bilateral Wilms' tumor:
  - Approximately 5% of patients
  - 20% have family history of other GU malignances.
- Anaplastic Wilms' tumor:
  - Associated with poorer prognosis.

Associated anomalies

- Sporadic aniridia:
  - Incidence in general population: 1/50 000 births
  - Incidence in Wilms' tumor: 1/70 cases (1.1%)
  - Patients with aniridia have a 33% risk of developing Wilms' tumor.
- WAGR syndrome:
  - **W**ilms' tumor, **A**niridia, **G**U anomalies, Mental **R**etardation
  - Usually presents before age 3
  - Associated with an 11p13 deletion
  - Ear deformities, inguinal/umbilical hernias, renal hypoplasia, ectopia/fusions/duplications, hypospadias, cryptorchidism, pseudohermaphroditism.
- Hemihypertrophy:
  - Incidence in general population: 1/14 000 births
  - Incidence in Wilms' tumor: 1/32 cases
  - Associated with embryonal carcinoma, pigmented nevi, and hemangiomata.
- Beckwith–Wiedemann syndrome:
  - Have a 4–10% chance of developing Wilms' tumor
  - Associated abnormalities include visceromegaly, hemihypertrophy, omphalocele, abdominal wall defects, microcephaly, mental retardation, macroglossia.
- Denys–Drash syndrome:
  - Associated with an 11p13 mutation
  - Associated abnormalities include male pseudohermaphroditism, renal mesangial sclerosis, nephroblastoma, and end-stage renal disease.

Biology

- Abnormal proliferation of metanephric blastema without normal differentiation into tubules or glomeruli.[1]
- Nephrogenic rest is a focus of abnormally persistent nephrogenic cells that can be secondarily induced to form a Wilms' tumor.
  - Histological appearance may be indistinguishable from Wilms' tumor[1]
  - Nephroblastomatosis: diffuse presence of nephrogenic rests.

Genetics

- Associated with loss of allelic heterogeneity of chromosome 11p, implicating WT1 (11p13 loss of heterozygosity in 33% of cases).[2]
- Loss of 11p15 (WT2) associated with Beckwith–Wiedemann syndrome.[3]
- p53, FWT1 (17q), FWT2 (19q), 16q, and 1p may also be involved.
- Knudson and Strong: '2-hit' hypothesis:[4]
  - Subpopulation predisposed to tumor formation due to germline primary 'hit' to one of the alleles
  - Tumor develops if renal cells later acquire 2nd 'hit' to the remaining normal allele.

Pathology

- Typically associated with a pseudocapsule.
- Favorable histology:
  - Classic triphasic pattern: epithelial/blastemal/stromal
  - Tubules/clusters of small blue cells with mature mesodermal elements.
- Unfavorable histology:
  - Associated with 10% of all cases but >50% of all deaths
  - Anaplasia
  - Rhabdoid/clear cell type.

Presentation

- Healthy-appearing child with abdominal mass.
  - Abdominal mass or increasing abdominal girth present in 75%[1]
  - Palpably smooth tumor which rarely crosses midline.
- 15% have other congenital abnormalities.
- <25% have microhematuria.
- 25–63% have renin-mediated hypertension.

Evaluation

- Renal ultrasound:
  - Screening test to assess IVC, establish tissue of origin, and discriminate solid vs cystic mass.
- CT:
  - Good for imaging liver, smaller tumors, and lymph nodes.
- MRI:
  - Useful for vascular mapping.

Staging

Based on US surgical practice and European imaging.
- Stage I: totally resected, specimen-confined tumor with no spillage or residual tumor.
- Stage II: gross total resection with regional spread (positive surgical margins, capsular penetration, biopsy, and/or tumor spill).
  - Extrarenal vessels may have thrombus or infiltration.
- Stage III: incomplete resection or unresectable primary, large tumor spill, positive lymph nodes.
- Stage IV: distant metastases.
- Stage V: synchronous bilateral tumors at the time of diagnosis.

Treatment

- By stage (in the United States, per NWTS protocol):
  - Stage I in patients <2 years with tumors <550 g: nephrectomy, then observation
  - Stages I and II (favorable histology) in older children: nephrectomy, then chemotherapy
  - Stage I with anaplasia or stages III and IV with favorable histology: nephrectomy, then radiation and chemotherapy

24

GENITOURINARY ONCOLOGY

- Stages II–IV with anaplasia or otherwise unfavorable histology: nephrectomy, then radiation and chemotherapy
- Stage V: bilateral biopsies, then chemotherapy, then clinical reassessment.
- Nephrectomy:
  - Chevron incision utilized with contralateral renal exploration and biopsy performed
  - Lymphadenectomy: no survival advantage, but important for staging[5]
  - May consider biopsy instead of nephrectomy if adjacent organ injury appears inevitable with resection.
- Bilateral tumors:
  - Must balance disease control vs preservation of functional renal mass
  - At second look after initial treatment; may excise if >2/3 renal mass can be preserved
  - May have to consider complete nephrectomy for unfavorable histology or chemotherapy failure.
- Consider partial nephrectomy if:
  - Bilateral Wilms' tumor
  - Solitary kidney
  - Renal insufficiency.
- Chemotherapy:
  - Consider preoperative chemotherapy when tumor is bilateral, intracaval, and/or unresectable
  - Preoperative chemotherapy or radiotherapy may lower intraoperative morbidity[6] but will probably not influence long-term survival.[7]
- Prognosis (based on overall survival from National Wilms' Tumor Study – 3): Table 24.1.[8]

CONGENITAL MESOBLASTIC NEPHROMA[9]

- Most common renal tumor in infants.
- Mean age at diagnosis is 3.5 months.
- Characterized by a solitary hamartoma which infiltrates renal stromal cells.
- May have hypercalcemia, vomiting, and polyuria.
- Almost always unilateral, rarely malignant, frequently in males.
- Frequently associated with polyhydramnios.
- Treatment is complete surgical excision.

TABLE 24.1

PROGNOSIS FOR WILMS' TUMOR

Stage	Histology	Survival (%)
I	Favorable	97
	Unfavorable	68
II	Favorable	92
	Unfavorable	68
III	Favorable	84
	Unfavorable	68
IV	Favorable	83
	Unfavorable	55

MULTILOCULAR CYSTIC NEPHROMA[9]

- Uncommon, benign renal tumor, usually unilateral.[10,11]
- 50% occur in young children, primarily males.
  - Also occurs in young adult women.
- Surgery is curative.
  - May have recurrence with incomplete resection.

CLEAR CELL SARCOMA

- Usually unilateral.
- Mean age at presentation is 3.5 years.[9]
- Classic histopathological pattern: polygonal cells with round oval nuclei.[12]
- Predictors of increased survival: lower stage, younger age at diagnosis, absence of tumor necrosis, and treatment with doxorubicin.[13,14]
  - Doxorubicin improves overall survival and relapse-free survival.
- 98% survival rate for stage I.[9]
- Long-term follow-up is needed.
  - 30% of relapses occur >3 years after diagnosis and treatment.
- Associated with bone and brain metastases.
- Treatment is radiotherapy and chemotherapy.
- Prognosis is generally poor.

RHABDOID[9]

- The most aggressive and lethal renal tumor of childhood.
- 2% of tumors registered to National Wilms' Tumor Study Group.[15]
- Median age at diagnosis is 16 months.
- May metastasize to brain, lungs, abdomen, and liver.[16]
- Treatment is radiotherapy and chemotherapy.
- Typically has poor survival.

TUMORS OF THE ADRENAL AND RETROPERITONEUM

NEUROBLASTOMA

Epidemiology

- Most common malignant tumor of infancy, second most common solid tumor of childhood.
- 50% of cases diagnosed at <2 years, 75% <4 years.[17]
- Slight male predominance.[18]
- Higher incidence in Turner's syndrome, Hirschsprung's disease, and neurofibromatosis type I.
- 55% of cases are abdominal; of those, 66% are adrenal.

Genetics

- May be hereditary or sporadic.
- Deletion in chromosome 1p with loss of heterozygosity associated with poor prognosis.[19,20]
- N-myc oncogene amplification correlated with advanced stages of disease, rapid progression, and poor outcomes.[21]
- Deletions of 11q and/or 14q detected in 25–50%.[22]

24

GENITOURINARY ONCOLOGY

Pathology

- Arises from neural crest cells.
- Gross appearance: highly vascular, purple mass.
- Microscopic appearance: small, round, blue cells.
- Shimada histological grading system determines prognosis.[23]

Clinical presentation and diagnosis

- Typically presents as a firm, irregular mass that may extend across midline.
- Paravertebral sympathetic ganglia may yield 'dumbbell' tumor growth through intervertebral foramen causing spinal cord compression.
  - Chemotherapy is associated with an excellent prognosis in this setting.
- 70% of patients present with metastases.[24,25]
  - Younger patients classically present with subcutaneous nodules and liver involvement, older patients with bony metastases.
- Tumor may secrete catecholamines, causing flushing, hypertension, and palpitations.

Evaluation

- Bone marrow aspiration (70% positive).[26]
- 24-hour urine for VMA (vanillylmandelic acid) and HVA (homovanillic acid) levels (elevated in 95%).
- CT:
  - Classically shows speckled calcifications in a suprarenal mass.
- MRI:
  - Helps identify bone marrow and major vascular involvement.
- MIBG:
  - Images tumor by competing for uptake in adrenergic secretory vesicles.

Staging (International neuroblastoma staging system; Table 24.2)[27]

Prognostic factors

- Favorable prognosis: age <1 year, localized disease, low serum ferritin, adrenal location, and absent *N-myc* amplification.
- Diploid status of tumor associated with poor response to chemotherapy.[28]

Treatment

- Surgery:
  - Excision is treatment of choice in localized cases
  - Postoperative chemotherapy and radiation therapy may shrink residual masses.

TABLE 24.2

INTERNATIONAL NEUROBLASTOMA STAGING SYSTEM[27]

Stage	Description
1	Localized, complete excision
2A	Localized, incomplete excision
2B	Localized with ipsilateral positive lymph nodes
3	Unresectable, crosses midline or contralateral N+
4	Distant metastases
4S	1, 2A, or 2B with liver/skin/bone marrow metastases (limited to infants <1 year)

- Chemotherapy:
  - Neuroblastoma is chemoresponsive
  - Reserved for patients with unresectable tumors and/or with respiratory/bowel compromise
  - May be used as neoadjuvant therapy in patients with unresectable, but otherwise favorable, disease.
- Radiation:
  - Neuroblastoma is radiosensitive, but radiation is not a curative modality
  - Reserved for unresectable tumors or progressive tumors unresponsive to chemotherapy
  - Primary role: palliation of pain, bone marrow transplant protocol, or for visible metastases.[29]
- Bone marrow transplant:
  - Performed in unfavorable disease following chemotherapy and total body irradiation.[30]

TUMORS OF THE TESTIS

GENERAL INFORMATION

- Older studies cite incidence ~0.5–2 per 100 000; some recent estimates suggest 2–3 per 1 000 000. [31]
- Majority <2 years old at presentation.
- Represent only 1–2% of pediatric neoplasms.
- Frequency by type:
  - Yolk sac tumors: 62%
  - Teratoma: 16%
  - Juvenile granulosa tumors: 4%
  - Gonadal stromal tumors: 3%.
- Extragonadal tumors are considered intermediate to high risk.

YOLK SAC TUMOR/ENDODERMAL SINUS TUMOR[31,32]

- Most common prepubertal testicular tumor.
- Occurs primarily in infants.
- Pathology:
  - Gross apperance: pale gray, mucoid, friable, encapsulated, and well-circumscribed
  - Microscopic appearance: Schiller–Duval bodies.
- Presentation and diagnosis:
  - Asymptomatic scrotal mass
  - 10% associated with hydrocele
  - 3% have a history of associated trauma
  - >90% are localized
  - Lung is the most common site of metastasis.[33]
- Staging (Table 24.3).

24

GENITOURINARY ONCOLOGY

TABLE 24.3

STAGING OF YOLK SAC TUMOR

Stage	Description
I	Complete resection, normalized AFP, negative imaging
II	Positive microscopic margins, persistent ↑AFP, positive RPLNs (<2 cm)
III	+RPLNs (>2 cm) without distant metastases
IV	Distant metastases

AFP = α-fetoprotein; RPLNs = retroperitoneal lymph nodes.

- Evaluation:
  - Serum AFP (α-fetoprotein): increased in 90% (note AFP is normally elevated in newborns up to 9 months of age!)
  - If pure yolk sac tumor, β-hCG (β-human chorionic gonadotropin) should be negative.
- Treatment:
  - Radical inguinal orchiectomy is usually curative (survival >85% for stage I)
  - Retroperitoneal lymph node dissection is not routine
  - Chemotherapy for persistent/recurrent disease: platinum-based regimens associated with >90% survival.

LEYDIG CELL TUMOR[31,34]

- Most common gonadal stromal tumor.
- Peak incidence at ages 4–5 years.
- Accounts for 10% of precocious puberty in males <9 years.
- Typically unilateral and benign.
- Typically produce testosterone.
  - Also may produce corticosteroids, progesterone, and/or estrogens.
- Presentation:
  - Precocious puberty with painless testicular mass, elevated testosterone, and elevated urine 17-ketosteroids
  - Differentiated from primary pituitary lesions by low LH/FSH (luteinizing hormone/follicle-stimulating hormone) from feedback inhibition.
- Pathology:
  - Reinke crystals are rare in children.
- Treatment:
  - Inguinal orchiectomy is usually curative.

TERATOMA[31]

- Second most common prepubertal testis tumor.
- Usually well-differentiated.
- Benign in children <2 years.
- Scrotal ultrasound shows heterogeneous intratesticular mass with internal echoes.
- Treatment:
  - Tumor enucleation (i.e. testis-sparing).

RHABDOMYOSARCOMA[1,35,36]

Epidemiology

- The most common soft tissue sarcoma of childhood.
- Genitourinary disease comprises ~20% of all rhabdomyosarcomas.
- Incidence peaks at:
  - 2–6 years
  - 15–19 years.
- 50% occur before age 5 years, 70% occur before age 10 years.
- Types:
  - Embryonal: majority (90%) of cases, typically occurs in younger children
  - Sarcoma botryoides – a polypoid form
  - Alveolar: typically occurs in adolescents/young adults.
- Associated with Li–Fraumeni syndrome and neurofibromatosis.
- Embryonal associated with translocation between chromosome 1 (or 2) and 13, resulting in chimeric protein PAX7 (or 3) fused to FKHR.
- Alveolar associated with loss of heterozygosity on chromosome 11p15.

Pathology[31]

- Tumor of mesenchymal origin with elements of skeletal muscle.
- Grossly, is nodular and firm. Typically infiltrates into adjacent tissue.
- Alveolar:
  - Anaplastic, undifferentiated
  - Cleft-like spaces lined with rhabdomyoblasts.

Clinical groups (Table 24.4)

Treatment

General principles

- Obtain tissue diagnosis with biopsy and stage with T2-weighted MRI.
  - Note that nearly 20% of patients present with retroperitoneal lymph node metastases.[37]
- Combination of surgery, chemotherapy, and/or radiation therapy.
  - Increased rates of bladder salvage with primary chemotherapy[38]
  - Surgery is diagnostic; adjuvant therapy is aimed at organ preservation.
- VAC chemotherapy is the mainstay.
- Residual masses require biopsy and meticulous radiological and clinical follow-up.[31]

24

GENITOURINARY ONCOLOGY

TABLE 24.4

RHABDOMYOSARCOMA

Group	Description
I	Localized disease, complete resection
II	Gross total resection, evidence of regional spread
a	Microscopic residual disease
b	Regional disease with involved lymph nodes, completely resected
c	Regional disease with involved lymph nodes, grossly resected with microscopic residual (i.e. most distant node microscopically involved)
III	Incomplete resection with gross residual disease
IV	Distant metastases

Bladder/prostate

- Prostatic involvement is a significant, independent predictor of poor outcome.
- Partial cystectomy is indicated for tumors of the dome and lateral wall that persist despite chemotherapy.

Paratesticular

- Arise in distal cord; may invade testis or surrounding tissues.
- Usually present as unilateral, painless, scrotal swelling or supratesticular mass.
- 60% are stage I at diagnosis and 90% are embryonal, which confers a favorable prognosis.[39]
- Treatment is radical inguinal orchiectomy and chemotherapy.
  - If older than 10 years at time of presentation, consider ipsilateral retroperitoneal lymph node dissection prior to chemotherapy.[40]

Vaginal and vulvar

- Typically presents with vaginal bleeding, discharge, and/or vaginal mass.
- Evaluation includes cystoscopy and vaginoscopy.
- Pathology is typically embryonal or botryoid, both of which are associated with excellent prognosis.[41]
- Vulvar:
  - Although often presents with alveolar histology, generally presents as a localized tumor with overall reasonable prognosis.
- Primary treatment: chemotherapy.
  - Conservative surgery as needed.

Uterine

- Typically presents with cervical or abdominal mass and/or vaginal bleeding.
- Mean age at diagnosis is 5.5 years.
  - Evaluation may include cystoscopy and vaginoscopy, CT of the chest, abdomen, and pelvis, and bone marrow aspirate.
- 90% are embryonal.[42]
- Primary treatment: chemotherapy.
  - Conservative surgery as needed.

REFERENCES

1 Kirsh AJ, Snyder HM: What's new and important in pediatric urologic oncology. AUA Update Series, Vol XVII, Lesson 11, 1998.
2. Hoffman M: One Wilms' tumor is cloned. Are there more? Science 246:1387, 1989.
3. Manners M, Slater RM, Heyting C et al: Molecular nature of genetic changes resulting in loss of heterozygosity of chromosome 11 in Wilms' tumors. Hum Genet 81:41–8, 1988.
4. Knudson AG, Strong LC: Mutation and cancer: a model for Wilms' tumor of the kidney. J Natl Cancer Inst 48:313, 1972.
5. Fortner J, Nicastri A, Murphy ML: Neuroblastoma: natural history and results of treating 133 cases. Ann Surg 167:132, 1968.
6. Lemerle J, Voute PA, Tournade MF et al: Preoperative versus postoperative radiotherapy, single versus multiple courses of actinomycin D, in the treatment of Wilms' tumor: preliminary results of a controlled clinical trial conducted by the International Society of Pediatric Oncology (SIOP). Cancer 38:647, 1976.

7. Lemerle J, Voute PA, Tournade MF et al: Effectiveness of preoperative chemotherapy in Wilms' tumor: results of an International Society of Pediatric Oncology (SIOP) clinical trial. J Clin Oncol 1:604, 1983.
8. Green DM, Brewslow NE, Beckwith JB et al: Comparison between single dose and divided dose administration of dactinomycin and doxorubincin for patients with Wilms' tumor: a report from the National Wilms' Tumor Study Group. J Clin Oncol 16:237–48, 1998.
9. Ritchey M: Pediatric urologic oncology. In: Walsh PC, Retik AB, Vaughan ED, Wein AJ, eds. Campbell's Urology, 8th edn. Philadelphia: WB Saunders, 2002, p 2493.
10. Johnson DE, Ayala AG, Medellin H, Wilbur J: Multilocular renal cystic disease in children. J Urol 109:101–3, 1973.
11. Banner MP, Pollack HM, Chatten J, Witzleben C: Multilocular renal cysts: radiologic-pathologic correlation. AJR Am J Roentgenol 136:239–47, 1981.
12. Schmidt D, Beckwith JB: Histopathology of childhood renal tumors. Hematol Oncol Clin North Am 9:1179–200, 1995.
13. D'Angio GJ, Breslow N, Beckwith JB et al: Treatment of Wilms' tumor: results of the Third National Wilms' Tumor Study. Cancer 64:349–60, 1989.
14. Argani P, Perlman EJ, Breslow NE et al: Clear cell sarcoma of the kidney: a review of 351 cases from the National Wilms' Tumor Study Group Pathology Center. Am J Surg Pathol 24:4–18, 2000.
15. D'Angio GJ, Evans AE et al: The treatment of Wilms' tumor: results of the Second National Wilms' Tumor Study. Cancer 47:2302–11, 1981.
16. D'Angio GJ, Rosenberg H, Sharples K et al: Position paper: imaging methods for primary renal tumors of childhood: cost versus benefits. Med Pediatr Oncol 21:205–12, 1993.
17. Fortner J, Nicastri A, Murphy ML: Neuroblastoma: natural history and results of treating 133 cases. Ann Surg 167:13, 1968.
18. Miller RW, Fraumeni JF, Hill JA: Neuroblastoma: epidemiologic approach to its origin. Am J Dis Child 15:253, 1968.
19. Brodeur GM, Fong CT: Molecular biology and genetics of human neuroblastomas. Cancer Genet Cytogenet 41:153–74, 1989.
20. Perri P, Longo L, McConville C et al: Linkage analysis in families with recurrent neuroblastoma. Ann NY Acad Sci 963:74–84, 2002.
21. Brodeur GM, Seeger RC, Sather H et al: Clinical implications of oncogene activation in human neuroblastomas. Cancer 58:541–5, 1986.
22. Srivastsan ES, Ying YL, Seeger RC: Deletion of chromosome 11 and of 14q sequences in neuroblastoma. Genes Chromosomes Cancer 7:32, 1993.
23. Silber JH, Evans AE, Fridman M: Models to predict outcome from childhood neuroblastoma: the role of serum ferritin and tumor histology. Cancer Res 51:1426–33, 1991.
24. Gross RE, Farber S, Martin LW: Neuroblastoma sympatheticum: a study and report of 217 cases. Pediatrics 23:1179, 1959.
25. Ritchey M: Pediatric urologic oncology. In: Walsh PC, Retik AB, Vaughan ED, Wein AJ, eds. Campbell's Urology, 8th edn. Philadelphia: WB Saunders, 2002, p 2470.
26. Finkelstein JR, Echert H, Isaacs H et al: Bone marrow metastases in children with solid tumors. Am J Dis Child 119:49, 1970.
27. Brodeur GM, Pritchard J, Berthold F et al: Revision of the international criteria for neuroblastoma diagnosis, staging and response to treatment. J Clin Oncol 11:1466, 1993.
28. Gansler T, Chatten J, Varello N et al: Flow cytometric DNA analysis of neuroblastoma. Cancer 58:2453–8, 1986.
29. Coplen DE, Evans AE: Neuroblastoma update. AUA Update Series. Volume XII, Lesson 35, p 278, 1993.
30. Dini G, Lamino E, Garaventa A et al: Myeloablative therapy and unpurged autologous bone marrow transplantation for poor prognosis neuroblastoma: report of 34 cases. J Clin Oncol 9:962–9, 1991.
31. Brosman SA: Testicular tumors in prepubertal children. Urology 13:581, 1979.

24

GENITOURINARY ONCOLOGY

32. Ritchey M: Pediatric urologic oncology. In: Walsh PC, Retik AB, Vaughan ED, Wein AJ, eds. Campbell's Urology, 8th edn. Philadelphia: WB Saunders, 2002, pp 2495–6.

33. Haas RJ, Schmidt P, Gobel U, Harms D: Testicular germ cell tumors, an update. Results of the German cooperative studies 1982–1997. Klin Padiatr 211:300–4, 1999.

34. Ritchey M: Pediatric urologic oncology. In: Walsh PC, Retik AB, Vaughan ED, Wein AJ, eds. Campbell's Urology, 8th edn. Philadelphia: WB Saunders, 2002, p 2498.

35. Sutow WW, Sullivan MP, Ried HL, Taylor HG, Griffith KM: Prognosis in childhood rhabdomyosarcoma. Cancer 25:1384–90, 1970.

36. Maurer HM, Moon T, Donaldson M et al: The Intergroup Rhabdomyosarcoma Study: a preliminary report. Cancer 40:2015–26, 1977.

37. Lawrence W Jr, Hays DM, Moon TE: Lymphatic metastases with childhood rhabdomyosarcoma. Cancer 39:556–9, 1977.

38. Hays DM, Raney RB, Crist W et al: Improved survival and bladder preserving among patients with bladder-prostate rhabdomyosarcoma primary tumors in Intergroup Rhabdomyosarcoma Study III. Abstract 119. Proc Am Soc Clin Oncol 10:318, 1991.

39. deVries JD: Paratesticular rhabdomyosarcoma. World J Urol 13:213–18, 1995.

40. Kattan J, Culine S: Paratesticular rhabdomyosarcoma in adult patients. 16 year experience at Institut Gustav-Roussy. Ann Oncol 4:871–5, 1993.

41. Andrassy RJ, Hays DM, Raney RB et al: Conservative surgical management of vaginal and vulvar pediatric rhabdomyosarcoma. A report from the Intergroup Rhabdomyosarcoma Study III. J Pediatr Surg 30:1034–7, 1994.

42. Corpron C, Andrassy RJ, Hays DM et al: Conservative management of uterine rhabdomyosarcoma. A report from the Intergroup Rhabdomyosarcoma Studies II and IV Pilot. J Pediatr Surg 30:942–4, 1998.

Exstrophy–epispadias complex

Benjamin H Lowentritt

SUMMARY

- Exstrophy–epispadias complex is a spectrum of congenital abnormalities of the genitourinary and gastrointestinal tracts.
- Epispadias is a condition in which the urethra lies open along its dorsal aspect.
- Bladder exstrophy is a condition in which the bladder lies open along its anterior aspect.
- Epispadias may occur alone, but bladder exstrophy normally occurs in association with epispadias.
- Cloacal exstrophy is a condition in which epispadias and bladder exstrophy occur in association with a midline omphalocele and prolapsed terminal ileum.
- Bladder exstrophy is associated with vesicoureteral reflux and lateral displacement of the penile nerves on the corporal bodies.
- There are two main approaches to the surgical repair of bladder exstrophy: staged and complete repair.

DEFINITIONS

Exstrophy–epispadias complex is a spectrum of congenital abnormalities occurring in the development of the genitourinary and gastrointestinal tracts. There are three basic disorders.

EPISPADIAS

- The least severe manifestation of the exstrophy–epispadias complex.
- The urethra fails to close – that is, to form into a complete tube – resulting in a dorsal midline urethral defect.
  - The defect typically begins in the distal urethral and extends proximally; the more severe the defect, the more proximal the extension
  - Note that in males the urethral defect occurs on the *side of the penis opposite the defect in hypospadias*
  - The genitalia (penis or clitoris) are divided (i.e. bifid) along the midline path of the defect, with each half typically lying on either side.
- Occurs in combination with bladder exstrophy or, less commonly, alone.
- Some defects (i.e. glanular epispadias) are minor and relatively easy to repair.

CLASSIC BLADDER EXSTROPHY

- The bladder fails to close – that is, to form into a complete sphere – resulting in an anterior bladder defect.
  - Exposed bladder mucosa is typically visible on the anterior abdominal wall
  - Normally occurs in association with epispadias, such that the urethral and bladder mucosa lie exposed along a single, continuous midline defect.

257

- In males, the prostate is also divided (i.e. bifid) along the path of the defect, with each half typically lying on either side.

CLOACAL EXSTROPHY

- Most severe manifestation of the exstrophy–epispadias complex.
- Malformation of the genitourinary tract, gastrointestinal tract, and anterior abdominal wall.
  - Epispadias and bladder exstrophy occur in association with a midline omphalocele and prolapsed terminal ileum.

VARIANTS

Multiple variants of these three basic disorders exist.[1]
- Epispadias with bladder prolapse:
  - Epispadiac urethra and genitalia with bladder prolapse through the superior aspect of the urethra.
- Pseudoexstrophy:
  - Intact bladder with associated musculoskeletal defects.
- Superior vesicle fissure:
  - Closed bladder except for an area below the umbilicus.
- Duplicate exstrophy:
  - Exstrophic bladder lies on the anterior abdominal wall while a second closed bladder lies within the abdomen; ureters can go to either or both.
- Covered exstrophy:
  - Thin membrane of skin overlies the bladder in association with musculoskeletal defects.
- Covered cloacal exstrophy:
  - Covered bladder occurring in association with duplicate bowel.
- Duplicate bladder:
  - Left–right duplication of the bladder often occurring in association with duplicate bowel.

INCIDENCE

- Isolated epispadias:
  - Approximately 1 in 140 000 live births.[2]
- Bladder exstrophy:
  - Approximately 1 in 40 000 live births[2]
  - Male:female ratio is approximately 2:1[3]
  - More common in whites than in other races.
- Cloacal exstrophy:
  - 1 in 200 000 live births
  - Incidence is the same for both males and females.

ETIOLOGY

- No consensus.
- Traditionally thought of as a 'wedge effect' of persistent cloacal membrane preventing mesoderm from closing in midline.[4]
  - Wedge potentially caused by persistence of caudal insertion of body stalk in embryo.[5]

- Another theory suggests alterations of apoptosis around the umbilicus as a potential cause.[6]

ASSOCIATED ANATOMICAL ANOMALIES[7]

- Divergent rectus muscles.
- Separation (termed 'diastasis') of the pubic symphysis.
- Penile corpora are short and wide.
- Exstrophic bladders have more type III collagen.
- The bony pelvis is externally rotated in both the anterior and posterior segments and sacroiliac joint.
- The pelvic musculature is abnormal, with more muscle distributed posteriorly compared with normals.
- **Vesicoureteral reflux is almost always present.**
- **Compared with normal individuals, the penile nerves are displaced laterally on the corporal bodies.**

OTHER ASSOCIATED ANOMALIES

- Epispadias and classic bladder exstrophy are not commonly associated with specific craniofacial, cardiac, or neurological anomalies.
- Cloacal exstrophy is often associated with:
  - Myelomeningocele
  - Short gut syndrome
  - Tethered cord
  - Hip dislocation
  - Clubfoot.

DIAGNOSIS

- Prenatal ultrasound:[8]
  - Primary finding is absence of the bladder
  - Other possible findings include a low-set umbilicus, widened pubic ramus, small genitalia, and conditions associated with cloacal exstrophy (see above).
- Neonatal period based on physical exam:
  - Relevant exam findings included exposed urethral and bladder mucosa, bifid genitalia, abdominal wall defects.

INITIAL MANAGEMENT OF CLASSIC BLADDER EXSTROPHY

- If possible, these patients should be delivered at and cared for in a tertiary care center with a multidisciplinary team available.
- Careful physical exam should be performed to evaluate for any associated anomalies.
- *The bladder mucosa should be protected by placing a plastic wrap over the exstrophic area to keep it moist.*
- Ultrasound should be performed to obtain a baseline evaluation of the kidneys.
- Prophylactic antibiotics should be started, since most patients have vesicoureteral reflux.

25

EXSTROPHY–EPISPADIAS COMPLEX

- Preliminary exam under anesthesia may be necessary to evaluate likelihood of successful bladder closure.
  - Multiple bladder polyps and small bladder size may indicate that bladder is not suitable for closure during the neonatal period.

SURGICAL THERAPY OF BLADDER EXSTROPHY

There are two main approaches to surgical repair: staged and complete repair.

STAGED REPAIR[9]

- Newborn period (typically first 72 hours of life) – closure of bladder, pubis, and abdominal wall:
  - If pubic separation is wide (>4 cm), osteotomies are performed to promote a tension-free closure
  - Patients will typically require 4–6 weeks of traction (Bryant's or Buck's traction) after initial closure to keep pelvis immobilized.
- Approximately 1 year of age – epispadias repair:
  - Cantwell–Ransley repair or penile disassembly
  - Care must be taken to avoid injury to the penile sensory nerves which course more laterally on the corpora.
- Approximately 4–5 years of age (or older) – ureteral reimplantation for reflux and (usually) a bladder neck reconstruction to improve urinary continence:
  - For bladder neck reconstruction, the child must be able to participate in continence training and should have a bladder capacity >85 ml
  - Young–Dees–Leadbetter bladder neck reconstruction most common technique for bladder neck reconstruction.

COMPLETE NEWBORN REPAIR[10,11]

- Newborn period – closure of bladder, pubis, fascia, *and* epispadias repair using penile disassembly:
  - Osteotomies and traction performed as with staged repair
  - Some patients may need additional reconstruction of the urethra during infancy.
- Approximately 4–5 years of age (or older) – ureteral reimplantation for reflux.

STAGED VS COMPLETE REPAIR: ADVANTAGES AND DISADVANTAGES

Staged repair

- Advantages: well-established, with excellent cosmetic and functional results.
- Disadvantages: requires multiple procedures; lack of urinary continence mechanism for first several years of life potentially adversely affects normal bladder growth.

Complete repair

- Advantages: early reconstruction of continence mechanism potentially allows for normal bladder cycling and growth at a younger age; in experienced hands, has excellent cosmetic and functional results.

- Disadvantages: technically challenging; associated with rare catastrophic complications to the genitalia; children may sometimes require the same number of surgeries as the staged approach.[12,13]

SURGICAL CHALLENGES

- If the newborn bladder is not large enough to close (<3 cm diameter):
  - Supportive measures are taken to preserve the mucosa and delayed closure is undertaken (usually at ~1 year of age) after additional bladder growth.[14]
- If a patient presents with a delayed or a failed closure:
  - Osteotomies and Buck's traction are usually necessary
  - Combined bladder closure and epispadias repair are often undertaken simultaneously, depending upon the patient's age and anatomy.[15]
- If a patient presents with poor bladder growth and/or refractory urinary incontinence after surgical repair:
  - Bladder augmentation or urinary diversion may be necessary.

MANAGEMENT OF CLOACAL EXSTROPHY

- Associated bowel and neurological abnormalities are usually more severe and potentially life threatening than genitourinary abnormalities.
  - Therefore, cloacal exstrophy is typically managed with a multidisciplinary surgical team of urologists, general surgeons, orthopedic surgeons, and neurosurgeons.
- The same general principles for management of the genitourinary abnormalities may be applied.
  - Successful bladder closure usually requires osteotomies and bladder augmentation.

OTHER ISSUES

- Fertility is possible, though long-term data (particularly for males) are scant.
  - Risk of inheritance is about 1 in 70.[3]
- ~1% of sibling births will have exstrophy.[16]
- Involvement of a multidisciplinary care team, with a child life specialist to provide psychosocial support, is essential throughout childhood and adolescence.
- Patient support groups exist to help families and patients with ongoing issues of self-image, particularly as patients enter adolescence.

REFERENCES

1. Lowentritt BH, Van Zijl PS, Frimberger D et al: Variants of the exstrophy complex: a single institution experience. J Urol 173(5):1732–7, 2005.
2. Nelson CP, Dunn RL, Wei JT: Contemporary epidemiology of bladder exstrophy in the United States. J Urol 173(5):1728–31, 2005.
3. Shapiro E, Lepor H, Jeffs RD: The inheritance of the exstrophy-epispadias complex. J Urol 132(2):308–10, 1984.
4. Muecke EC: The role of the cloacal membrane in exstrophy: the first successful experimental study. J Urol 92:659–62, 1964.
5. Mildenberger H, Kluth D, Dziuba M: Embryology of bladder exstrophy. J Pediatr Surg 23(2):166–70, 1988.

25

EXSTROPHY–EPISPADIAS COMPLEX

6. Vermeij-Keers C, Hartwig NG, van der Werff JF: Embryonic development of the ventral body wall and its congenital malformations. Semin Pediatr Surg 5(2):82–9, 1996.

7. Poli-Merol ML, Watson JA, Gearhart JP: New basic science concepts in the treatment of classic bladder exstrophy. Urology 60(5):749–55, 2002.

8. Gearhart JP, Ben Chaim J, Jeffs RD, Sanders RC: Criteria for the prenatal diagnosis of classic bladder exstrophy. Obstet Gynecol 85(6):961–4, 1995.

9. Mathews R, Gearhart JP: Modern staged reconstruction of bladder exstrophy – still the gold standard. Urology 65(1):2–4, 2005.

10. Mitchell ME: Bladder exstrophy repair: complete primary repair of exstrophy. Urology 65(1):5–8, 2005.

11. Hammouda HM, Kotb H: Complete primary repair of bladder exstrophy: initial experience with 33 cases. J Urol 172(4 Pt 1):1441–4, 2004.

12. Gearhart JP: Complete repair of bladder exstrophy in the newborn: complications and management. J Urol 165(6 Pt 2):2431–3, 2001.

13. Husmann DA, Gearhart JP: Loss of the penile glans and/or corpora following primary repair of bladder exstrophy using the complete penile disassembly technique. J Urol 172(4 Pt 2):1696–700, 2004.

14. Dodson JL, Surer I, Baker LA, Jeffs RD, Gearhart JP: The newborn exstrophy bladder inadequate for primary closure: evaluation, management and outcome. J Urol 165(5):1656–9, 2001.

15. Gearhart JP, Peppas DS, Jeffs RD: The failed exstrophy closure: strategy for management. Br J Urol 71(2):217–20, 1993.

16. Ives E, Coffey R, Carter CO: A family study of bladder exstrophy. J Med Genet 17(2):139–41, 1980.

Genitourinary trauma

Matthew E Nielsen

SUMMARY

- Degree of hematuria may not correlate with severity of renal injury.
- Management of renal trauma is guided by an imaging-based staging system.
- Ureteral trauma demands a high index of suspicion.
- Intraperitoneal bladder rupture requires urgent operative repair, whereas extraperitoneal rupture may be managed with catheter drainage.
- In the acute setting, posterior urethral trauma should be managed with endoscopic realignment or suprapubic diversion.

26

UPPER URINARY TRACT

RENAL TRAUMA

General information

- 90% is caused by blunt trauma secondary to motor vehicle accident (MVA), sports injuries, assault, etc.
- Associated clinical signs: history of rapid deceleration event or direct blow to flank, abdominal pain and/or tenderness, flank pain, flank ecchymosis, and rib and vertebral body fractures.
- Hematuria may not be present in up to 36% of major renal injuries.[1]

Indications for imaging

- For blunt trauma:[2]
  - Gross hematuria
  - Microscopic hematuria >5 RBC/hpf (red blood cells per high power field)
  - Shock: systolic blood pressure (SBP) <90 mmHg
  - History of rapid deceleration injury.
- For penetrating trauma:[3]
  - Any degree of hematuria
  - Suspicion of significant injury based on history and/or exam.
- For pediatric patients:
  - Most authors recommend liberal imaging of pediatric patients.[4]
- Persistent or increasing hematuria during observation warrants imaging in patients with an otherwise low index of suspicion for serious renal trauma.

Imaging

- Computed tomography (CT) with IV contrast is the principal imaging modality for diagnosis.
- Single-shot intraoperative intravenous pyelography (IVP) may also be useful: 2 ml/kg IV contrast bolus followed by a single 10-minute film.[5]

Radiological staging system

- Based upon CT findings.
- *Grade I:* contusion or non-expanding subcapsular hematoma. No laceration.

- *Grade II:* non-expanding perirenal hematoma. Cortical laceration <1 cm deep without urinary extravasation.
- *Grade III:* cortical laceration >1 cm deep without extravasation.
- *Grade IV:*
  - Laceration through the corticomedullary junction and into the collecting system (often with frank extravasation) *or*
  - Injury to segmental renal artery or vein with contained hematoma.
- *Grade V:*
  - Laceration with shattered kidney *or*
  - Substantial renal pedicle injury or avulsion.

Other points related to injury staging

- 'Cortical rim sign:' associated with renal artery thrombosis of >8 hours:
  - Merits consideration of a conservative approach, as likelihood of kidney salvage will be low.
- Ureteropelvic junction (UPJ) disruption:
  - May be difficult to diagnose
  - May occur in the absence of retroperitoneal hematoma
  - Classic sign is non-visualization of ureter (may require delayed images; rapid-sequence trauma CT often not adequate).
- Forniceal rupture:
  - Urine extravasation with good ureteral visualization
  - Intact renal cortex
  - No hematoma.

Treatment by mechanism of injury

Blunt injury

- Most blunt injuries may be managed conservatively with bedrest, broad-spectrum antibiotics, serial complete blood counts (CBCs), and follow-up CT scan within 72 hours.
- Indications for renal exploration include: hemodynamic instability; grade V injury; grade IV injury with urinary extravasation and >20% devitalized parenchyma; vascular thombosis of a solitary kidney; UPJ disruption; and large or pulsatile retroperitoneal hematoma found at laparotomy.[6]
- Persistent urinary extravasation from an otherwise viable kidney often responds to stent placement and/or percutaneous drainage.
- Arteriography with selective embolization to control hemorrhage is reasonable if there is no other indication for immediate surgery.[6]

Penetrating injury

- Treatment is more often surgical than with blunt: injuries tend to be more extensive and less predictable, and are frequently associated with other injuries (i.e. bowel) that require abdominal exploration.
- However, over 50% of renal stab wounds and roughly 25% of renal gunshot wounds have been managed non-operatively in carefully selected and staged patients.[7]
- May consider the same indications for operative intervention as with blunt (although threshold may be lower for intervention).

Principles of renal reconstruction[6,7]

- Early vascular control is important.
- If arterial occlusion is necessary, warm ischemia time should be less than 30 minutes.
- Debride and oversew lacerations with 4-0 absorbable capsular sutures. Oversew large segmental vessels and exposed collecting system with fine absorbable suture.
- Use absorbable bolsters and/or fibrin sealant to close defects; also consider coverage with perirenal fat or omental pedicle flap.
- Use a dependent, non-vacuum drain (i.e. Penrose drain).
- Nephrectomy is rarely required but may be a lifesaving maneuver.

URETERAL TRAUMA

General information

- Though rare (<1% of urological trauma), injuries may be associated with significant morbidity due to coexisting injuries to other viscera.[8]
- Only rarely occur as isolated injuries.
- Should be suspected with penetrating injury to common iliac vessels and/or bladder.
- May occur as a complication of gynecological (0.5–1.5% of cases) or abdominoperineal colorectal procedures (0.3–5.7% of cases).[9]
- Hematuria absent in >30% of cases.

Diagnosis

- No single test reliably excludes.
- Methods of diagnosis:
  - Direct inspection during exploration: methylene blue injection (antegrade or retrograde) may aid with visualization
  - CT with IV contrast: 1–2 hour delayed films may be useful for decreasing rates of false-negative results[10]
  - Retrograde pyelogram: useful but rarely practical.
- Delayed diagnosis:
  - Classically presents with fever, leukocytosis, and peritonitis
  - If <5 days from injury and clinically stable, consider immediate open repair vs ureteral stent placement
  - If >5 days or clinically unstable, place nephrostomy tube or ureteral stent and plan for delayed reconstruction.

Principles of exploration and repair

- Immediate diagnosis with immediate repair is best.
- May attempt stent placement if contusion is suspected.
  - Use caution because of potential for later stricture.
- Avoid excessive mobilization of the ureter to preserve adventitial blood supply.
- Debride to a bleeding edge to assure viable blood supply.
- Ureter may be anatomically divided into proximal, mid, and distal segments when considering reconstruction options.

GENITOURINARY TRAUMA 26

- Proximal:
  - Ureteroureterostomy: 5-0 absorbable suture should be used and the anastomosis should be tension-free, spatulated, watertight, end-to-end, and stented
  - Ileal interposition
  - Autotransplantation.
- Mid:
  - Ureteroureterostomy
  - Transureteroureterostomy.
- Distal:
  - Reimplant (ureteroneocystostomy) with submucosal tunnel: use 6-0 monofilament suture at reimplant site and stent
  - Psoas hitch: may add 5 cm of length; psoas anchoring suture should be placed longitudinally to prevent injury to the genitofemoral nerve
  - Boari bladder flap: may add 10–15 cm of length.

LOWER URINARY TRACT

BLADDER

General information

- Accounts for <2% of blunt abdominal injuries requiring surgery.
- Associated with pelvic fractures, especially of the pubic arch.[11,12]
- Coexisting urethral injury may be seen in 10–29% of cases.[13]
- Penetrating bladder injuries are commonly associated with major abdominal or pelvic vascular injuries and hemodynamic instability.
- Hematuria is the cardinal sign, with gross hematuria occurring in >95% of cases, and is an indication for imaging.
- Classification of bladder perforation (percentage of cases):
  - Extraperitoneal (62%)
  - Intraperitoneal (25%)
  - Both intra- and extraperitoneal (13%).

Diagnosis

- Cystogram:
  - Nearly 100% accurate when filling and drainage films are obtained
  - *Do not underfill*, which may be associated with false-negative results. Gently instill 300–350 ml or until patient is uncomfortable.
- CT cystogram:
  - Follow same principles as above, since passive filling of bladder from kidneys may miss a significant injury[14]
  - Requires dilution of contrast to 2–4%.[15]

Treatment

- Extraperitoneal perforation:
  - Most common type of perforation
  - Predominant treatment is catheter drainage alone[16]
  - However, since complications associated with catheter drainage may be as high as 26%,[17] may also consider open repair[18]

- Indications for open repair include bone fragment projecting into bladder (rare),[19] rectal perforation, and poor drainage of bladder secondary to blood clots.
- Intraperitoneal perforation:
  - Open repair in two layers is indicated
  - Although a suprapubic tube may be placed to facilitate postoperative drainage, a urethral catheter alone may suffice.[20]

URETHRA

Posterior

26

GENITOURINARY TRAUMA

- Commonly occurs in association with pelvic fractures.[21,22]
- 98% of patients are males, although girls <17 years have an increased risk compared with older females.[23,24]
- Associated with bladder rupture in 10–17% of cases.
- Signs:
  - Blood at urethral meatus (50% of cases); severity does not correlate with injury severity
  - Inability to urinate
  - Palpable bladder
  - 'High-riding prostate' (34% of cases); false positives are common, since pelvic hematoma may render prostate non-palpable on digital rectal examination (DRE)[25]
  - Perineal hematoma.[26]
- Diagnosed with retrograde urethrography:[27]
  - 14F Foley catheter placed 1–2 cm into fossa navicularis, balloon inflated with 1–2 ml of water, and Hypaque-M gently injected in 10 ml increments
  - Fluorography is desirable, but static lateral decubitus films are acceptable.
- Colapinto and McCallum classification system:
  - *Type I:* urethral stretch injury
  - *Type II:* urethral disruption proximal to genitourinary diaphragm
  - *Type III:* urethral disruption both proximal and distal to genitourinary diaphragm.
- Other staging systems have described complete vs partial rupture, but lack of consistent meaningful radiological differences limits utility of distinction.[28]

Management

- *Primary open realignment is to be avoided* due to increased rates of impotence, incontinence, stricture formation, and intraoperative blood loss.[29–31]
- Endoscopic realignment should be the first line of treatment.
- If realignment is not possible and/or patient is unstable, then a suprapubic catheter should be placed.
- Endoscopic realignment:
  - If successful, will heal without stricture in 50–65% of cases;[32,33] most strictures that do occur are mild[34]
  - Urethral stricture occurs in >95% of cases initially treated with suprapubic tube drainage alone (although subsequent treatment with posterior urethroplasty in experienced hands is highly successful)[35]

GENITAL SKIN LOSS

Etiology

- Burns:
  - Involve perineum 1% of the time and are often full-thickness burns.
- Other:
  - Fournier's gangrene (necrotizing fasciitis)
  - Constricting bands placed around penis
  - Mechanical avulsion from machinery.

Management

- Burns:
  - Eschar resection and debridement
  - Silvadene dressings for partial-thickness burns
  - Frequent wet-to-dry gauze dressing changes
  - Skin graft coverage if needed.
- Skin coverage – penis:
  - May use foreskin grafts if uncircumcised
  - Split-thickness skin grafts are appropriate
  - Avoid meshed grafts in potent patients
  - Hair-bearing scrotal rotation flaps may yield unacceptable cosmetic results[54]
  - Dress with a bulky gauze dressing soaked in mineral oil, which will stiffen when dry and act as a splint[53]
  - Graft placement may require removal of subcoronal skin to minimize circumferential lymphedema.[55]
- Skin coverage – scrotum:
  - Loss involving <50% of scrotal skin may be closed primarily[55]
  - Meshed 2:1 split-thickness skin grafts are associated with excellent results – construct a pouch for the testicles
  - Thigh flaps are another alternative, particularly if testes have already been placed in thigh pouches.[56]

REFERENCES

1. Cass AS: Renovascular injuries from external trauma. Urol Clin North Am 16:213–20, 1989.
2. Miller KS, McAninch JW: Radiographic assessment of renal trauma: our 15-year experience. J Urol 154:352–5, 1995.
3. Carroll PR, McAninch JW: Operative indications in penetrating renal trauma. J Trauma 25:587–92, 1985.
4. Brown SL, Elder JS, Spirnak JP: Are pediatric patients more susceptible to major renal injury from blunt trauma? A comparative study. J Urol 160:138–40, 1998.
5. Morey AL, McAninch JW, Tiller BK et al: Single shot intraoperative excretory urography for the immediate evaluation of renal trauma. J Urol 161:1088–92, 1999.
6. McAninch JW, Carroll PR, Klosterman PW et al: Renal reconstruction after injury. J Urol 145:932–7, 1991.
7. McAninch JW, Carroll PR: Renal trauma: kidney preservation through improved vascular control – a refined approach. J Trauma 22:285–9, 1982.
8. Medina D, Lavery R, Ross SE, Livingston DH: Ureteral trauma: preoperative studies neither predict injury nor prevent missed injuries. J Am Coll Surg 186:641–4, 1998.
9. St. Lezin MA, Stoller ML: Surgical ureteral injuries. Urology 38:497–506, 1991.

10. Kawashima A, Sandler CM, Corriere JN Jr et al: Ureteropelvic junction injuries secondary to blunt abdominal trauma. Radiology 205:487–92, 1997.
11. Cass AS, Luxenberg M: Features of 164 bladder ruptures. J Urol 138:743–5, 1987.
12. Carroll PR, McAninch JW: Major bladder trauma: mechanisms of injury and a unified method of diagnosis and repair. J Urol 132:254–7, 1984.
13. Cass AS, Gleich P, Smith C: Simultaneous bladder and prostatomembranous urethral rupture from external trauma. J Urol 132:907–8, 1984.
14. Haas CA, Brown SL, Spirnak JP: Limitations of routine spiral CT in the evaluation of bladder trauma. J Urol 162:51–2, 1999.
15. Peng MY, Parisky YR, Cornwell EE et al: CT cystography versus conventional cystography in evaluation of bladder injury. AJR Am J Roentgenol 173:1269–72, 1999.
16. Hayes EE, Sandler CM, Corriere JN Jr: Management of the ruptured bladder secondary to blunt abdominal trauma. J Urol 129:946–8, 1983.
17. Kotkin L, Koch MO: Morbidity associated with nonoperative management of extraperitoneal bladder injuries. J Trauma 38:895–8, 1993.
18. Cass AS, Luxenberg M: Management of extraperitoneal ruptures of the bladder caused by external trauma. Urology 33:179–83, 1989.
19. Corriere JN Jr, Sandler CM: Mechanisms of injury, patterns of extravasation and management of extraperitoneal bladder rupture due to blunt trauma. J Urol 139:43–4, 1988.
20. Volpe MA, Pachter EM, Scalea TM et al: Is there a difference in outcome when treating traumatic intraperitoneal bladder rupture with or without a suprapubic tube? J Urol 161:1103–5, 1999.
21. Colapinto V, McCallum RW: Injury to the male posterior urethra in fractured pelvis: a new classification. J Urol 118:575–80, 1977.
22. Lowe MA, Mason JT, Luna GK et al: Risk factors for urethral injuries in men with traumatic pelvic fractures. J Urol 140:506–7, 1988.
23. Routt ML, Simonian PT, Defalco AJ et al: Internal fixation in pelvic fractures and primary repairs of associated genitourinary disruptions: a team approach. J Trauma 40:784–90, 1996.
24. Hemal AK, Dorairajan LN, Gupta NP: Posttraumatic complete and partial loss of urethra with pelvic fracture in girls; an appraisal of management. J Urol 163:282–7, 2000.
25. Elliott DS, Barrett DM: Long-term follow-up and evaluation of primary realignment of posterior urethral disruptions. J Urol 157:814–16, 1997.
26. Koraitim MM, Marzouk ME, Atta ME, Orabi SS: Risk factors and mechanism of urethral injury in pelvic fractures. Br J Urol 77:876–80, 1996.
27. Sandler CM, Corriere JN Jr: Urethrography in the diagnosis of acute urethral injuries. Urol Clin N Am 16:283–9, 1989.
28. Morehouse DD, Belitsky P, Mackinnon K: Rupture of the posterior urethra. J Urol 130:898–902, 1972.
29. Webster GD, Mathes GL, Selli C: Prostatomembranous urethral injuries: a review of the literature and a rational approach to their management. J Urol 130:898–902, 1983.
30. Coffield KS, Weems WL: Experience with management of posterior urethral injury associated with pelvic fracture. J Urol 117:722–4, 1977.
31. Koraitim MM: Pelvic fracture urethral injuries; the unresolved controversy. J Urol 161:1433–41, 1999.
32. Morehouse DD, Mackinnon K: Management of prostatomembranous urethral disruption: 13-year experience. J Urol 123:173–4, 1980.
33. Asci R, Sarikaya S, Buyukalpelli R et al: Voiding and sexual dysfunctions after pelvic fracture urethral injuries treated with either initial cystotomy and delayed urethroplasty or immediate primary realignment. Scand J Urol Nephrol 33:228–33, 1999.
34. Al-Ali IH, Husain I: Disrupting injuries of the membranous urethra – the case for early surgery and catheter splinting. Br J Urol 55:716–20, 1983.
35. Herschorn S, Thijssen A, Radomski SB: The value of immediate or early catheterization of the traumatized posterior urethra. J Urol 148:1428–31, 1992.

26

GENITOURINARY TRAUMA

36. Devine CJ, Jordan GH, Devine PC: Primary realignment of the disrupted prostatomembranous urethra. Urol Clin N Am 16:291–5, 1989.
37. Jackson DH, Williams JL: Urethral injury: a retrospective study. Br J Urol 46:665–76, 1974.
38. Kotkin L, Koch MO: Impotence and incontinence after immediate realignment of posterior urethral trauma: result of injury or management? J Urol 155:1600–3, 1996.
39. Jepson BR, Boullier JA, Moore RG et al: Traumatic posterior urethral injury and primary endoscopic realignment: evaluation of long-term followup. Urology 53:1205–10, 1999.
40. Patterson DE, Barrett DM, Myers RP et al: Primary realignment of posterior urethral injuries. J Urol 129:513–16, 1983.
41. Porter JR, Takayama TK, Defalco AJ: Traumatic posterior urethral injury and early realignment using magnetic urethral catheters. J Urol 158:425–30, 1997.
42. Miles BJ, Poffenberger RJ, Farah RN et al: Management of penile gunshot wounds. Urology 36:318–21, 1990.
43. Gomez RG, Castanheira AC, McAninch JW: Gunshot wounds to the male external genitalia. J Urol 150:1147–9, 1993.
44. Aboseif S, Gomez R, McAninch JW: Genital self-mutilation. J Urol 145:1267–70, 1991.
45. Romilly CS, Isaac MT: Male genital self-mutilation. Br J Hosp Med 55:427–31, 1996.
46. McAninch JW, Santucci RA: Genitourinary trauma: In: Walsh PC, Retik AB, Vaughan ED, Wein AJ, eds. Campbell's Urology, 8th edn. Philadelphia: WB Saunders, 2002, p 3733.
47. Orvis BR, McAninch JW: Penile rupture. Urol Clin North Am 16:369–75, 1989.
48. Zargooshi J: Penile fracture in Kermanshah, Iran: report of 172 cases. J Urol 164:364–6, 2000.
49. Fergany AF, Angermeier KW, Montague DK: Review of Cleveland Clinic experience with penile fracture. Urology 54:352–5, 1999.
50. Nicolaisen GS, Melamud A, Williams RD et al: Rupture of the corpus cavernosum: surgical management. J Urol 130:917–19, 1983.
51. Nolan JF, Stillwell TJ, Sands JP: Acute management of the zipper-entrapped penis. J Emerg Med 8:305–7, 1990.
52. Schuster G: Traumatic rupture of the testicle and review of the literature. J Urol 127:1194–6, 1982.
53. McAninch JW, Santucci RA: Genitourinary trauma. In: Walsh PC, Retik AB, Vaughan ED, Wein AJ, eds. Campbell's Urology, 8th edn. Philadelphia: WB Saunders, 2002, p 3739.
54. Horton CE, Dean JA: Reconstruction of traumatically acquired defects of the phallus. World J Surg 14:757–62, 1990.
55. Bertini JE Jr, Corriere JN Jr: The etiology and management of genital injuries. J Trauma 28:1278–81, 1988.
56. McDougal WS: Scrotal reconstruction using thigh pedicle flaps. J Urol 129:757–9, 1983.

Priapism

Mohamad E Allaf and Trinity J Bivalacqua

SUMMARY

- Ischemic priapism is a urological emergency.
- Prompt treatment is the key to the resolution of ischemic priapism and the maintenance of subsequent erectile function.
- Ischemic priapism is treated in a stepwise fashion starting with aspiration and intracavernosal sympathomimetic injection and progressing towards invasive surgical shunts.
- Color duplex ultrasonography is helpful in the evaluation of non-ischemic priapism.
- If expectant management fails, non-ischemic priapism is treated with selective embolization.
- Stuttering priapism is best treated with systemic therapy aimed at the prevention of recurrence.
- Prospective multi-institutional trials are needed to assess the safety and efficacy of treatments in this poorly understood disease.

27

INTRODUCTION

GENERAL INFORMATION

- Definition:
  - Persistent penile erection that continues for >4 hours in duration and is unrelated to sexual stimulation.[1]
- Three types:
  - Ischemic (veno-occlusive, low flow)
  - Non-ischemic (arterial, high flow)
  - Stuttering (intermittent).

EVALUATION

- History:
  - Erection duration
  - Previous episodes
  - Intracavernous injections
  - Trauma
  - Pain
  - Medications (prescribed, over-the-counter, and illicit drugs)
  - Hematological malignancy or sickle cell
  - Baseline erectile function.
- Physical examination:
  - Penis, perineum, abdomen, pelvis, digital rectal examination, lymph node assessment
  - Copora cavernosa are rigid while corpus spongiosum and glans penis are soft.

TABLE 27.1

CORPORAL BLOOD GAS PARAMETERS IN PRIAPISM

Source	Appearance	Po$_2$ (mmHg)	Pco$_2$ (mmHg)	pH
Arterial blood	Bright red	>90	40	7.40
Ischemic priapism	Dark/thick	<40	>60	<7.30
Non-ischemic priapism	Bright red	>90	40	7.40
Normal flaccid penis	Dark	40	50	7.35

- Laboratory/imaging tests:
  - Corporal blood gas is key to distinguishing ischemic from non-ischemic priapism (Table 27.1)
  - Color duplex ultrasonography (in lithotomy or frog leg position) can document flow status of cavernosal arteries and evaluate for anatomical anomalies (fistulae, pseudoaneurysm, etc.)
  - Complete blood count (CBC) should be obtained on all patients
  - Consider reticulocyte count, hemoglobin electrophoresis, and peripheral smear (sickle trait, thalassemia, etc.)
  - Toxicology screen can implicate legal and illicit drugs as etiologies.

ISCHEMIC PRIAPISM

DEFINITION AND PATHOPHYSIOLOGY

- No (or little) blood flow through cavernosal arteries – *compartment syndrome of penis*.
- Decreased venous outflow causes erection and impedes arterial inflow, resulting in a prolonged erection, local hypoxia, and acidosis.
- Prospect of further injury and permanent erectile dysfunction (ED) increases with duration.

CAUSES

- Sickle cell disease and trait.
- Malignant infiltration (e.g. prostate cancer).
- Hematological conditions (e.g. leukemia, thalassemia).
- Drugs (e.g. trazodone, intracavernosal injection therapy for ED, cocaine, phenothiazines, alcohol).
- Spinal cord injury.

TREATMENT

- First step is intracavernous intervention: aspiration (+/− irrigation) and intracavernous injection of sympathomimetic drugs.
  - Aspiration alone or in conjunction with irrigation is equally effective (approximately 30% success rate).[1]

Aspiration and irrigation

- Prep and drape penis in sterile fashion.
- Anesthesia via penile block.
- Administer prophylactic antibiotics.

- Puncture corpus cavernosum at 2 or 10 o'clock position in the shaft near the base of the penis with a 19-gauge needle connected to long tubing and syringe.
- Tubing allows exchange of syringe so that only one puncture is used.
- Puncture of only one side is necessary since corpora communicate.
- Aspirate 20–30 ml of blood, may then inject 20–30 ml of sterile saline if irrigation is performed (repeat process).
- To inject sympathomimetics (see below), use same needle and exchange syringe (make sure to account for length of tubing to ensure accurate dosing):
  - Injection of sympathomimetics increases chances of success and reduces risk of subsequent ED
  - Phenylephrine is the drug of choice due to limited systemic effects (epinephrine, norepinephrine, and ephedrine are other sympathomimetics)
  - Phenylephrine is unlikely to work in patients with priapism of >48 hours' duration
  - Dilute phenylephrine with normal saline to concentrations of 100 500 µg/ml and inject 1 ml every 3–5 minutes for 1 hour before deeming treatment a failure[1]
  - High-risk cardiovascular patients should be monitored (cardiac monitor and frequent blood pressure checks)
  - Low-risk patients must be observed for systemic side effects (hypertension, reflex bradycardia, headache, arrythmias).

Shunts

- **If sympathomimetics and aspiration fail, then the next step is a surgical shunt.**
- Cavernoglanular shunts (distal) are attempted first and proximal shunts are only attempted after failure of all other measures.
- Distal shunts:[2]
  - Al-Ghorab shunt: through a transverse glanular incision both tips of the corpora cavernosa are excised
  - Winter shunt: percutaneous insertion of a large biopsy needle through the glans and corpora cavernosa with extraction of multiple cores creating a shunt
  - Ebbehoj shunt: scalpel is inserted through glans and corpora cavernosa.
- Proximal shunts:[2]
  - Quackels shunt: through a perineal or penile shaft incision the corpora cavernosa and corpus spongiosum are incised and anastomosed to each other (urethral fistulae and purulent cavernositis are among serious complications)
  - Grayhack shunt: involves mobilization of saphenous vein and anastomosis to corpus cavernosum (time consuming and technically challenging).

Other

- Oral terbutaline may be of use in men with prolonged erections due to self-injection therapies for ED (especially for erections of durations <4 hours).[3]
- Data are lacking regarding the ED rates following therapy; it is generally accepted that the risk of ED increases as the invasiveness of therapy increases.

27

PRIAPISM

- Treatment of the primary process (e.g. sickle cell disease, leukemia, etc.) should occur concurrent to the above algorithm and not instead of it.

NON-ISCHEMIC PRIAPISM

DEFINITION AND PATHOPHYSIOLOGY

- **Not an emergency.**
- Associated with unregulated arterial inflow.
- Exam:
  - Tumescent copora cavernosa without full rigidity and tenderness (in contrast to ischemic priapism).
- Causes:
  - Most common cause is perineal trauma with cavernous artery injury
  - In some patients it is idiopathic
  - In rare circumstances may occur following resolution of ischemic priapism episode (cause is unknown).[4]

TREATMENT

- Aspiration is used for diagnosis only.
- There is no role for sympathomimetic injections.
- Initially, expectant management is recommended as spontaneous resolution may occur.
- Case series level data suggest that ice and compression may aid in resolution of episode.
- Limited data also suggest that intracavernous injection of methylene blue, which inhibits guanylate cyclase, may be efficacious.[5]
- Selective embolization after a trial of observation is the treatment of choice.
  - Autologous clot and absorbable gels should be used in preference to permanent materials such as coils (lower risk of erectile dysfunction).
- Surgical management with arterial ligation is used if all fails (erectile dysfunction rates up to 50%).
- Prior to embolization or surgical intervention, color duplex ultrasonography is the study of choice to localize and document the pathology (angiogram is more invasive but remains the gold standard).

STUTTERING PRIAPISM

DEFINITION AND PATHOPHYSIOLOGY

- Often occurs in patients with sickle cell disease.
- Mechanism is unknown.

TREATMENT

- Acute episodes are approached with the ischemic priapism protocol as described above.
- Goal in the management of patients with stuttering priapism is the prevention of future episodes.
- Systemic therapies proposed for the prevention of recurrent priapism include: hormonal agents,[6-9] sildenafil,[10] baclofen,[11] digoxin,[12] and terbutaline.[13]

- Gonadotropin-releasing hormone (GnRH) agonists or antiandrogens may be used in the management of recurrent priapism (SHOULD NOT BE USED IN PATIENTS WHO HAVE NOT REACHED SEXUAL AND PHYSICAL MATURITY).
- GnRH agonists may decrease libido but most patients are still able to engage in sexual activity.
- GnRH agonists may have a contraceptive effect and thus should be discontinued if the patient is planning to conceive a child.
- Early home management with phenylephrine self-injection intracavernosal therapy can be used in patients who fail (or cannot tolerate) systemic therapy – this is a treatment and not a prevention modality.

27

PRIAPISM

REFERENCES

1. Montague DK, Jarow J, Broderick GA et al: American Urological Association guideline on the management of priapism. J Urol 170:1318, 2003.
2. Hinman FJ, Donley S, Sempen P: Atlas of Urologic Surgery, 2nd edn. Philadelphia: WB Saunders, 1998, pp 177–228.
3. Lowe FC, Jarow JP: Placebo-controlled study of oral terbutaline and pseudoephedrine in management of prostaglandin E1-induced prolonged erections. Urology 42:51, 1993.
4. Seftel AD, Haas CA, Brown SL et al: High flow priapism complicating veno-occlusive priapism: pathophysiology of recurrent idiopathic priapism? J Urol 159:1300, 1998.
5. Steers WD, Selby JB, Jr: Use of methylene blue and selective embolization of the pudendal artery for high flow priapism refractory to medical and surgical treatments. J Urol 146:1361, 1991.
6. Dahm P, Rao DS, Donatucci CF: Antiandrogens in the treatment of priapism. Urology 59:138, 2002.
7. Levine LA, Guss SP: Gonadotropin-releasing hormone analogues in the treatment of sickle cell anemia-associated priapism. J Urol 150:475, 1993.
8. Javed MA: Priapism associated with fluoxetine therapy: a case report. J Pak Med Assoc 46:45, 1996.
9. Serjeant GR, de Ceulaer K, Maude GH: Stilboestrol and stuttering priapism in homozygous sickle-cell disease. Lancet 2:1274, 1985.
10. Champion HC, Bivalacqua TJ, Takimoto E, Kass DA, Burnett AL: Phosphodiesterase-5A dysregulation in penile erectile tissue is a mechanism of priapism. Proc Natl Acad Sci USA 102:1661, 2005.
11. Rourke KF, Fischler AH, Jordan GH: Treatment of recurrent idiopathic priapism with oral baclofen. J Urol 168:2552, 2002.
12. Gupta S, Salimpour P, Saenz de Tejada I et al: A possible mechanism for alteration of human erectile function by digoxin: inhibition of corpus cavernosum sodium/potassium adenosine triphosphatase activity. J Urol 159:1529, 1998.
13. Ahmed I, Shaikh NA: Treatment of intermittent idiopathic priapism with oral terbutaline. Br J Urol 80:341, 1997.

Testicular torsion

David J Hernandez

SUMMARY

- Torsion of the spermatic cord is a surgical emergency caused by twisting and impedance of arterial blood flow to the testicle.
- There are two types of testicular torsion: extravaginal, which occurs in neonates; intravaginal, which typically occurs in adolescents.
- Intravaginal torsion presents as acute onset of testicular pain. Exam may show high-riding testis with transverse lie, absence of cremasteric reflex, and continued pain despite scrotal elevation.
- Diagnosis should be based primarily on history and physical exam. Scrotal ultrasound with color Doppler flow may aid diagnosis.
- Treatment is scrotal exploration with detorsion of the affected testicle. If the testicle is necrotic, it is excised. If it is viable, it is secured in place. The contralateral testicle is also explored and secured in place.

28

GENERAL INFORMATION AND EPIDEMIOLOGY

Torsion of the spermatic cord is a surgical emergency which can result in irreversible ischemic injury to the testicle in as little as 4 hours.

DEFINITION

- Twisting of the testis and spermatic cord around a vertical axis, resulting in venous obstruction, progressive swelling, arterial compromise, testicular ischemia, and eventually infarction.

TYPES OF TORSION

Extravaginal

- Occurs in neonates (often in utero).
- Associated with incomplete attachment of the gubernaculum and testicular tunics to the scrotal wall, therefore leaving the testis, epididymis, and tunica vaginalis free to twist within the scrotum.
- Accounts for approximately 10% of all cases of testicular torsion.

Intravaginal

- Testis twists within the tunica vaginalis.
- Results from lack of normal fixation of the testis and epididymis to the fascial and muscular coverings that surround the cord within the scrotum.

BELL-CLAPPER DEFORMITY

- An abnormally mobile testis, associated with intravaginal torsion, that hangs freely within the tunical space.

- An abnormally narrowed testicular mesentery and a tunica vaginalis that completely surrounds the entire testis and epididymis facilitates twisting of the testis about its vascular pedicle.

INCIDENCE

- Acute scrotal pain makes up approximately 0.5% of all complaints presenting to the Emergency Room.
  - The most common diagnoses for scrotal pain are testicular torsion and epididymitis.
- One estimate of testicular torsion incidence: 1 in 4000 males before age 25 years, accounting for 25–35% of acute pediatric scrotal disease.

ETIOLOGY

- The inciting event is thought to be sudden contraction of the cremasteric muscle, which initiates a rotational effect on the testis as it is pulled upward.
- Usually, the anterior surface of each testis turns toward the midline (>2/3).
- In addition to duration, the degree of rotation and residual torsion after manual detorsion correlate to clinical outcome.

PRESENTATION

EXTRAVAGINAL

- Typically presents as a hard, non-tender testis which is fixed to the overlying scrotal skin of a neonate. The overlying skin is often discolored.

INTRAVAGINAL

- Typically, patients are adolescents who present with acute onset of scrotal pain and swelling.
- However, can appear more gradually and at any age.
- Usually occurs spontaneously, but can occur in association with trauma or athletic activity.
- Often associated with nausea and vomiting as well as referred pain to the ipsilateral lower quadrant of the abdomen.
- Dysuria and other lower urinary tract symptoms are usually absent (unlike epididymitis).
- Patients may report prior episodes of severe, self-limited scrotal swelling and pain which likely represent *intermittent torsion* with spontaneous detorsion (see below).
- Physical examination:
  - Tender, high-riding testis (secondary to foreshortening of the spermatic cord as a result of twisting) with an abnormal, transverse lie
  - May have associated hydrocele and/or scrotal edema
  - Absence of a cremasteric reflex (i.e. stroking the ipsilateral medial thigh fails to produce contraction of the affected testicle)
  - Unlike epididymitis, elevation of the scrotum will *not* relieve the pain (negative Prehn's sign)

- 'Blue dot sign' is a small, dark blue spot on the skin that may occur with torsion of a testicular appendage (appendix testis or epididymis) but not testicular torsion.
- *Intermittent torsion* is a kind of intravaginal torsion characterized by acute and intermittent sharp testicular pain and scrotal swelling, interspersed by symptom-free intervals.
  - Physical findings may include horizontal or very mobile testes, an anteriorly located epididymis, or bulkiness of the spermatic cord from partial twisting.

DIAGNOSIS AND EVALUATION

HISTORY AND PHYSICAL EXAM

- These are key components of the diagnosis.
- Threshold should always be low for performing surgical exploration based on history and physical exam.

DIFFERENTIAL DIAGNOSIS

- Torsion of the appendix testis or appendix epididymis.
- Epididymitis:
  - Age: torsion usually occurs around puberty, whereas epididymitis more often occurs in older individuals
  - Urinalysis: typically negative in torsion, positive (i.e. presence of RBCs, WBCs, bacteria) in epididymitis
  - Scrotal ultrasound
  - Note: epididymitis is rare in pediatric patients. Diagnosis should prompt thorough pediatric urological evaluation.
- Trauma.
- Inguinal hernia.
- Testicular tumor.

ULTRASOUND

- Doppler sonography is usually diagnostic:
  - Characteristic finding is decreased or absent arterial flow to the affected testicle.
- Should not be relied on as the one and only discriminator in cases of testicular torsion, because:
  - It is operator-dependent
  - Arterial flow may not accurately reflect the overall perfusion of the testis
  - Blood flow imaging is most sensitive when blood flow to the testis is missing and infarction is present or impending, which may occur late after initial twisting of the cord.

TESTICULAR SCAN (NUCLEAR SCINTIGRAPHY)

- Often difficult to obtain, but is generally an accurate and reliable method to distinguish between epididymo-orchitis and testicular torsion.

TREATMENT

EXTRAVAGINAL

- Although the testicle is rarely salvageable, most clinicians agree that emergency scrotal exploration (see below) of neonatal torsion is safe and prudent, and may result in higher testicular salvage rates.

INTRAVAGINAL

Manual detorsion

- A potential method of quickly relieving pain and restoring blood flow to the testicle prior to definitive surgical repair.
- May be attempted after performing a spermatic cord block.
- The testicle is manually rotated (untwisted) in a medial-to-lateral and caudal-to-cranial direction, like opening the pages of a book.
- Even if successful, scrotal exploration should still be promptly initiated.

Scrotal exploration

- A median raphe incision allows for exploration of both sides. The affected side should be explored first so as to achieve detorsion quickly.
- The affected testicle should be untwisted (see above). If viability is unclear after untwisting, the testicle may be wrapped in warm, saline-soaked sponges for several minutes and then re-examined.
- Intraoperative ultrasound may be used to assess for arterial flow and viability.
- If the testicle is necrotic, it is excised.
- Viable testes must be placed into a dartos pouch or secured in place in at least 3 points with non-absorbable, monofilamentous sutures ('3-point fixation').
- The contralateral hemiscrotum is explored and the testis secured in the same manner to prevent future torsion.
- When intermittent torsion with spontaneous detorsion of the spermatic cord is suspected, elective scrotal exploration should be performed with fixation of both testes to prevent future torsion.

TORSED APPENDAGE (APPENDIX TESTIS OR APPENDIX EPIDIDYMIS)

- May be treated non-operatively with restricted activity, nonsteroidal anti-inflammatory agents, and observation.
- If surgery is performed, the infarcted appendage may simply be excised.

PROGNOSIS

- Long-term follow-up studies have shown that patients who undergo successful detorsion and fixation of a viable testicle within 8 hours of the onset of symptoms will have a normal-sized testicle and only slight changes in testicular morphology.
- However, other data suggest that even when patients undergo detorsion of a viable testicle within 4 hours of the onset of symptoms, subsequent exocrine function of the affected testicle may decrease in up to 50% of cases.

FURTHER READING

Allen TD, Elder JS: Shortcomings of color Doppler sonography in the diagnosis of testicular torsion. J Urol 154(4):1508–10, 1995.

Baker LA, Sigman D, Mathews RI et al: An analysis of clinical outcomes using color doppler testicular ultrasound for testicular torsion. Int J Cancer 71(4):517–20, 1997.

Bartsch G, Frank S, Marberger H, Mikuz G: Testicular torsion: late results with special regard to fertility and endocrine function. J Urol 124(3):375–8, 1980.

Dresner M: Torsed appendage. Diagnosis and management: blue dot sign. Urology 1(1):63–6, 1973.

Levy OM, Gittleman MC, Strashun AM et al: Diagnosis of acute testicular torsion using radionuclide scanning. J Urol 129(5):975–7, 1983.

Nagler H, White R: The effect of testicular torsion on the contralateral testis. J Urol 128(6):1343–8, 1982.

Paltiel HJ, Connolly LP, Atala A et al: Acute scrotal symptoms in boys with an indeterminate clinical presentation: comparison of color Doppler sonography and scintigraphy. Radiology 207(1):223–31, 1998.

Pinto K, Noe H, Jerkins GR: Management of neonatal testicular torsion. J Urol 158(3 Pt 2):1196–7, 1997.

Rabinowitz R: The importance of the cremasteric reflex in acute scrotal swelling in children. J Urol 132(1):89–90, 1984.

Schneck FX, Bellinger MF: Abnormalities of the testes and scrotum and their surgical management. In: Walsh PC, Retik AB, Vaughan ED, Wein AJ, eds. Campbell's Urology, 8th edn. Philadelphia: WB Saunders, 2002.

Sessions AE, Rabinowitz R, Hulbert WC et al: Testicular torsion: direction, degree, duration and disinformation. J Urol 169(2):663–5, 2003.

Stillwell TJ, Kramer SA: Intermittent testicular torsion. Pediatrics 77(6):908–11, 1986.

Williamson RC: Torsion of the testis and allied conditions. Br J Surg 63(6):465–76, 1976.

28

TESTICULAR TORSION

Acute gross hematuria: etiology and management

Christopher A Warlick

SUMMARY

- Acute gross hematuria is usually self-limiting.
- Intractable, severe hematuria from the bladder may require treatment.
- Invasive treatments should be utilized after failure of the simplest and least morbid approaches.
- Finasteride is effective for treatment of persistent hematuria associated with benign prostatic hyperplasia.

29

GENERAL PRINCIPLES

- Acute gross hematuria is a common reason for urological consultation.
- Most cases are mild, self-limiting, and require only observation and reassurance.
- Intractable hematuria from the bladder may be refractory to conservative management, life-threatening, and require transfusion and/or intense supportive care.[1]
  - Several treatments are available
  - In general, *invasive treatments should be attempted only after failure of the simplest and least morbid treatments.*

COMMON CAUSES OF ACUTE GROSS HEMATURIA

- Traumatic urethral catheter insertion or removal.
- Recent urinary tract instrumentation or surgery.
- Bladder, ureteral, or renal cancer.
- Prostate cancer.
- Urinary stones.
- Benign prostatic hyperplasia.
- Severe bladder infection.
- Severe prostatitis.
- Anticoagulation therapy.
- Radiation cystitis.
- Cyclophosphamide-induced hemorrhagic cystitis:
  - Caused by the metabolite acrolein.
- BK virus-induced hemorrhagic cystitis.

INITIAL EVALUATION AND MANAGEMENT

- Initial evaluation and treatment should include:
  - History, physical exam, and laboratory evaluation
  - Evaluation of need for bladder clot evacuation and/or continuous bladder irrigation
  - Identification and treatment of underlying cause, if possible.

- History should consider:
  - Prior episodes
  - Identification of potential inciting or precipitating events
  - Duration
  - Prior or current urinary tract diseases
  - Symptoms of anemia and/or hemodynamic instability
  - Presence of other urinary symptoms and/or flank pain
  - Prior or current non-urological malignancy
  - Prior treatment with cyclophosphamide
  - Current use of anticoagulation therapy.
- Physical exam should include:
  - Vital signs to evaluate for hemodynamic instability
  - Abdominal exam with evaluation for bladder distension suggesting urinary retention
  - Rectal exam to approximate prostate size and assess for prostate and/or bladder cancer.
- Further evaluation should include:
  - Serum hemoglobin and/or hematocrit
  - Serum creatinine
  - Coagulation parameters
  - Urine cultures
  - Urine cytology (may be non-diagnostic in the acute setting)
  - Cystoscopy
  - Ultrasound, CT, or MRI of upper urinary tract.
- Gross hematuria may be observed as long as the patient is hemodynamically stable, maintains a stable blood count, and is not in urinary retention.
- Manual clot evacuation and/or continuous bladder irrigation with a 22F or larger 3-way catheter should be instituted if urinary obstruction is present or likely to occur. Clots may be evacuated at the bedside or in the Operating Room.[1]

MANAGEMENT OPTIONS FOR INTRACTABLE HEMATURIA OF BLADDER ORIGIN

If conservative management fails, the following treatments are available, in order from least to most invasive/drastic.

PENTOSAN POLYSULFATE SODIUM (ELMIRON)

Mechanism of action

- Postulated to replenish protective glycosaminoglycans layer at urine–bladder interface.[2]

Dose

- 100 mg PO tid.

Contraindications and warnings[3]

- Contraindications: pentosan polysulfate allergy.
- Warnings: None.

Comment

- Some investigators have recommended it as first-line therapy for radiation- or chemotherapy-induced cystitis.[4]
- Highly effective in several uncontrolled case series.[2,4-6] No data available from randomized, controlled trials.
- May potentially prevent and/or reduce recurrent episodes if taken chronically.[2,4]
- May require up to 1–7 weeks of therapy before eliciting a response.
- Safe and well tolerated.

HYPERBARIC OXYGEN

Mechanism of action

- Reverses tissue hypoxia caused by radiation-induced endarteritis by inducing neovascularization of the bladder and increasing tissue oxygen tension.[7,8]

Protocol

- Requires access to a hyberbaric oxygen chamber.
- 20 daily sessions of 100% oxygen inhalation at 0.3 MPa, 90 minutes per session, 5–6 times per week.[1]
- Increase to 40 daily sessions as needed.

Complications (rare)

- CNS toxicity.
- Pulmonary barotrauma.
- Oxygen toxicity.
- Decompression sickness.

Contraindications

- Relative: significant pulmonary disease.
- Absolute: none.

Comment

- Has shown efficacy in up to 80–90% of patients with radiation-induced hemorrhagic cystitis.[9,10]
- There is no evidence that it will promote growth of malignancy.[1]

INTRAVESICAL PROSTAGLANDIN

Mechanism of action

- Postulated to improve the mucosal barrier by encouraging platelet aggregation, inducing vasoconstriction, and inducing smooth muscle contractions in mucosal and submucosal blood vessels.[11-13]

Protocol[13]

- Instill 50 ml of 4–8 mg/L carboprost tromethamine (PGF2α) for 1 hour; drain, repeat, and irrigate with saline.

- Repeat instillations (2 hours per instillation) 4 × per day for a total of 400 ml of agent for 8 hours over each 24-hour period.
- If no improvement occurs by the fourth course, may increase dose to 10 mg/L.
- Alternatively, run continuous bladder irrigation with 8–10 mg/L carboprost tromethamine at 100 ml/h for 10 hours.

Complications

- Bladder spasm.

Contraindications

- Relative: none.
- Absolute: none.

Comment

- Efficacy is questionable and clinical data are outdated.
- Agents are generally expensive and may be difficult to obtain.

INTRAVESICAL ALUM IRRIGATION

Mechanism of action

- Protein precipitation on cell surface and superficial interstitial spaces resulting in decreased capillary permeability, contraction of intercellular spaces, vasoconstriction, and hardening of the capillary endothelium.[14,15]

Protocol (for 1% alum continuous bladder irrigation)[16]

- Dissolve 50 g of alum (potassium aluminum sulfate) into 5 L sterile water.
- Irrigate bladder at 250–300 ml/h (slower rates may result in precipitation of alum).

Potential complications[1]

- Aluminum toxicity:
  - May occur in patients with renal impairment and/or large absorptive surface areas such as large bladder tumors
  - Discontinue *immediately* if suspected
  - Associated with encephalopathy, dementia, confusion, speech disorders, seizures, lethargy, nausea/vomiting, respiratory depression, metabolic acidosis, and renal impairment.
- Suprapubic pain.
- Bladder spasms.
- Ileus (rare).

Contraindications

- Relative: renal impairment, large bladder tumors, allergy to topical aluminum agents.
- Absolute: none.

Comment

- Generally safe and well tolerated.
- Toxicity is almost exclusively limited to those with renal insufficiency.
- Precipitation of agent may clog catheter, particularly at slower irrigation flow rates.

CYSTOSCOPIC FULGURATION

Mechanism of action

- Direct hemostasis of bleeding vessels.

Protocol

- Initiate spinal or general anesthesia.
- Evacuate clot.
- Fulgarate bleeding vessels and/or inflamed urothelium with electrocautery or neodymium (Nd):YAG laser.[17]

Potential complications

- Generally the same as for other cystoscopic procedures.

Contraindications

- Poor anesthesia risk.

Comments

- Potentially useful with discrete lesions (i.e. bladder tumor), but rarely successful with diffuse bleeding (i.e. radiation cystitis).[18]
- Visualization may be difficult.

INTRAVESICAL FORMALIN INSTILLATION

Mechanism of action

- Precipitates proteins on the mucosal surface and fixes and occludes telangiectatic tissue and small capillaries.[19,20]

Protocol[1]

- A preprocedure VCUG (voiding cystourethrogram) is required to evaluate for vesicoureteral reflux. If reflux is present, place a ureteral occlusion stent or Fogarty catheter[1] to occlude ureter prior to formalin instillation to prevent renal scarring.
- Initiate spinal or general anesthesia.
- Evacuate clot and fulgurate identifiable bleeding vessels.
- Do not allow formalin to come into unnecessary contact with patient: protect exposed skin and mucosa with Vaseline and pack the vagina.
- Irrigate bladder with 1% formalin at <15 cmH_2O for 10 minutes, or instill formalin 1% under gravity at <15 cmH_2O with catheter open at level just above pubic symphysis.
- If possible, monitor bladder pressure and discontinue if pressure >50 cmH_2O.
- Limit total formalin contact time to 15 minutes per instillation.
- Several instillations may be required. The formalin concentration may be slowly increased up to 10%, but complications increase with increasing concentration, and lower concentrations (<5%) are advised.
- Always verify formalin concentration with pharmacy: 100% formalin = 37% formaldehyde.

ACUTE GROSS HEMATURIA

29

Complications

- **Bladder fibrosis and scarring, with reduced capacity and/or complete defunctionalization – important in younger patients with long life expectancies.[1]**
- **Acute tubular necrosis (ATN) with anuria.**
- **Bladder rupture.**
- **Death.**
- Bladder spasm.
- Irritative voiding symptoms.
- Urinary incontinence.
- Vesicoureteral reflux.
- Ureteric stricture with obstruction.
- Vesicovaginal and vesicoileal fistula.
- Myocardial toxicity.
- Systemic absorption of formalin, resulting in increased levels of formic acid with subsequent inhibition of cholinesterase, succinate oxidation, anaerobic glycolysis, and hexokinase.

Contraindications

- Relative: small bladder capacity or severe voiding symptoms, young age, reflux.
- Absolute: none.

Comment

- Highly effective treatment for severe hematuria with reported success rates >80%, but with a high risk of severe complications.
- Should be attempted with caution and only after less-invasive treatments have failed.
- Formalin concentration and exposure time should be minimized.
- If successive treatments are administered, repeat VCUGs should be performed, as the treatment itself may result in new-onset reflux.

EMBOLIZATION[1]

Mechanism of action

- Thrombosis of the arterial supply to the bladder.

Procedure

- Consultation with interventional radiology.
- Embolization of vessels supplying the bladder, ranging from branches of the inferior and superior vesical arteries (superselective embolization) to occlusion of the entire internal iliac artery.

Complications

- Gluteal pain from occlusion of superior gluteal artery.
- Distal embolization and ischemia of lower limb arteries.
- Long-term bladder dysfunction secondary to fibrosis and scarring.
- Gangrene of the bladder (rare).
- Neurological deficit of one or both lower limbs (rare).

Contraindications

- Relative: severe peripheral vascular disease.
- Absolute: none.

Comment

- Effective, but results in infarction of viable tissue with potentially severe consequences.
- Should consider after failure of other procedures.

SURGERY[1]

Procedure

- Urinary diversion with or without simple cystectomy.

Complications

- Same as those for urinary diversion and cystectomy.
- For cystectomy, may be as high as 50–70% in patients with prior radiation therapy.[21]

Contraindications

- Relative: long life span, poor anesthesia risk.
- Absolute: none.

Comment

- An effective but drastic intervention.
- Consider only after failure of less-invasive procedures and/or presence of intractable, life-threatening hemorrhage.
- Temporary urinary diversion with packing of bladder has been described.[22]

MANAGEMENT OF RECURRENT HEMATURIA FROM BENIGN PROSTATIC HYPERPLASIA

FINASTERIDE (PROSCAR)

Mechanism of action

- Possibly through decreased expression of vascular endothelial growth factor (VEGF) in the prostate, with subsequent decreased angiogenesis and microvessel density.[23]

Dose

- 5 mg PO qd.

Potential side effects

- Reduced volume ejaculate.
- Loss of libido.
- Gynecomastia.

Contraindications and warnings[24]

- Contraindications: finasteride allergy.
- Warnings: pregnant women should not handle broken or crushed tablets; caution in patients with liver function abnormalities.

Comment

- Highly effective in uncontrolled case series, with up to 77% of patients responding.[25,26]
- Data on other 5α-reductase inhibitors are not currently available.

REFERENCES

1. Choong SKS, Walkden M, Kirby R: The management of intractable hematuria. BJU Int 86:951–9, 2000.
2. Parsons CL: Successful management of radiation cystitis with sodium pentosanpolysulfate. J Urology 111:603, 1986.
3. Pentosan Polysulfate Sodium: Mosby's Drug Consult. St Louis: Mosby, 2005.
4. Sandhu SS, Goldstraw M, Woodhouse CR: The management of haemorrhagic cystitis with sodium pentosan polysulphate. BJU Int 94:845–7, 2004.
5. Toren PJ, Norman RW: Cyclophosphamide induced hemorrhagic cystitis successfully treated with pentosanpolysulphate. J Urol 173:103, 2005.
6. Hampson SJ, Woodhouse CR: Sodium pentosanpolysulphate in the management of haemorrhagic cystitis: experience with 14 patients. Eur Urol 25:40–2, 1994.
7. Noordzij JW, Dabhoiwala NF: Hemorrhagic radiation cystitis. Int Urogynecol 4:160–7, 1993.
8. Kindwall EP: Hyperbaric oxygen treatment of radiation cystitis: management of chronic radiation wounds. Clin Plast Surg 20:589–92, 1993.
9. Bevers RFM, Bakker DJ, Kurth KH: Hyperbaric oxygen treatment for haemorrhagic radiation cystitis. Lancet 346:803–5, 1995.
10. Corman JM, McClure D, Pritchett R, Kozlowski P, Hampson NB: Treatment of radiation induced hemorrhagic cystitis with hyperbaric oxygen. J Urol 169:2200–2, 2003.
11. Jeremy JY, Mikhailidis DP, Dandona P: The rat urinary bladder produces prostacyclin as well as other prostaglandins. Prostagl Leukotr Med 16:235, 1984.
12. Konturek SJ, Brzozowski T, Piastucki I et al: Role of locally-generated prostaglandins in adaptive gastric cytoprotection. Dig Dis Sci 27:967, 1982.
13. Levine LA, Jarrard DF: Treatment of cyclophosphamide-induced hemorrhagic cystitis with intravesical carboprost tromethamine. J Urol 149:719–23, 1993.
14. Ostroff EB, Chenault OW: Alum irrigation for the control of massive bladder hemorrhage. J Urol 128:929–30, 1982.
15. Arrizabalaga M, Extramiana J, Parra JL et al: Treatment of massive haematuria with aluminous salts. Br J Urol 60:223–6, 1987.
16. Goel AK, Rao MS, Bhagwat AG et al: Intravesical irrigation with alum for the control of massive bladder hemorrhage. J Urol 133:956–7, 1985.
17. Gweon P, Shanberg A: Treatment of cyclophosphamide induced hemorrhagic cystitis with neodymium:YAG laser in pediatric patients. J Urol 157:2301–2, 1997.
18. Mathews R, Rajan N, Josefson L, Camporesi E, Makhuli Z: Hyperbaric oxygen therapy for radiation induced hemorrhagic cystitis. J Urol 161:435–7, 1999.
19. Shah BC, Albert DJ: Intravesical instillation of formalin for the management of intractable hematuria. J Urol 110:519–20, 1973.
20. McGuire EJ, Weiss RM, Schiff M, Lytton B: Hemorrhagic radiation cystitis: treatment. Urology 3:204–8, 1974.
21. Crew JP, Jephcott CR, Reynard JM: Radiation-induced haemorrhagic cystitis. Eur Urol 40:111–23, 2001.
22. Andriole GL, Yuan JJ, Catalona WJ: Cystotomy, temporary urinary diversion and bladder packing in the management of severe cyclophosphamide-induced hemorrhagic cystitis. J Urol 143:1006–7, 1990.

23. Pareek G, Shevchuk M, Armenakas NA et al: The effect of finasteride on the expression of vascular endothelial growth factor and microvessel density: a possible mechanism for decreased prostatic bleeding in treated patients. J Urol 169:20–3, 2003.
24. Finasteride: Mosby's Drug Consult. St Louis: Mosby, 2005.
25. Kearney MC, Bingham JB, Bergland R, Meade-D'Alisera P, Puchner PJ: Clinical predictors in the use of finasteride for control of gross hematuria due to benign prostatic hyperplasia. J Urol 167:2489–91, 2002.
26. Miller MI, Puchner PJ: Effects of finasteride·on hematuria associated with benign prostatic hyperplasia: long-term follow-up. Urology 51:237–40, 1998.

29

ACUTE GROSS HEMATURIA

Antimicrobial prophylaxis for urological procedures

Edward M Schaeffer

SUMMARY

- Antimicrobial prophylaxis is the prevention of a local or systemic infection by administration of an antimicrobial prior to and for a limited time after a surgical procedure.[1]
- Age, anatomical abnormalities, medical comorbidity, concurrent medications, and immune state influence risk for developing a surgical infection.[2]
- Patients with special considerations for antimicrobial prophylaxis include those at risk of endocarditis and those with certain types of indwelling orthopedic hardware.[3,4]

30

GENERAL PRINCIPLES OF SURGICAL PROPHYLAXIS

DEFINITIONS

Antimicrobial prophylaxis

- Prevention of a local or systemic infection by administration of an antimicrobial prior to and for a limited time after (<24 hours) the procedure.[1]

Antimicrobial treatment

- Treatment of a local or systemic infection with administration of an antimicrobial agent tailored to culture-documented organisms.[1]

RISK FACTORS FOR INFECTION

- Host factors that increase risk of surgical site infection:[2]
  - Young or advanced age
  - Anatomical abnormalities
  - Recent surgical reconstruction
  - Inhaled tobacco use
  - Chronic steroid use
  - Immune compromised state
  - Concurrent medication use.
- Host factors that increase the sequelae of a surgical site infection:[2–4]
  - Artificial heart valve
  - Prosthetic joint.
- Factors that increase the concentration and virulence of putative infectious organisms:[2]
  - Infection of distant site
  - Prolonged hospitalization or residence in a chronic care facility
  - Indwelling hardware
  - Infected endogenous or exogenous material.

- *Patients with such risk factors are at increased risk of developing a postprocedural/surgical infection and/or will incur increased morbidity if an infection occurs. Accordingly, antimicrobial prophylaxis is more strongly recommended.*

CORRECT ADMINISTRATION OF ANTIMICROBIAL AGENTS

- Prophylactic antimicrobial agents should be administered between 2 hours and 30 minutes prior to initiation of the procedure.[2]
- Intravenous infusions should be completed, at most, 30 minutes before starting the procedure.[2]
- Intravenous infusions should be re-dosed if the procedure lasts longer than the half-life of the drug.[2]
- Prophylactic antimicrobial agents should be continued for a limited time after the procedure:
  - Typically for <24 hours. Exceptions are discussed below.

CONTEMPORARY INDICATIONS FOR ANTIMICROBIAL PROPHYLAXIS FOR SPECIFIC UROLOGICAL PROCEDURES (TABLE 30.1)

URETHRAL CATHETERIZATION AND REMOVAL

- *Antimicrobial prophylaxis is not recommended in most hosts.*
- Risk of infection after single catherization is 1–2%.[5]
- Prolonged catheterization is associated with a 3–10% incidence of bacterial colonization per day.[1,6]
  - However, prophylactic antimicrobials are not recommended for the duration of urethral catheterization under most circumstances.
- Administration of antimicrobials at the time of catheter removal is poorly studied.
  - One study found a 25% incidence of urinary tract infection (UTI) in a group of women after catheterization for 4–6 days[7]
  - Therefore, antimicrobial treatment rather than prophylaxis may be indicated at the time of catheter removal
  - Send urine for culture prior to initiating antimicrobial treatment.
- Antimicrobial prophylaxis for changing of a chronic indwelling catheter is not routinely indicated.[1]
  - In at least one study, the incidence of bacteremia was low and no sequelae were noted when antimicrobials were withheld during routine catheter changes.[8]

TRANSRECTAL ULTRASOUND-GUIDED PROSTATE BIOPSY

- *Antimicrobial prophylaxis is recommended.*
- Prophylactic antimicrobials reduce the incidence of postprocedural UTI and sepsis.[9,10]
- 1–3 days of fluoroquinolones prior to the day of biopsy is appropriate. Bactrim has also been used.[10,11]

TABLE 30.1

GUIDE FOR ANTIMICROBIAL PROPHYLAXIS FOR COMMON UROLOGICAL PROCEDURES

Procedure	Antimicrobial recommendations	
	Patient – ideal	Patient with risk factors
Urethral catheter removal	None advised	Oral fluoroquinolone – single dose Bactrim DS – single dose
Extracorporal shock wave lithotripsy	Bactrim DS or oral fluoroquinolone – single dose	If stone infected, treat preoperatively for infection
Transrectal prostate biopsy	Oral fluoroquinolone – 1–4 days	Consider culture-directed treatment if infection suspected
Endoscopic procedures of the lower urinary tract		
Urethroscopy, cystoscopy	No absolute indication	Oral fluoroquinolone – single dose Bactrim DS – single dose
Urodynamics	No absolute indication	Oral fluoroquinolone – single dose Bactrim DS – single dose
Prostate resection	Ampicillin + gentamicin or oral/IV fluoroquinolone	Ampicillin + gentamicin or oral/IV fluoroquinolone; consider culture-directed treatment if infection suspected
Bladder tumor resection	Bactrim DS or fluoroquinolone or ampicillin + gentamicin	Bactrim DS or fluoroquinolone or ampicillin + gentamicin
Transrectal prostate biopsy	Oral fluoroquinolone – 1–4 day coverage	Consider culture-directed treatment if infection suspected
Endoscopic procedures of the upper urinary tract		
Percutaneous renal surgery	Fluoroquinolone or ampicillin + gentamicin	Fluoroquinolone or ampicillin + gentamicin; consider culture-directed treatment if infection suspected
Ureteroscopy	Ampicillin + gentamicin	Ampicillin + gentamicin
Open/laparoscopic surgery		
Renal surgery	Cefazolin, vancomycin, or clindamycin for β-lactam allergic	Cefazolin, vancomycin, or clindamycin for β-lactam allergic
Procedures with open, sterile urinary tract	Cefazolin, vancomycin, or clindamycin for β-lactam allergic	Cefazolin, vancomycin, or clindamycin for β-lactam allergic
Reconstruction with colon or appendix	Cefotetan or cefoxitin Clindamycin + gentamicin or azetreonam or ciprofloxacin for β-lactam allergic oral non-absorbable antimicrobial pre-op + mechanical bowel preparation	Cefotetan or cefoxitin Clindamycin + gentamicin or azetreonam or ciprofloxacin for β-lactam allergic oral non-absorbable antimicrobial pre-op + mechanical bowel preparation
Dirty wound, including trauma, abscess or non-directed genitourinary perforation	N/A	Treatment dose with broad coverage, narrowed and directed when cultures indicate

Drug doses: ampicillin, 25 mg/kg; gentamicin, 1.5 mg/kg; cefazolin, 25 mg/kg.
Adapted from Schaeffer EM, Schaeffer AJ: Infections of the urinary tract. In: Wein AJ, Novick AC, Patrin AW, Kavoussi LR, Peters CA, eds. Campbell-Walsh Urology, 9th edn. Philadelphia: WB Saunders, 2006.

30

ANTIMICROBIAL PROPHYLAXIS

EXTRACORPOREAL SHOCK WAVE LITHOTRIPSY (ESWL)

- *Antimicrobial prophylaxis should be considered.*
- The incidence of postprocedural UTI ranges from 0 to 28%.
- A systematic review demonstrated that prophylactic antimicrobial administration in patients with sterile urine reduces the incidence of postprocedural UTI from 5.7% to 2.1%.[12]
- Cost–benefit analysis suggests antimicrobial prophylaxis is financially sound prior to ESWL.[12]
- Patients with infected urine should be treated for a UTI prior to ESWL.

ENDOSCOPIC PROCEDURES OF THE LOWER URINARY TRACT

Diagnostic cystoscopy

- *Antimicrobial prophylaxis is recommended in hosts with increased risk factors for infection.*
- Most studies report 2–8% incidence of postprocedural UTI.[13,14]
- Risk of infection increases with history of prior infection.[13]
- Single-dose antimicrobials reduce infections to 1–5%.[13,14]

Urodynamics

- *Antimicrobial prophylaxis is recommended in hosts with increased risk factors for infection.*
- Associated with a 5–7% incidence of UTI in healthy patients.[15]
- This incidence does not decrease significantly with the use of prophylactic antimicrobial agents.[15]
- Comorbidities, including neurogenic bladder, spinal cord injury, and diabetes, will increase risk of postprocedural infection.
- Antimicrobial prophylaxis is advised in hosts with increased risk factors for infection.

Transurethral resection of the prostate

- *Antimicrobial prophylaxis is recommended.*
- Prophylactic antimicrobials reduce bacteriuria 3–5 days after procedure (from 26% to 9%)[16] and septicemia.
  - Note that in most studies, antimicrobials were continued throughout the duration that the catheter was in place (3–5 days).[16]
- Effective classes of antimicrobials include aminoglycosides, cephalosporins, fluoroquinolones, and bactrim.[16]

Bladder biopsy and transuretheral resection of bladder tumor

- *Antimicrobial prophylaxis is recommended.*
- Although not well studied, urothelial injury and use of pressurized, high-flow irrigation (especially in larger resections) increase the risk of local or systemic infection compared with simple cystoscopy.

ENDOSCOPIC PROCEDURES OF THE UPPER URINARY TRACT

Diagnostic ureteroscopy

- *Antimicrobial prophylaxis is recommended.*
- Although not well studied, the use of pressurized, high-flow irrigation increases the risk of infection.
- In one prospective study, single-dose flouroquinolone reduced infections.[17]

Ureteroscopy with lithotripsy or biopsy

- *Antimicrobial prophylaxis is recommended.*
- Urothelial injury, the use of pressurized irrigation, and the manipulation of potentially infectious material may increase the risk of infection.[17]

Percutaneous renal access

- *Antimicrobial prophylaxis is recommended.*
- Pyrexia and bacteremia can occur after percutaneous renal access.
- Degree of risk is associated with the type of procedure, the duration of the procedure, and the volume of irrigant used.[18]

OPEN AND LAPAROSCOPIC PROCEDURES

- **Surgical sites are classified by the CDC into four categories:**[2]
  - *Clean*: wound uninfected, no inflammation, closed drainage. No entry into urinary or alimentary tracts
  - *Clean contaminated*: wound uninfected with controlled entry into urinary or alimentary tracts
  - *Contaminated*: wound uninfected, major break in sterile technique, gross unanticipated spillage from alimentary tract *or* open fresh accidental wound
  - *Dirty/infected:* wound with pre-existing clinical infection or perforated viscera or old, devitalized tissue.
- Procedures without entry into the urinary tract are considered clean (includes radical nephrectomy):
  - Antimicrobial prophylaxis is not absolutely indicated for these procedures as long as entry into the urinary tract does not occur[2]
  - Note that inguinal surgery (hernia, radical orchiectomy, etc.), although technically clean, is considered a clean contaminated procedure due to the location of the surgical site.
- Procedures with controlled entry into a sterile urinary tract are considered clean contaminated:
  - *Prophylaxis is recommended.*
- Procedures with entry into the gastrointestinal tract for urinary reconstruction are considered clean contaminated:
  - *Prophylaxis is recommended*
  - For lower intestinal (colon) reconstruction, broadened anaerobic coverage is recommended[2]
  - The administration of oral non-absorbable antimicrobials and mechanical bowel preparation to reduce the density of colonized bacteria are also recommended.

SPECIAL CONSIDERATIONS

PROPHYLAXIS AGAINST ENDOCARDITIS[3]

General principles

- Urinary tract is the second most common site of entry of organisms that cause endocarditis.
- *Enterococcus faecalis* is the most common organism causing endocarditis after a urological procedure.

Patients at risk for endocarditis[3]

- High risk cardiac conditions – *prophylaxis is recommended*:
  - Prosthetic heart valves
  - Cyanotic congenital heart disease
  - Systemic–pulmonary shunts of conduits
  - Previous endocarditis.
- Moderate-risk cardiac conditions – *prophylaxis is recommended*:
  - Congenital malformations except for those listed below under 'low risk'
  - Acquired valvular disease
  - Hypertrophic cardiomyopathy
  - Mitral valve prolapse with valvular regurgitation or thicken leaflets.
- Low-risk cardiac conditions – *prophylaxis is not recommended*:
  - The following congenital malformations: isolated secundum atrial septal defects, surgically repaired atrial septal defects, ventricular septal defects, and patent ductus arteriosus
  - Previous coronary artery bypass surgery
  - Benign heart murmurs
  - Previous Kawasaki disease or rheumatic fever
  - Implanted pacemaker or defibrillator.
- See Table 30.2 for AHA-recommended antimicrobial regimens.[3]

TABLE 30.2

ANTIMICROBIAL REGIMENS FOR PATIENTS AT RISK FOR ENDOCARDITIS

Patient type	Antimicrobial recommendation
High risk	Ampicillin 2.0 g IM or IV + gentamicin 1.5 mg/kg (not exceeding 120 mg) 30 minutes prior to procedure and ampicillin 25 mg/kg or amoxicillin 25 mg/kg PO 6 hours after procedure
High risk with allergy to ampicillin or amoxicillin	Vancomycin 1.0 g over 1–2 hours and gentamicin 1.5 mg/kg (not to exceed 120 mg) within 30 minutes of starting procedure
Moderate risk	Amoxicillin 2.0 g PO 1 hour prior to procedure
Moderate risk with allergy to ampicillin or amoxicillin	Vancomycin 1.0 g IV over 1–2 hours, within 30 minutes of completed infusion

Adapted from the AHA 1997 recommendations.[3]

PROPHYLAXIS AGAINST SEEDING OF INDWELLING ORTHOPEDIC HARDWARE[4]

- *Antimicrobial prophylaxis is recommended* for patients with total joint replacements <2 years old or patients with altered risk factors (see criteria above).
- *Antimicrobial prophylaxis is not recommended* for patients with total joint replacements ≥2 years old, pins, plates, or screws.

See Table 30.3 for AUA-recommended antimicrobial regimens.[4]

30

TABLE 30.3	
ANTIMICROBIAL REGIMENS FOR PATIENTS WITH INDWELLING ORTHOPEDIC HARDWARE	
Patient type	**Antimicrobial recommendation**
Total joint inserted >2 years ago; pins, plates, screws + no host risk factors	Not recommended empirically
Total joint inserted <2 years or abnormal host factor	Oral quinolone or ampicillin 2 g IV + gentamicin 1.5 mg/kg IV 30–60 minutes prior to the procedure Substitute vancomycin 1 g IV over 1–2 hours prior to procedure for ampicillin if allergic

Adapted from the AUA advisory statement.[4]

ANTIMICROBIAL PROPHYLAXIS

REFERENCES

1. Schaeffer A: Infections of the urinary tract. In: Walsh PC, Retik AB, Vaughan ED, Wein AJ, eds. Campbell's Urology, Philadelphia: WB Saunders, 2002.
2. Bratzler DW, Houck PM: Antimicrobial prophylaxis for surgery: an advisory statement from the National Surgical Infection Prevention Project. Clin Infect Dis 38:1706–15, 2004.
3. Dajani AS, Taubert KA, Wilson W et al: Prevention of bacterial endocarditis: recommendations by the American Heart Association. JAMA 277:1794–801, 1997.
4. American Urological Association and American Academy of Orthopaedic Surgeons: Antibiotic prophylaxis for urological patients with total joint replacements, 2002.
5. Turck M, Goffe B, Petersdorf RG: The urethral catheter and urinary tract infection. J Urol 88:834–7, 1962.
6. Larsen EH, Gasser TC, Madsen PO: Antimicrobial prophylaxis in urologic surgery. Urol Clin North Am 13:591–604, 1986.
7. Harding GK, Nicolle LE, Ronald AR et al: How long should catheter-acquired urinary tract infection in women be treated? A randomized controlled study. Ann Intern Med 114:713–19, 1991.
8. Polastri F, Auckenthaler R, Loew F, Michel JP, Lew DP: Absence of significant bacteremia during urinary catheter manipulation in patients with chronic indwelling catheters. J Am Geriatr Soc. 38:1203–8, 1990.
9. Sieber PR, Rommel FM, Agusta VE et al: Antibiotic prophylaxis in ultrasound guided transrectal prostate biopsy. J Urol 157:2199–200, 1997.
10. Raaijmakers R, Kirkels WJ, Roobol MJ, Wildhagen MF, Schrder FH: Complication rates and risk factors of 5802 transrectal ultrasound-guided sextant biopsies of the prostate within a population-based screening program. Urology 60:826–30, 2002.
11. Sabbagh R, McCormack M, Peloquin F et al: A prospective randomized trial of 1-day versus 3-day antibiotic prophylaxis for transrectal ultrasound guided prostate biopsy. Can J Urol 11:2216–19, 2004.
12. Pearle MS, Roehrborn CG: Antimicrobial prophylaxis prior to shock wave lithotripsy in patients with sterile urine before treatment: a meta-analysis and cost-effectiveness analysis. Urology 49:679–86, 1997.

13. Clark KR, Higgs MJ: Urinary infection following out-patient flexible cystoscopy. Br J Urol 66:503–5, 1990.
14. Manson AL: Is antibiotic administration indicated after outpatient cystoscopy? J Urol 140:316–17, 1988.
15. Cundiff GW, McLennan MT, Bent AE: Randomized trial of antibiotic prophylaxis for combined urodynamics and cystourethroscopy. Obstet Gynecol 93:749–52, 1999.
16. Berry A, Barratt A: Prophylactic antibiotic use in transurethral prostatic resection: a meta-analysis. J Urol 167:571–7, 2002.
17. Knopf HJ, Graff HJ, Schulze H: Perioperative antibiotic prophylaxis in ureteroscopic stone removal. Eur Urol 44:115–18, 2003.
18. Dogan HS, Sahin A, Cetinkaya Y et al: Antibiotic prophylaxis in percutaneous nephrolithotomy: prospective study in 81 patients. J Endourol 16:649–53, 2002.

Guide to radiological procedures and nerve blocks

J Kellogg Parsons and Peter Pinto

RADIOLOGICAL PROCEDURES

CYSTOGRAM[1,2]

Indications

- Suspected bladder injury/perforation.

Procedure

- Insert a 16F or 18F Foley catheter into the bladder.
- Gently instill at least 350 ml (or until perception of pain) of 30% contrast solution into the bladder.
  - If performing computed tomography (CT) cystogram, use 2–4% contrast only
  - If bladder perforation is suspected, using <250 ml of contrast may be associated with false-negative results.
- Clamp the Foley catheter to prevent contrast leakage.
- Obtain one anteroposterior (AP) image.
- *Optional: place the patient in a steep oblique position using a soft bump or rolled-up towel and obtain additional images.*
- Unclamp the Foley catheter and drain the bladder.
- Obtain post-drainage image.

RETROGRADE URETHROGRAM[3]

Indications

- Suspected urethral injury/perforation.
- Urethral stricture.
- Congenital abnormalities.

Procedure

- Place the patient in steep oblique position with a soft bump or rolled-up towel.
- Insert a 14F Foley catheter ~3 cm into the urethra.
  - Use minimal lubrication to prevent migration of the catheter tip out of the urethral meatus.
- Gently inflate the catheter balloon with 1–2 ml of saline.
- Gently inject 25 ml of 30% contrast solution through the catheter.
- Obtain one or more AP images during active injection.
  - If available, consider using fluoroscopy.

SINGLE-SHOT INTRAVENOUS PYELOGRAPHY (IVP)[4]

Indications

- Suspected upper urinary tract injury after penetrating or blunt trauma.

Procedure

- Administer 2 ml/kg IV contrast as a single bolus.
- Wait 10 minutes.
- Obtain a single AP view.

NERVE BLOCKS

PENILE BLOCK (FIGURE 31.1)[5]

Indications

- Manual reduction of paraphimosis.
- Irrigation/aspiration for priapism.
- Any procedure involving reconstruction or excision of penile tissue.

Procedure

- Palpate the symphysis pubis at the base of the penis.
- Insert a 22-gauge needle to one side of the midline at the 2 o'clock position along the inferior portion of the symphysis, aiming toward the caudal border of the symphysis on the left side. As the needle is advanced toward the symphysis, aspirate to insure extravascular placement, and then inject 1–2 ml of 2% lidocaine or 0.25% Marcaine (bupivacaine).
- Advance until the bone may be gently palpated with the needle tip. Withdraw the needle slightly, aim caudally, and then pass the needle tip immediately underneath the symphysis.

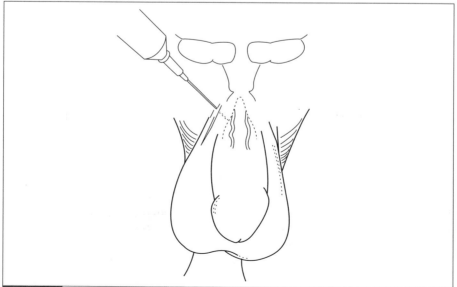

FIGURE 31.1

Penile block. The needle tip passes through Buck's fascia at the base of the penis at the 10 and 2 o'clock positions.

- Advance until experiencing a 'pop' (i.e. sudden loss of resistance), indicating that the needle tip has passed through Buck's fascia.
- Aspirate to insure extravascular placement, then inject 3 ml of 2% lidocaine or 0.25% Marcaine.
- Repeat the procedure on the right side at the 10 o'clock position.

SPERMATIC CORD BLOCK (FIGURE 31.2)[5]

Indications

- Vasectomy.
- Orchiectomy, orchidopexy, and other testicular procedures.

Procedure

- Stand on the patient's right-hand side.
- At the top of the scrotum, grasp the right spermatic cord with the left hand by placing the thumb lateral to (that is, in front of) the cord and the index finger medial to (that is, behind) the cord. Hook the index finger and thumb securely under the cord and pull it superficially. Insure that all the components of the cord have been drawn upward.
- Insert a 25-gauge needle obliquely into the cord, aiming toward the tip of the index finger.
- Aspirate to insure extravascular placement, then infiltrate the cord with 3–5 ml of 2% lidocaine or 0.25% Marcaine.
- Remain on the patient's right side and repeat the procedure for the left spermatic cord by grasping it with the left index finger lateral and the left thumb medial to the cord.

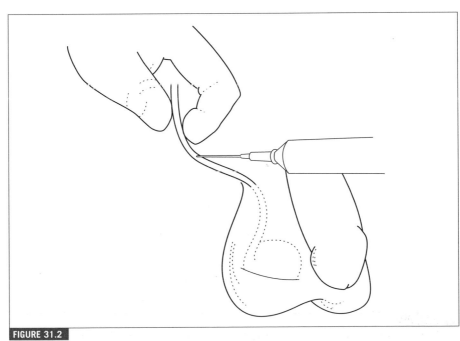

FIGURE 31.2
Spermatic cord block. The cord is grasped securely with the thumb and index finger and infiltrated obliquely.

- For left-handed surgeons, this same procedure may be followed by reversing all of the sides.

PROSTATE BLOCK (FIGURE 31.3)[6,7]

Indications

- Transrectal ultrasound-guided prostate needle biopsy.

Procedure

- Place the patient in the left lateral decubitus position.
- *Optional: prior to probe insertion, instill 10 ml of 2% lidocaine jelly mixed with 1 ml of sodium bicarbonate into the rectum and allow to sit for 5–10 minutes.*
- Insert the ultrasound probe.
- Using a 22-gauge 7-inch spinal needle, inject 1–2 ml of 1% lidocaine at three locations on each side of the prostate: at the junction between the base and seminal vesicle; in the mid-region; and at the apex. Proper placement of anesthetic is verified by a hypoechoic wheal that should appear along the prostate capsule at each location.

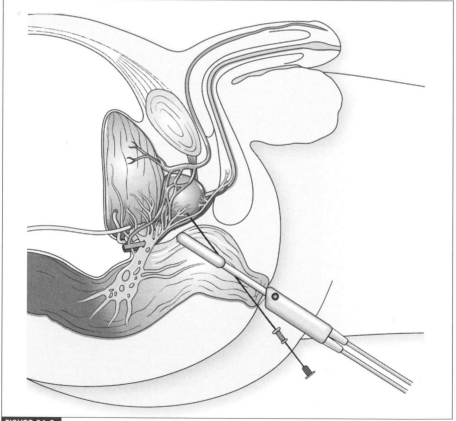

FIGURE 31.3

Prostate block. Using ultrasound guidance and a 22-gauge 7-inch spinal needle, 1–2 ml of 1% lidocaine are injected at the base, mid-region, and apex on each side of the prostate.

REFERENCES

1. Cass AS, Luxenberg M: Features of 164 bladder ruptures. J Urol 138:743–5, 1987.
2. Peng MY, Parisky YR, Cornwell EE 3rd, Radin R, Bragin S: CT cystography versus conventional cystography in evaluation of bladder injury. AJR Am J Roentgenol 173:1269–72, 1999.
3. Sandler CM, Corriere JN Jr: Urethrography in the diagnosis of acute urethral injuries. Urol Clin North Am 16:283–9, 1989.
4. Morey AF, McAninch JW, Tiller BK, Duckett CP, Carroll PR: Single shot intraoperative excretory urography for the immediate evaluation of renal trauma. J Urol 161:1088–92, 1999.
5. Hinman F: Methods of nerve block. In: Hinman F, ed. Atlas of Urologic Surgery. Philadelphia: WB Saunders, 1998, pp 75–80.
6. Shinohara K, Master VA, Thomas C, Carroll PR: Prostate needle biopsy techniques and interpretation. In: Vogelzang NJ, Scardino PT, Shipley WU, Debruyne FMJ, Linehan WM, eds. Genitourinary Oncology. Philadelphia: Lippincott, Williams & Wilkins, 2005, pp 111–19.
7. Soloway MS: Do unto others – why I would want anesthesia for my prostate biopsy. Urology 62:973–5, 2003.

31

GUIDE TO RADIOLOGICAL PROCEDURES AND NERVE BLOCKS

Index

Page numbers in *italics* indicate figures or tables.

INDEX